THE CAMBRIDGE HISTORY OF MEDICINE

Against the backdrop of unprecedented concern for the future of health care, *The Cambridge History of Medicine* surveys the rise of medicine in the West from classical times to the present. Covering both the social and scientific history of medicine, this volume traces the chronology of key developments and events, while at the same time engaging with the issues, discoveries, and controversies that have beset and characterised medical progress. The authors weave a narrative that connects disease, doctors, primary care, surgery, the rise of hospitals, drug treatment and pharmacology, mental illness and psychiatry. This volume emphasises the crucial developments of the past 150 years, but also examines classical, medieval, and Islamic and East Asian medicine. Authoritative and accessible, *The Cambridge History of Medicine* is for readers wanting a lively and informative introduction to medical history.

Roy Porter (1946–2002), Professor Emeritus of the Social History of Medicine at the Wellcome Trust Center for the History of Medicine at the University College London, was the author of more than 200 books and articles, including *Doctor of Society: Thomas Beddoes and the Sick Trade in Late Enlightenment England* (1991), *London: A Social History* (1994), *The Greatest Benefit to Mankind: A Medical History of Humanity* (1997), and *Bodies Politic: Disease, Death and Doctors in Britain, 1650–1900* (2001).

THE CAMBRIDGE HISTORY OF
MEDICINE

Edited by

Roy Porter

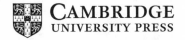
CAMBRIDGE
UNIVERSITY PRESS

CAMBRIDGE UNIVERSITY PRESS
Cambridge, New York, Melbourne, Madrid, Cape Town, Singapore, São Paulo, Delhi

Cambridge University Press
32 Avenue of the Americas, New York, NY 10013-2473, USA

www.cambridge.org
Information on this title: www.cambridge.org/9780521682893

First published 2006
Reprinted 2009

A catalog record for this publication is available from the British Library.

Library of Congress Cataloging in Publication Data

Rev. ed. of: The Cambridge illustrated history of medicine / edited by
Roy Porter.
p. cm – (Cambridge illustrated history).
ISBN 978-0-521-86426-8
1. Medicine – History. I. Porter, Roy, 1946–2000. II. Series.
R131.C232 1996
610'.9–dc20 95-38000

ISBN 978-0-521-86426-8 hardback
ISBN 978-0-521-68289-3 paperback

Transferred to digital printing 2008

Contents

Introduction 1

1. The History of Disease 10
Kenneth F. Kiple

2. The Rise of Medicine 46
Vivian Nutton

3. What Is Disease? 71
Roy Porter

4. Primary Care 103
Edward Shorter

5. Medical Science 136
Roy Porter

6. Hospitals and Surgery 176
Roy Porter

7. Drug Treatment and the Rise of Pharmacology 211
Miles Weatherall

8. Mental Illness 238
Roy Porter

9. Medicine, Society, and the State 260
John Pickstone

10. Looking to the Future (1996) 298
Geoff Watts

Contents

Addendum: Looking to the Future Revisited 331
Geoff Watts

Reference Guide 341
    Chronology   343
    Major Human Diseases   357
    Notes   363
    Further Reading   369

Index of Medical Personalities 383
General Index 394
Map Acknowledgements 408

Introduction

Never have people in the West lived so long, or been so healthy, and never have medical achievements been so great. Yet, paradoxically, rarely has medicine drawn such intense doubts and disapproval as today. No-one could deny that the medical breakthroughs of the past 50 years – the culmination of a long tradition of scientific medicine – have saved more lives than those of any era since the dawn of medicine. So blasé have we become about medical progress, that it is worth taking stock of just some of the tremendous innovations taken for granted today yet unavailable a century or two ago. These advances are discussed and explained at length in the chapters that follow. By way of introduction, here is a brief summary of the most dramatic changes that have occurred during the second half of the twentieth century.

At the outbreak of the Second World War, penicillin was still at the laboratory stage and remained rationed for several years. Before the advent of such antibiotic 'magic bullets', pneumonia, meningitis, and similar infections were still frequently fatal. Tuberculosis – dubbed the 'white plague' to contrast it with the Black Death (and because sufferers had a characteristic pallor) – was long the single most important cause of death in the developed world. But that was given the *coup de grâce* by the introduction of the BCG vaccine and streptomycin in the 1940s. The 1950s extended the 'first pharmacological revolution' on to a broad front. The new biological drugs beat the bacteria, improved the control of deficiency diseases, and produced effective medications (such as the psychotropic drug chlorpromazine) for mental illnesses. The first vaccines against polio arrived at the same time.

Other drug breakthroughs, notably steroids such as cortisone, made it feasible to capitalize on the growing understanding of the immune system. By tackling the rejection problem, the development of immunosupressants opened up vast new fields for plastic and transplant surgery. Cardiology also blossomed. One milestone was the first surgical intervention in 1944 for 'blue babies' born with congenital heart disease; thereafter, paediatric cardiology forged ahead. Open-heart surgery dates from the 1950s; bypass operations, another leap forward, began in 1967.

By that time, surgery was beginning to resemble space travel, and it was also capturing the public's imagination; it seemed to know no bounds. Organ replacement was developed, first with kidneys. Transplants became banner headlines in 1967 when Christiaan Barnard sewed a woman's heart into Louis Washkansky, who lived for 18 days. By the mid-1980s, hundreds of heart transplants were being conducted each year in the USA alone, with two-thirds of the recipients surviving for 5 years or more. During the past 50 years, surgery has not just grown: its nature has been transformed. Early in the twentieth century, its essence lay in extirpation: locate the lesion and cut it out (often effective but rather crude). Now, its philosophy has become far more sophisticated: that of continuous repair and (perhaps endless) replaceability.

Alongside these practical leaps forward in intervention, science has been contributing to healing. Such technological breakthroughs as electron microscopes, endoscopes, computerized axial tomography (CAT), positron emission tomography (PET), magnetic resonance imaging (MRI), lasers, tracers, and ultrasound have created a revolution in medicine's diagnostic capacities. Lasers brought microsurgery. Iron lungs, kidney-dialysis machines, heart-lung machines, and pacemakers have all taken their place in medicine's armoury. Meanwhile, research in basic science has transformed our understanding of the body and its battles with disease. In particular, genetics and molecular biology developed rapidly after Francis Crick and James Watson's discovery of the double-helical structure of DNA and the cracking of the genetic code in 1953. Genetic screening and engineering have been making great headway. At the same time, brain chemistry opened new horizons for medicine: research on endorphins has been laying bare and mastering the secrets of pain; synthetic manipulation of neurotransmitters such as L-dopa has provided treatments for Parkinson's disease and other disorders of the central nervous system. So long a Cinderella, clinical science – the application of scientific methods to the actual experience of sickness – has come into its own, thanks partly to the randomized clinical trial, developed from the mid-1940s.

Such advances in science and therapeutics have not blossomed in a desert. They have arisen from the vast endowment of medicine as a social utility (discussed in Chapter 9). In the UK, the creation of the National Health Service (NHS) in 1948 remains a red-letter day, but nations worldwide have been devoting ever larger public and private resources to medicine. In the USA and several European Union nations, more than 10 per cent of gross national product now goes on health. The World Health Organization (WHO) continues to expand. Its programmes of disease prevention and eradication, especially in developing countries, have had some striking successes, notably the global eradication of smallpox in 1977.

To put developments in a nutshell, two facts give powerful (if conflicting) evidence of the growing significance of medicine. First, the doubling of world population in the past 50 years (from around 2,500 million in 1950 to an estimated 6,250 million in the year 2000), no small percentage of which has been caused by new medical interventions and preventions. Second, the introduction of the contraceptive pill, which, in theory at least, paved the way for a safe and simple means to control that population. These developments are well known, but familiarity does not detract from the achievement. Many revolutions have occurred in human history – the introduction of agriculture, the growth of cities, printing, the great scientific advances in the seventeenth century, and the industrial revolutions. But not until the last half of the twentieth century has there been a medical revolution with dramatic therapeutic implications, if we take as our yardstick the dependable ability to vanquish life-threatening disease on a vast scale. The healthiness and longevity of the rich world, and the populousness of the poor world, alike attest this.

A major aim of this volume is to set those changes in medicine in their historical context. We trace the long tradition that arose out of Ancient Greece, which first set medicine on a rational and scientific foundation. We examine the transformations stimulated by the Renaissance and the Scientific Revolution, which presented medicine with the triumphs of physics and chemistry. And we consider the remarkable contribution of nineteenth-century medical science, with its advances in public health, cell biology, bacteriology, parasitology, antisepsis, and anaesthetic surgery. Major advances were made early in the twentieth century: X-rays, immunology, the understanding of hormones and vitamins, chemotherapy, even psychoanalysis.

As the following chapters show, a historical understanding of medicine is far more than a cavalcade of triumphs. It involves the attempt to explain the more distant and indirect antecedents of modern changes, to show why one path was taken and not another, to examine the interconnections of the theoretical and practical aspects of medicine, science, and healing, and doctor and patient; to analyse the relations between the broad trends and leading individuals; and, not least, to lay bare the thinking – often to our minds bizarre and unscientific – that lay behind the physiological and therapeutic systems of the past.

But *The Cambridge History of Medicine* also attempts to go beyond simply telling the story of the rise of medicine and its interplay with science, society, and the public. It aims, through historical analysis, to put medicine under the microscope, and to raise questions about the great forces that have fuelled medical change over the centuries and continue to do so. Who has controlled medicine? Has it been shaped by supply or by demand, by money and market forces? How adequately has it met the needs of the sick? How responsive has it been to the wishes of the medical profession? What has been the role of the state in financing and directing healing?

The volume thus poses questions about medicine's social and political roles. For if healing has, obviously, been medicine's task, has it also had hidden programmes, which, as some critics have alleged, may have an unsavoury side? The involvement of German doctors and scientists with the Nazi final solution, from unethical and deadly human experimentation to the supervision of the gas chambers at Auschwitz and elsewhere, needs to remembered alongside the selfless dedication of innumerable other physicians and health professionals. Partly by way of recoil from the atrocities of the Second World War, doctors have been conspicuous in humanitarian movements during the past 50 years, including campaigns for nuclear disarmament and against torture.

Questioning the roles of medicine is important, not for any cynical reasons but because if we are to understand the directions medicine is taking now – its priorities, funding, and regulation – it is crucial that we have a historical perspective on how it has come to be. That is why it is helpful to return to the paradoxical state of medicine today.

In spite of all the tremendous advances, an atmosphere of disquiet and doubt now pervades medicine. The flag-waving optimism of the 1960s has disappeared. Euphoria bubbled up over penicillin, over the coming of heart transplants, and over the first test-tube baby, Louise Brown, in 1978. Now, fears are growing over the strange powers that medicine might assume as genetic engineering and biotechnology expand. At the same time, as health costs get out of hand, prospects loom of real medical cutbacks in major Western societies. Will the development of scientific medicine make it unaffordable to many people? Will it succumb to an inverse square law – growing costs and complexity entailing diminishing utility?

Now that the big battles have been won, medicine is more open to criticism. Setbacks, major and minor, naturally do not help. For example, thalidomide proved disastrous; iatrogenic (doctor-caused) illness has grown; research on cancer, schizophrenia, multiple sclerosis, Alzheimer's, and other degenerative diseases creeps forwards at a snail's-pace; and doubts remain about the medical basis of psychiatry. In Britain, the NHS has been turned into a political football and faces disintegration or possible dismantling; in the USA, insurance and litigation scandals dog the profession. In rich countries, the needy still get a poor medical deal. In the developing world, for lack of international will, malaria and other tropical diseases remain rampant, while diphtheria and tuberculosis, once thought to have been routed, are resurgent in the former USSR and other industrialized nations. Not least, the pandemic of AIDS (acquired immunodeficiency syndrome) destroyed any naive faith that disease itself has been conquered.

Medicine is arguably going through a serious crisis, one that is in large part the price of progress and unrealistically high expectations that have been whipped up by the media and indeed by the medical profession itself. Medicine may appear to be losing its way, or rather having to redefine what its goals are. In 1949, in an article in the *British Medical Journal*, the distinguished physician Lord Horder posed the question: 'Whither Medicine?', and returned the answer direct: 'Why, whither else but straight ahead'.[1] Today, who even knows where 'straight ahead' lies?

For centuries, the medical enterprise was too paltry to attract radical critiques of itself. It had its mockers, yet those who could invariably called the doctor when sick. As Edward Shorter suggests in Chapter 4, in what might paradoxically be called the good-old-bad-old-days, things were simple: people did not have high expectations of medicine, and when the Old Doc typically achieved rather little, his patients did not blame him too much. Medicine was a profession, but it carried no great prestige and had rather little power. In the twentieth century, by contrast, medicine has claimed greater authority, and has become immensely costly. Once medicine grew mighty, it drew critics. And once it proved effective, the scourge of pestilence was forgotten, and the physician became exposed to being viewed primarily as a figure of authority, the tool of patriarchy, or the servant of the state.

In one other key respect, medicine has become the prisoner of its own success. Having finally conquered many grave diseases and provided relief for suffering, its goals have ceased to be so clear and its mandate has become muddled. What are its aims? Where is it to stop? Is its prime duty to keep people alive as long as possible, whatever the circumstances? Is its charge to make people lead healthy lives? Or is it but a service industry, to fulfil whatever fantasies its clients may frame for their bodies – for instance, a facelift or cosmetic remodelling?

In the particular case, many of these quandaries can be resolved reasonably satisfactorily with the aid of common decency, good will, and a sensible ethics committee. But in the wider world, who can decree for the directions medicine may now be taking? Now that (in the rich world at least) medicine has accomplished most of its basic targets as understood by Hippocrates, William Harvey, or Lord Horder, who decides its new missions?

In this situation, public alarm is bound to grow over the high-tech 'can do, will do' approach apparently embraced by scientific medicine at the cutting edge – medicine led by an elite that sometimes seems primarily interested in extending its technical prowess, with scant regard for ends and values, or even the individual sufferer. Where patients are seen as 'problems' and reduced to biopsies and lab tests, no wonder sections of the public vote with their feet, and opt for styles of holistic medicine that present themselves as more humane.

What may be more disquieting than the switch to alternative treatments is the public's fixation on medicine. Ironically, the healthier Western society becomes, the more medicine it craves; indeed, it comes to regard maximum access to medicine as a political right and a private duty. Especially in the USA, where a free market operates, intense pressures are created – by, for example, the medical profession, medi-businesses, the media, and compliant (or susceptible) individuals – to expand the diagnosis of treatable illnesses. Scares about new diseases and conditions arise. People are bamboozled into more and more lab tests, often of dubious reliability. Thanks to 'diagnostic creep', ever more disorders are revealed, or, as many would say, concocted. Extensive and expensive treatments are then urged. In the USA, the physician who chooses not to treat leaves himself exposed to accusations of malpractice. Anxieties and interventions spiral upwards. Practitioners, lawyers, and pharmaceutical companies do well, even if patients don't get well; and medicine is increasingly blown off course.

To understand the roots of the trouble, particularly in the USA but elsewhere too, we need to examine these elements in the light of historical change. The problem is endemic to a system in which an expanding medical establishment, faced with a healthier population of its own creation, is driven to medicating normal life events (such as the menopause), to converting risks into diseases, and to treating trivial complaints with fancy procedures. Doctors and 'consumers' alike are becoming locked within a fantasy that unites the creation of anxiety with gung-ho 'can-do, must-do' technological perfectibilsm: everyone has something wrong with them, everyone can be cured. Medical success may be creating a Frankenstein's monster, what has been called by Ivan Illich, a critic of modern medicine, the 'medicalization of life'. To air these predicaments is not antimedical spleen – a churlish reprisal against medicine for its victories – but simply a realization of medical power that is growing not exactly without responsibility but with dissolving goals. Even though this may be in medicine's finest hour, it might also be the dawn of its dilemmas.

For centuries medicine was impotent and hence unproblematic. From the Greeks to the First World War, its job was simple: to struggle with lethal diseases and gross disabilities, to ensure live births, and to manage pain. It performed these uncontroversial tasks mostly with meagre success. Today, with mission accomplished, medicine's triumphs are dissolving in disorientation. The task facing medicine in the twenty-first century will be to redefine its limits even as it extends its capacities.

The triumphs and trials of modern medicine can be understood only in a historical framework. That understanding must be based on proper scholarship. All too often oversimplified and caricatured visions of the rise of medicine are reproduced in books and newspapers. For example, the late and extremely distinguished American physician, Lewis Thomas, wrote that

The history of medicine has never been a particularly attractive subject in medical education and one reason for this is that it is so unbelievably deplorable . . . bleeding, purging, cupping and the administration of infusions of every known plant, solutions of every known metal, every conceivable diet including total fasting, most of them based on the weirdest imaginings about the cause of disease, concocted out of nothing but thin air – this was the heritage of medicine until a little over a century ago.[2]

One understands the emotions behind Professor Thomas's statements. His view, however, amounts to extremely bad history: almost every statement contained in the quotation above will be shown, somewhere in this volume, to be untrue. If we reduce the history of medicine to a travesty, through gross oversimplification, how can we expect to achieve more than a superficial grasp of trends at work now? One of the main aims of this volume is to create the sense that

8

medicine has been constantly remaking itself, demolishing old dogmas, building on the past, forging new perspectives, and redefining its goals. In one respect, of course, medicine has always been about the same thing: healing the sick. But what that has entailed – imaginatively, organizationally, scientifically, humanely – has forever been (as this volume shows) in a state of transformation.

A few further words of explanation are due. This volume does not attempt to be a universal history of medicine worldwide, and some topics – such as primary care, surgery, and psychiatry – are covered in more detail than, for example, tropical medicine, dentistry, medical jurisprudence, and complementary therapies. The book is essentially a history of the roots, rise, and present state of the major specialities of Western medicine, or, as it might be called, scientific medicine. Very little is said about the medical systems to be found in the hundreds of tribal societies the world over; nor are there chapters on Chinese medicine, Islamic medicine, the Ayurvedic medicine of India, and the many medical systems that have flourished in Asia. The omission of those traditions is not a comment on their historical importance or value. To have done such subjects justice – and to have included more detail on other subjects – would have doubled the length of the work. These topics have been sacrificed for coherence and concentration. We have chosen instead to examine in detail the historical roots of Western scientific medicine, which, to a greater or lesser degree, is now becoming the dominant system of the world. Why this is so is one of the questions we address in this volume.

As the story told here shows, we are today living through momentous times for medicine but ones also full of doubt. During the past two centuries, and especially in recent decades, medicine has grown ever more powerful and successful. Yet there is deep personal anxiety and public debate about many of the directions in which medicine may be heading. The paradox involved (better health and longer life, but greater medical anxieties) may be understood, if not resolved, by the historical perspectives that this volume offers.

Roy Porter

1. The History of Disease

Kenneth F. Kiple

Humans have been fighting the diseases of 'civilization' since they began congregating in large numbers. There is written and pictorial evidence of this from Egypt and Mesopotamia around 1000 BC, India about 750 BC, Greece of the sixth century BC, and China about 100 BC. Yet, as the Canadian physician and historian William Osler commented, 'Civilization is but a filmy fringe on the history of man'. By this he meant that the past four or five millennia represent a tiny fraction of 1 per cent of the time since human ancestors first appeared on earth. There is, of course, no recorded history of the ailments of people before the emergence of civilizations and thus before the diseases that they spawned, but we can make informed guesses about them from skeletons and other archaeological remains.

Before Farming

For at least 4.5 million years, human ancestors (hominids) were hunters and gatherers. They lived in scattered groups of perhaps 50 to 100 individuals. The low numbers and low densities of the populations reduced the incidence of viral and bacterial infections so that people were not troubled by contagious diseases such as small-pox or measles, whose pathogens require large and dense populations for survival. Moreover, the lifestyle of hunter-gatherers spared them other illnesses. They were restless folk, often on the move, and thus not tied to a neighbourhood long enough to pollute water sources with human wastes that transmit disease, nor to pile up refuse that attracts disease-carrying insects. Finally, hunter-gatherers had no domesticated animals. Tamed animals helped to create civilizations with their meat, hides, milk, eggs, and bones but also transmitted many diseases.

Our hunting, fishing, and gathering ancestors did not escape diseases altogether but they were less exposed to them than are modern humans. There were two principal sources of disease in those far-off times, one of them wild animals. Infections (zoonoses) were acquired by eating or just being in contact with animals. The second threat of disease came from organisms that were present in pre-hominid ancestors and continued to evolve with humans. In this second category were numerous worms, lice, and bacteria such as *Salmonella* and *Treponema* (the agent of yaws and syphilis).

The zoonotic illnesses in the first category may have included trichinosis, sleeping sickness, tularaemia (rabbit fever), tetanus, schistosomiasis (bilharziasis), and leptospirosis (Weil's disease). Other possibilities are one or more of the various forms of typhus, malaria, and even yellow fever. Encounters with these infections would have been mostly incidental and individual and would seldom, if ever, have affected many members of a group, especially in view of the mobility of hunter-gatherers and their tendency to abandon areas when food became short.

Such mobility also put hunter-gatherers within reach of a wide range of wild plant and animal food that presumably helped establish the kinds and quantities of the nutrients that humans need today. Studies of the few remaining hunter-gatherers of present times point to the consumption of a truly astounding variety of foodstuffs. If such variety was characteristic of hunter-gatherer diets of the past, it may partly explain anomalies of modern humans, such as the ability to develop scurvy if food contains insufficient vitamin C (ascorbic acid). Humans and only a few other animals cannot synthesize their own ascorbic acid. Because of the importance of vitamin C to metabolic processes, it seems unlikely that an ability to synthesize it would have been lost in evolution, unless it had been rendered superfluous – unnecessary because ascorbic acid had been well supplied by the diet over hundreds of thousands of years.

If, however, early humans were blessed with nutritional plenty and a life relatively untroubled by disease, why is it that they remained hunter-gatherers for more than 99.5 per cent of the 2.5 million years that 'cultural' (that is, toolmaking) people have been on earth? Why did human populations not quickly mushroom in just a few thousand of those years to the point where people could no longer feed themselves with hunting and gathering strategies?

Such population crises may, in fact, have occurred countless times. Famine must often have intervened to bring population size back into line with the available food supply. Doubtless, too, many lives were lost in high-risk, high-return endeavours associated with scavenging and hunting of large animals. Doubtless many were lost in the higher-risk, higher-return business of killing fellow humans. Other checks on population growth may also have operated to permit hunting and gathering to continue for so long. Childbirth was risky and many infants probably died from natural causes. Infanticide may also have been practised. Indeed, viewed within the context of the restlessness of hunter-gatherers on the one hand, and the fact that, when moving, they had to carry everything they owned, on the other, it is difficult to believe that infanticide was not an important factor in checking the growth of ancient populations.

In spite of these restraints, populations grew. If a hunter-gatherer band became too large to function efficiently, it split into two. This kind of multiplication took ancient humans into every corner of the Old World after 1.8 million–1.5 million years ago. From their ancestral home in Africa, *Homo erectus* populations expanded into the tropical regions of Asia and later into more temperate zones, continuing their peripatetic existence. Even the first modern humans (*Homo sapiens*), with brains the size of ours, continued as hunter-gatherers for some 100,000 years.

The advent of a sophisticated tool culture around 40,000 years ago led to efficiencies in hunting and food preparation but there was no major change in the nomadic lifestyle until 12,000–10,000 years ago at the end of the last ice age. This presents us with another puzzle, especially for those who believe that replacing hunting and gathering with the domestication of plants and animals was a major improvement in the human condition.

American anthropologist Mark Cohen has argued that people were wise enough to know when they were well off – they became farmers only because increasing population pressure left them little choice. By at least 50,000 years ago, humanity had spilled over from the Old World to Australasia and sometime before 12,500 years ago to the Americas as well. During the coldest parts of the ice age it was possible to walk over to these new continents on land. When the ice caps melted 12,000 to 10,000 years ago and the seas rose to seal off this kind of migration, there was simply no place to absorb surplus populations. Stone Age technology was strained to its utmost to support people in all the habitable parts of the Old World, and in the words of an American historian, Alfred Crosby, humankind was now faced with the choice of becoming 'either celibate or clever. Predictably, the species chose the latter course': people settled down and took up producing their own food.

Farming and Disease

Once set on that course, events moved with dizzying speed – at least when measured against the 5 million to 6 million years that the human family has been around. As Mark Cohen has remarked, around 10,000 years ago almost everybody lived exclusively on wild food; by 2,000 years ago, most people were farmers. Such a transition was indisputably the most important event ever engineered by humankind.

Wild grasses were tamed and tinkered with until they became domesticated varieties of wheat, rye, barley, and rice. Dogs were probably the first animals to be domesticated (around 12,000 years ago) and over the next few thousand years they were followed by cattle, sheep, goats, pigs, horses, and fowl. The few square miles that a hunter-gatherer band might have quickly picked clean were thus transformed into a base that could support many more people indefinitely. The population expanded dramatically because those who surrendered their mobile lifestyle were no longer constrained in the number of offspring they might have. Rather, the more people there were, the more hands for the fields and security for the elderly. It was from this crucible of the agricultural revolution that people began learning to manipulate the planet – to rearrange its ecological systems, not to mention the genes of the plants and animals within those systems. They began the enterprise of undoing

13

a self-regenerating nature without knowing what they were doing, an unthinking process that has continued to the present.

The agricultural revolution thus had ecological downsides, the depths of which we cannot yet fathom. One of these downsides embraces the many realms of parasites. By inventing agriculture, humans also cultivated disease. Pathogens of domesticated animals now found their way into human bodies and began adapting to them as well. According to William McNeill, an American historian, humans share some 65 diseases with dogs, 50 with cattle, 46 with sheep and goats, 42 with pigs, 35 with horses, and 26 with poultry. These animals joined with humans in fouling drinking water with their bodily wastes. Humans scattered those wastes on the cultivated land, which maximized the opportunities of parasitic worms and attracted disease-spreading insects.

Permanent dwellings attracted other domesticates, albeit self-appointed ones. Mice and rats learned to take shelter with humans, enjoy their warm surroundings, and eat the same food. After several thousand years of co-evolution the day has long passed when these small, furry animals could live without humans, to which they have become adapted so well. All too often, however, these commensals have helped spread disease.

Permanent settlements attracted mosquitoes and other assorted blood-sucking insects, which now had many human bodies to feed on. Mosquito breeding sites were available in forest clearings and in stagnant water near dwellings. Faeces-feeding houseflies flourished in these new settlements and their 'dirty feet' on food intended for the human stomach insured a variety of self-perpetuating diarrhoeal diseases and bacillary dysentery. Fleas and lice colonized the outside of the human body, and amoebas, hookworms, and countless other parasitic worms moved into its interior. All would proliferate easily because people lived in close proximity.

In spite of such disease-producing squalor, human breeding ability insured that the festering villages became home for increasing numbers of people. Infant and child mortality rates doubtless increased but birth rates soared even higher, which meant more and more individuals living within spitting, coughing, and sneezing distance of one another to lay the groundwork for a myriad of airborne illnesses.

Farming itself also promotes disease. Irrigation farming in the early river valley civilizations, such as that of the Yellow River (Huang He) in China and the Nile, especially the flooding of lands for the cultivation of rice, had the desired effect of killing off competing plant species. But in the warm, shallow waters of the paddy fields lurked parasites able to penetrate the skin and enter the bloodstream of wading human rice farmers. Foremost among these is a blood fluke called *Schistosoma* that uses aquatic snails as an intermediate host through successive stages of development and produces the debilitating, and often deadly disease called schistosomiasis (or bilharziasis). Evidence of the presence of the disease has been found in Egypt in the kidneys of 3,000-year-old Egyptian mummies.

Slash-and-burn agriculture – a method of land clearance in which vegetation is cut, allowed to dry, and then burned before crop-planting – created niches in which relatively small populations of parasites could breed into very large ones. In Africa south of the Sahara, for example, it has been shown that this type of cultivation led to the proliferation of the mosquito *Anopheles gambiae* that spreads falciparum malaria, the most dangerous of malarial diseases.

Finally, just the act of breaking the sod for cultivation brought humans into new and intimate contact with numerous insects and worms, not to mention bacteria, viruses, protozoans, and the rickettsias (microorganisms intermediate between bacteria and viruses) carried by ticks, fleas, and lice.

Clearly, then, the establishment of permanent settlements from about 12,000 years ago and the cultivation of land around them did human health no good. But, even worse, disease came from the domestication of animals. Cattle contributed their poxes to the growing pool of pathogens; pigs, birds, and horses, their influenzas. Measles is probably the result of rinderpest, or canine distemper, oscillating back and forth between humans and cattle or dogs; smallpox is probably the product of a long evolutionary adaptation of cowpox to humans.

One says 'probably' because, although there is little doubt that humans acquired most of their diseases after they became farmers, one can only speculate about distant evolutionary changes. It was a process in which viruses and bacteria ricocheted back and forth between various domesticated animal species that had never before been in close contact and between those animals and their human owners. In this new pathogenic crucible, microorganisms incubated, combined, altered, perished, and prospered. Their prosperity was often a function of still more evolutionary trial and error, in which pathogens found their way to intermediary hosts, which served as staging areas for later assaults on humans. Similarly, it probably took other microorganisms a long time to acquire vectors to shuttle them about from intermediary host to people as well as from person to person.

Some diseases such as smallpox and measles were so perfectly adapted to humans when they emerged from this crucible that they no longer needed their old host or hosts to complete their life cycle. They were also so contagious that they spread with remarkable ease from human to human. Indeed, the appearance of these 'new' diseases that require only human hosts – but many of them – is testimony to the population explosion that occurred after people gave up hunting and gathering. This happened in spite of the declining health of people. As small settlements grew into large ones they became even more squalid, and population pressure dictated the concentration of the diet on fewer and fewer foodstuffs. In other words, people became nutritionally impoverished as disease became more ubiquitous, opening the door to a synergistic union of malnutrition and pathogens.

The Rise of New Diseases

The roundworm (*Ascaris*), which was probably acquired from pigs, and the hookworm, both spread by faecal pollution of soil, would have joined in this assault on the human body. These worms live in the gut and compete with their human hosts for protein, causing anaemia. Deprived of nutrients important in combating disease, early farmers, especially their children, would have been less able to withstand the next wave of pathogens to invade them: and so the cycle continued.

Ironically, then, as humans switched their activities from living off nature to vigorously manipulating it, they were increasingly parasitized by microorganisms with a vigour of their own. The microorganisms had a clear advantage because they reproduce with lightning speed and can go through several thousand life cycles while humans are still working their way from infancy to reproductive age.

Humans were not totally defenceless in this apparently uneven struggle. Those that survived a disease were, at best, left with an ability to escape completely its next visitation or, at worst, with some immunity against its ravages. Humans hence began developing sophisticated immune systems to enable them to live with their invaders. Pathogens co-operated in this immunological development. Although the most susceptible humans they infected died out, so, too, did the most virulent pathogens, which killed themselves by killing their hosts. Thus invader and invaded reached a compromise: the host survived but passed on the pathogens to other hosts.

Immunities, developed by mothers against diseases they encountered, were delivered across the placenta, which provided the newborn with some defence against the inevitable invasion of germs. Some individuals are also protected genetically from disease. In the case of the dangerous falciparum malaria, for example, individuals with the sickle-cell trait, a deficit in energy metabolism called glucose-6-phosphate dehydrogenase (G6PD) deficiency, beta-thalassaemia, or several other blood anomalies have increased resistance to the disease. Genes for such traits have proliferated in malarious areas. Where parasitic worms are widespread, people develop a tolerance for the worms – or, as it were, a partial immunity to them. Indeed, the rule seems to be that those who live in close proximity to a particular pathogen for long enough develop an ability to 'live' with the disease that the pathogen provokes.

Other diseases are, however, far more difficult to live with. These are the pathogens that first emerged when human numbers increased sufficiently to support them in their new form. Speculation about when and where these new plagues of humankind first manifested themselves is fascinating but is little more than guesswork, given the dearth of archaeological data and the frequently contradictory nature of what there is. It was certainly not much before 3000 BC. Around that time, cities with populations as large as 50,000 were springing up in Mesopotamia and Egypt. In the Indus

Valley in the Indian subcontinent, too, large populations were also emerging. These had substantial cattle herds, from which several pathogens, including perhaps that of smallpox, spread to humans. Evidence to strengthen the suspicion that smallpox was present quite early in southern Asia lies in the existence of ancient Indian temples that appear to have been erected to worship a smallpox deity. In addition, smallpox inoculation seems to have been practised in India in ancient times. Focusing a little nearer present times, William McNeill decided that the period beginning about 500 BC was when pathogens began to have an impact on the growth of civilizations in Asia and Europe. These were the microparasites that trigger smallpox, diphtheria, influenza, chickenpox, mumps, and numerous other illnesses. They pass quickly and directly from human to human and need no intermediary carrier. These new illnesses changed the course of human history. Populations in which a particular disease had arisen presumably developed some immunity against it, just as they had developed resistance to the older diseases in their immediate locale. But marauders, merchants, missionaries, and marching armies did not long permit civilizations to flourish in exotic isolation. Moving from one place to another, they also linked their pools of pathogens. Thus, one people's familiar disease became another people's plague.

The immediate consequence of an invasion by novel pathogens would have been a massive epidemic and a dramatic fall in population as the most susceptible individuals were eliminated. The survivors would have then begun the painful process of population recovery, only to be set upon by another new disease, and yet another. Populations that had grown large enough to host such illnesses would have suddenly become too small to do so. With almost everybody immune and few non-immune individuals being born, the illnesses themselves would have disappeared, only to return after the populations had grown large again and were full of people with low resistance.

While one group enjoyed an epidemiological respite, the new diseases attacked other populations that had grown large, often near the limits of their food supplies. In short, the new diseases became important in preventing human overpopulation while immunologically tempering those that survived them.

Cities as Magnets for Disease

By limiting population growth, such diseases also made possible the agricultural surpluses that sped the growth of cities. These in turn became magnets for pathogens as well as people. Until relatively recently, cities were generally so unhealthy that their populations could not replace themselves by reproduction. They maintained their numbers or grew in size only because of migration from the surrounding countryside. Many who were attracted to gregarious living perished from the gauntlet of disease that accompanied city life. But those that survived joined a growing immunological elite of urbanites – a teeming infectious multitude that was acutely dangerous to less immunologically developed neighbours. When such biologically dangerous peoples had the urge to expand their territories, their pathogens often spearheaded the effort.

Hence, wherever armies marched pathogens flourished. The Peloponnesian war (431–404 BC) was one of the earliest and best examples of this. Before the war we know from the Hippocratic treatises that, whereas the ancient Greeks suffered from malaria and probably tuberculosis, diphtheria, and influenza as well, they seemed to have been spared killer epidemic diseases such as small-pox. However, growing populations, especially that of Athens, helped to kindle the flames of imperial ambition. Those flames were abruptly extinguished during Athens's war with Sparta and the sudden advent of epidemic disease.

The famous description by the Greek historian Thucydides tells us much about this epidemic that reputedly began in Africa, spread to Persia, and reached Greece in 430 BC. He claimed that initially it killed 25 per cent of the Athenian forces; then lingered in southern Greece for the next 4 years, killing up to 25 per cent of the civilian population. On the basis of the symptoms described, plague, smallpox, measles, typhus, or even syphilis and ergotism have been proposed as likely candidates. Whatever the disease was it seems to have destroyed the Greek people's ability to host it by killing or immunizing them. Whereupon it disappeared, leaving in its wake the wreckage of Athenian dreams of hegemony, which has been called a 'turning point' in the history of Western civilization.

Disease occasioned other turning points. Roman conquest knitted together much of the known world and most of its deadly pathogens by successively embracing Macedonia and Greece (146 BC), Seleucid Asia (64 BC), and finally Egypt (30 BC). Disease began affecting the Empire and Rome from the second century AD onwards. The first widespread epidemic, the so-called Antonine plague, may have killed from a quarter to a third of the populations in infected areas between AD 165 and 180, whereas a second, which struck between 211 and 266, scourged both Rome and the countryside. In short, after AD 200 epidemics and barbarians joined in first battering and ultimately bringing down the Roman Empire. A shrinking world also resulted in wider and wider pools of diseases shared by more and more people in South Asia, the Middle East, and East Asia; that is, centres from which diseases rotated outwards to draw other Old World populations into their vortices. The example of Japan is a classic in this regard. Before AD 552, the Japanese seem to have escaped the epidemic diseases that had long scourged mainland populations. In that year, however, Buddhist missionaries from Korea visited the Japanese court, and shortly after many Japanese died from what may have been smallpox.

In 585 – after a new, non-immune generation had arisen in Japan – there was another outbreak of disease that seems clearly to have been smallpox or measles. Once again many died. Then a century seems to have elapsed without notable outbreaks of illness. The seventh century, however, was brought abruptly to an end with the beginning of Japan's 'age of plagues' (700–1050). During the eighth century, the country was rocked with thirty-four epidemics; in the ninth century, it suffered through thirty-five; in the tenth century, twenty-six; and in the eleventh century, twenty-four, sixteen of which had occurred by mid-century.

In the forefront of the diseases known to have triggered these epidemics were smallpox and measles, although influenza, mumps, and dysentery were also well represented. All continued to pound Japan during the period 1050–1260 but not with the same intensity, and the population finally began to grow after stagnating for centuries. Much of the reason for this renewed growth may be found in the fact that, by about 1250, smallpox and measles had come to be regarded as childhood diseases.

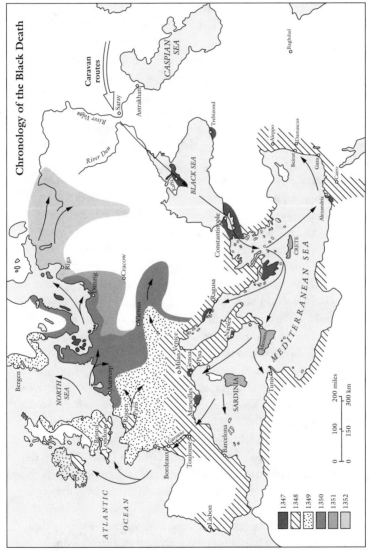

Map 1. An approximate chronology of the Black death as it spread across Europe from Asia in the middle of the fourteenth century.

Viewed from the present day, such a transformation of plagues into childhood illnesses stands out as a large milestone in the epidemiological history of humankind. In the case of the Japanese, it meant that almost all of the adults had already suffered illnesses that they could not get again. But it also meant that they were producing enough non-immune children to hold onto the illnesses so that they dwelled generation after generation in the bodies of the young – and did not escape to return at a later date as devastating plagues. Epidemic diseases that became endemic diseases were not only substantially less disruptive of political, social, and economic life, they were also less wasteful of human life because many epidemic diseases tend to affect the young less severely than they do adults.

Yet, if larger populations had the effect of taming many of the epidemic diseases, such populations remained exposed to other serious infections. These were diseases against which its members were immunologically defenceless because they were diseases of animals, not usually of humans. One such illness is bubonic plague, which has assaulted humans with extreme ferocity whenever and wherever populations have accidentally been caught in a crossfire of disease transmission involving rats, fleas, and the plague bacillus.

As had happened so often in the past, a killer disease (in this case, plague) made its appearance when populations were enjoying a substantial period of growth, and in Europe the next few centuries witnessed demographic stagnation with populations reasserting themselves at different rates. After the Great Plague of London in 1665, for example, the disease withdrew from north-western Europe but not the Mediterranean. Spain, which had suffered cruelly from epidemics in 1596–1602 and 1648–52, also endured another 9 years of plague from 1677 to 1685. The timing of these epidemics seems especially significant when one recalls the rise in English fortunes during this period and the decline of those of Spain.

In the fifteenth and sixteenth centuries, however, not even plague was able to stop the inhabitants of the Iberian Peninsula from engineering the beginning of the European expansion. The Portuguese followed up the capture of Ceuta in 1415 (the year their queen, Philippa, died of plague) with the voyages of trade and exploration that would ultimately take them into the Indian Ocean and on to the threshold of a huge East Indies empire. Meanwhile the Spaniards were also active in waters off the African coast as they conquered the Canary Islands. There, the native resistance of the Guanches, although initially stiff, crumbled in the face of diseases that eventually annihilated them. Sugar plantations were operated by black slaves brought from the African coast to replace the dying Guanches. All of this constituted awful and eerie harbingers of events soon to transpire in the Americas.

It is important to note that, plague notwithstanding, the Iberians who were poised to reunite the New with the Old World were as immunologically fit as any people on earth. For aeons they had been in touch with the outside world in a way that few others had. Iberians had gone to Rome as emperors and Iberian soldiers had marched in Roman legions. From 710 onwards they were intimately involved with invading Arabs and thus with the greater Muslim empire. Indeed, Iberia became something of a melting pot of Christians, Arabs, and incoming Jews. Crusaders paused at Iberian ports on their way to and from the Holy Land (sometimes for lengthy periods as they were drawn into local political or military disputes). Iberians traded from the North Sea to the eastern Mediterranean, and their fishing fleets covered the North Atlantic. By the fourteenth century, the Catalans had built a Mediterranean empire that stretched all the way to Greece. In the fifteenth century, the Portuguese drew Africa and Africans into the Iberian sphere of pathogenic propinquity.

In short, the cities of Spain and Portugal, especially those with harbours, were clearing houses of diseases as well as bank drafts, and in them, as in other Renaissance centres, diseases flourished. Bathing was frowned upon, and clothing was coarse and changed infrequently. Hence the human body was a veritable nest of lice and fleas. Human wastes were flung into the streets to mingle with those of dogs and horses. All of this was paradise for flies that flitted from faeces to food. Water for drinking and cooking was practically a soup of microorganisms. Rats, mice, and other assorted vermin burrowed, crawled, slithered, and skulked their way through houses, shops, warehouses, churches, and taverns. The corpses of dogs, cats, and even horses were, more often than not, left to rot, adding to the stench of the streets, and providing sustenance for still more vermin.

Clearly, survivors of this milieu were equipped with very alert and agile immune systems. To reach adulthood they not only ran a gauntlet of childhood diseases, such as smallpox, measles, diphtheria and the like, but also had to weather a gamut of gastrointestinal infections along with an appalling variety of other afflictions of the skin, blood, bones, and organs seldom seen today outside of the poorest countries. The explorers and conquerors of the Americas, then, can be viewed as a sort of immunological elite, which made for a breathtaking (and deadly) contrast between them and those they conquered.

Disease Conquers the New World

The ancestors of those who came to be known as Amerindians were hunters and gatherers. At least 12,500 years ago, some traversed the Bering Straits from Asia to Alaska on a land bridge created by the last ice age, which had substantially lowered the levels of the world's oceans and exposed the shallow continental shelf between Asia and North America. On the basis of genetic evidence it has recently been suggested that others may have come from Polynesia. Crossing the Bering Straits was not a sunny outing. The land bridge was bleak, foggy, and cold, prompting some scholars to suspect that population pressure made such expeditions not so much a matter of human restlessness but one of human survival. In other words, the successive waves of migrants may well have been pushed into adventure.

As we have portrayed them, hunter-gatherers were relatively disease-free, and the rigours of the Bering crossing would doubtless have eliminated any that were diseased or weak. Moreover, the pioneers left the Old World before the domestication of animals, which means that (save perhaps for the dog in the later waves) they brought no other portable disease-carriers except themselves and they encountered no humans, diseased or otherwise, after their arrival.

The ice age came to a close about 10,000 years ago. Ice caps melted and seas rose to cover the land bridge and seal off the new Americans. At the same time the great glaciers covering much of North America melted, opening up an entire continent to the arrivals. If the hunter-gatherers had dreamed of paradise, this was it. The new land, however, had a few nasty surprises. First, the Americas had a few unique illnesses to offer. Rocky Mountain spotted fever, for example, is an American rickettsial disease found today from Brazil to Canada. Although the illness, which is transmitted by ticks, was really identified only in the twentieth century, it is conceivable that it affected the continent's early pioneers as well as its modern inhabitants. Those who pushed into South America may have encountered mucocutaneous leishmaniasis (uta), a protozoan disease transmitted by blood-sucking sandflies. Those reaching the Andes region risked Carrión's disease (also called Oroya fever and verruga Peruana). This illness is also spread by sandflies and its disfiguring impact is seemingly depicted on pottery thousands of years old. Another native illness of South America is Chagas' disease or American trypanosomiasis, which probably had its origin in Brazil. It is caused by a trypanosome protozoan carried by guinea-pigs and other animals and transmitted to humans by blood-sucking bugs.

In addition, there were diseases of wild animals such as trichinosis and tularaemia to contend with, and, later, some diseases of civilization made their appearance as a New World agricultural revolution got underway. The Maya, the Aztec, the Inca, and the Mississippian peoples of North America settled into sedentary agriculture and built complex civilizations complete with cities and many of the attendant problems of health that, as we have seen, accompany such a lifestyle. Some kinds of tuberculosis developed and intestinal parasites and hepatitis passed from person to person through water and food. Pinta, one of several diseases caused by *Treponema* bacteria, seems to have been a problem wherever it was warm enough for scanty dress to permit easy skin-to-skin transmission. Other treponemal infections seem to have been present, including some sort of (apparently) non-venereal syphilis.

But the New World peoples, who were named 'Indians' by Christopher Columbus and his fellow adventurers, were 'virgin soil' for the avalanche of diseases that arrived from Europe. They had been dangerously exempted from the disease pools of the Old World, which the American scholar Alfred Crosby has listed

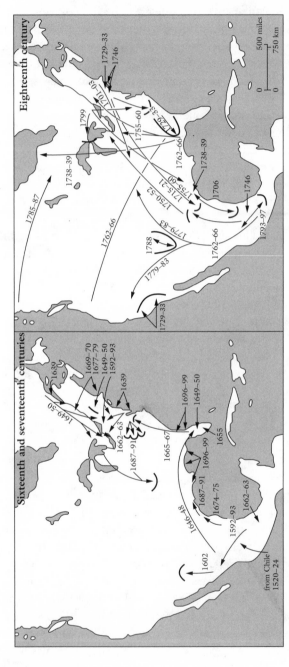

Map 2. The native populations of the Americas were devastated by an avalanche of infectious diseases that European colonizers brought with them from the fifteenth century onwards. Smallpox arrived in the Caribbean in 1518, and entered Mexico and South America soon afterwards, killing millions in epidemic after epidemic. Later, the disease spread to North America. This is one interpretation of the spread of smallpox in North America in the sixteenth to eighteenth centuries.

as including smallpox, measles, diphtheria, trachoma, whooping cough, chickenpox, bubonic plague, malaria, typhoid fever, cholera, yellow fever, dengue fever, scarlet fever, amoebic dysentery, influenza, and helminthic infestations. To this list one might add illnesses such as typhus, brucellosis, erysipelas, filariasis, mumps, onchocerciasis, relapsing fever, leprosy, and probably hookworm disease.

No one knows how many native Americans were present when Columbus and disease arrived and thus no one knows for certain the numerical magnitude of the demographic disaster they endured. Indeed, questions about the size of American populations at European contact have been among those most hotly contested by historical demographers and anthropologists throughout the twentieth century, and the subject of keen debate in the Quincentennial scholarship of 1992. But whether one is inclined to accept high estimates, of around 100 million, or a more conservative 50 million or less, there is some agreement that the hurricane of disease that swept the Americas ultimately claimed about 90 per cent of the 1492 populations.

The first American epidemic, which struck the island of Hispaniola in 1493, may well have been swine influenza. Other unnamed diseases followed so that West Indian populations were in decline even before smallpox made its official Caribbean debut in 1518. Smallpox accompanied Hernando Cortés to Mexico and raced ahead of the Pizarros into Peru, greatly expediting both conquests, while radiating outwards to kill other untold millions that the Spanish never had to conquer. Following this, epidemic after epidemic rained on the New World. One of the worst to be recorded was the typhus epidemic that reportedly killed some 2 million in the Mexican highlands towards the end of the sixteenth century.

One can only imagine the horror: young adults are frequently the chief victims of epidemics, meaning that few are left to plant, and cook, and clean, and care for children and the old. The epidemics frequently descended in pell-mell fashion, providing no time for populations to recover and immune systems to adjust. Social, political, economic, and religious life crumbled, and the wonder is that anyone managed to survive to develop immunities and pass them on. But they did, and the mainland populations of Mexico and the Andean region gradually recovered.

Population decline (and recovery) came later in North America. It took a particularly nasty downward turn in the Caribbean and in parts of Brazil where decline actually meant obliteration. The reason for these differing demographic circumstances, however, does not lie among Eurasian illnesses but rather in another group of Old World diseases whose cradle lay in sub-Saharan Africa.

African Diseases Enter the New World

The arrival of Africans in the Americas was a tragedy begotten by another New World tragedy, the establishment of black slavery, which, in turn, was the consequence of the fall in the indigenous population. The Iberian conquerors had counted on the labour of the Amerindians to colonize the vastness of the Americas. But the rapid decline in numbers of native Americans meant that they had to look elsewhere for such assistance. By 1518 the transatlantic slave trade was well underway.

The arriving Africans bore many of the same immunities as the Europeans because, for millennia, most Eurasian illnesses had regularly found their way into sub-Saharan Africa in desert caravans and across the Indian Ocean. In addition, Africans were resistant to the resident tropical illnesses of their own part of the world, which most other peoples were not. One of these was falciparum malaria, the most dangerous of the malarial types and also a relatively new one, which, as we have seen, was spawned by the development of sedentary agriculture in Africa. It had not remained strictly an African disease and at some time in the past it had moved north to parts of the Mediterranean. Indeed, this was another lethal force that some have credited with contributing significantly to the decline of the Roman Empire. Evidence that at one time falciparum malaria was of considerable prevalence in southern Italy and Greece can be found today in the blood anomalies of many Mediterranean people that we know are genetic defences against the disease.

The incidence of such protective anomalies as the sickle-cell trait and glucose-6-dehydrogenase (G6PD) deficiency is far greater among Africans, and is testimony to their long and intimate association with falciparum malaria. Such defences also testify to an extensive and extended experience with another, more ubiquitous malarial type, vivax malaria, which has virtually disappeared from Africa. Vivax malaria is believed to be among the oldest of the malarial types. Like the other forms it originated in Africa where the protozoan *Plasmodium*, the cause of all malarias, parasitized thousands of generations of humans. In such a process, however, close to 100 per cent of Africans acquired a genetic trait that protects them against vivax malaria and probably against falciparum malaria as well.

With few human carriers of vivax malaria in Africa, the disease changed locales to become a scourge of much of the rest of the world, including Europe. Hence, Europeans were the carriers of vivax malaria to the New World; the more serious falciparum malaria arrived with Africans. Anopheline mosquitoes were present in the Americas to spread the protozoan infections and add them to the list of microbes slaughtering the native Americans.

Yellow fever, that other great tropical killer to emanate from Africa, was slower to make an American appearance because its principal vector, the *Aedes agypti* mosquito, was not immediately on hand. Entomological evidence suggests that slave ships brought *Aedes* from Africa, along with the yellow-fever virus. From 1647, when an epidemic in Barbados spread throughout the Caribbean, yellow fever so scourged American coastal cities that it came to be regarded as an American disease.

In discussing the fall in the Amerindian populations, it is important to note the impact of this second – African – wave of diseases. In the highland areas of the Andes and central Mexico, the native populations staggered under the assault of Eurasian diseases, but they ultimately recovered. This was, at least in part, because they were spared the African illnesses – the mosquito vectors do not thrive at altitudes significantly above sea level. The populations of the low-lying areas of the Caribbean and the Amazon basin, however, were seriously affected by both the Eurasian and the African diseases and were almost obliterated. Other less-lethal, but nonetheless formidable, African diseases also arrived on the slave ships, among them dracunculiasis, filariasis, onchocerciasis, hookworm disease (caused by the misnamed *Necator americanus*), yaws (allied to pinta), and even leprosy, which had previously disappeared from Europe.

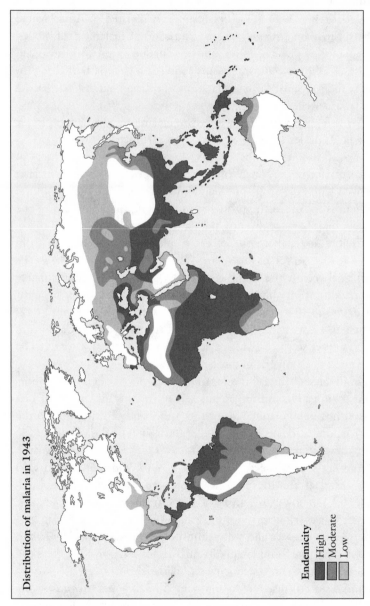

Distribution of malaria in 1943

Endemicity
High
Moderate
Low

Map 3. World distribution of malaria before the era of mass travel.

New Worlds, New Pathogens?

The abrupt linking of the disease environments of Europe, the Americas, and Africa has come under much scrutiny by scholars. Their suspicion is that it did more than simply scatter known diseases more widely – that it, in fact, spawned some new diseases for the world. From a European viewpoint, some new diseases did seem to appear around the time of the Columbian voyages. Typhus was one of these. It appeared in Europe during the last of the wars of the reconquest, as Spain finally conquered Granada in 1492; the disease seems to have reached Spain from the Arab world. In this case, therefore, Columbus is exonerated.

Like syphilis, smallpox presents historians of medicine with a puzzle. It seems to have varied considerably in its virulence over time. There were two types of smallpox before the disease finally disappeared in the second half of the 1970s: variola major, which had mortality rates of up to 25–30 per cent, and variola minor, a much milder disease with mortality rates of 1 per cent or less. Doubtless, strains intermediate between the two also existed. Before about 1500 – in Europe at least – smallpox was not a virulent killer, but around that date it became so, causing some 10 to 15 per cent of all deaths in some countries. Investigators have occasionally voiced the suspicion that the most virulent form of smallpox originated in sub-Saharan Africa, not Asia. Recently, the argument has been advanced that it was with the Atlantic slave trade that this most deadly strain was unleashed.

These new, or newly modified, diseases served to enrich the already sizable swarm of pathogens that swept over other 'newly discovered' peoples, who, like the Amerindians, were so brutally united with the larger world. Vasco da Gama, in leading the Portuguese into the Indian Ocean (1498) and an eastern empire, also inadvertently spearheaded the spread of syphilis as far east as Japan. The voyage of Ferdinand Magellan (1519–22) finished what Columbus started by sailing west and taking the Spanish into the East. And in the wake of his ships came diseases with the crews of the Manilla galleons, as well as other explorers, missionaries, traders, and, in the eighteenth century, British and American whalers.

The inhabitants of many Pacific islands had suffered from malaria, filariasis, and tropical skin afflictions before the arrival of Europeans. But these populations of Asian horticulturalists, in many cases separated from the larger world for thousands of years, were 'virgin soil' for the infectious foreign diseases. However, the relative smallness of their populations, on the one hand, and isolation, on the other, would have caused most epidemics to burn out quickly.

Some idea of the thousands of small holocausts of disease that must have occurred among these populations can be gained by viewing the example of the Hawaiian Islands. First settled around AD 300, they remained 'undiscovered' until the arrival of Captain James Cook in 1778. Cook's surgeon wrote that the following year the crew deliberately introduced syphilis to the islands. Whether true or not, syphilis, along with smallpox and other illnesses, reportedly reduced the native population by 90 per cent within a century.

A similar precipitous decline of the native populations of Australia got underway after the start of English settlement in 1788. Smallpox erupted almost immediately (1789) among the Aborigines in the eastern half of the continent and, according to British estimates, destroyed half of those with any contact with Port Arthur (Sydney). After this, the disease spread into the interior with unknown consequences. A young Charles Darwin in 1836 had clearly absorbed much of this sort of mournful history when he wrote in his *Beagle* diary '[w]herever the European has trod, death seems to pursue the aboriginal'.

While Europeans were establishing their empires and carrying death to aboriginal peoples, they themselves were caught in a crossfire of disease at home. Epidemics of plague punished areas of the south and east; malaria was on the increase; in the sixteenth century, at least three severe influenza epidemics swept the continent and virulent smallpox appeared; syphilis was increasingly virulent; there were epidemics of diphtheria and scarlet fever; and typhus began to make regular appearances among armies. In fact, it was disease (in this case typhus rather than syphilis) that once more was decisive in spoiling French hopes of conquering the Kingdom of Naples. Typhus broke out among the French soldiers just as victory over Charles V seemed assured. Some 30,000 of them died before the remnants of the army were withdrawn.

On the other side of the world, new diseases such as syphilis, scarlet fever, and diphtheria entered China to join smallpox, measles, malaria, and other old ailments. Cholera was described by Westerners for the first time when the Portuguese visited sixteenth-century India, where, it seems, plague was also raging. In Japan, the first Westerners to visit in 1543 arrived during a period of great population growth, the Japanese having come to immunological terms with their most important diseases. The only new illness in their environment was syphilis, which had reached the islands from China where Europeans had introduced it somewhat earlier. The Japanese called it the 'Chinese pox'.

Europe and China were now to enjoy their own rise in population. In Europe, the winds of change stirred up by the Renaissance signalled an end to feudalism, while fostering the rise of capitalism, predatory nation states, empires, and increasingly authoritarian governments. There were strides towards industrialization and urbanization, stimulated on the one hand by growing governmental bureaucracies and on the other by the needs and fruits of empire – or by the determined quest for those fruits.

It is within this array of historical circumstances that the populations of Britain and northern Europe gradually escaped from the age-old tyranny of disease and its check on population growth. Growing cities exposed more people to disease, and increasing numbers became immunized in the process. Strong governments, by establishing quarantine measures directly, and indirectly, with the inspection of ships for tax collection, helped to keep plague and other diseases at bay. Moreover, governments launched public-health campaigns that reduced the populations of vermin and insects, especially houseflies. Finally, attempts were made in the early eighteenth century to reduce outbreaks of smallpox by variolation, a technique that may have originated in China. Variola in pus from the pustules of infected persons was inserted into scratches on people unaffected, which gave them a mild form of the disease. The procedure sometimes proved fatal, and even resulted in epidemics, but after the 1760s safer inoculation methods were found. The strongest blow against smallpox came with the cowpox vaccination introduced in England by Edward Jenner in 1796. This was quickly adopted throughout Europe and within a few years had reached the Spanish colonies in South America and Asia.

Nutrition and Declining Mortality

Another important factor in this momentous demographic turnaround has to do with nutrition. If the Americas offered few pathogens to the rest of the world, they provided much in the way of foodstuffs. The increasingly widespread cultivation of the potato, which was introduced to Europe in the sixteenth century (along with squash), helped to make a better life for many, especially the poor. In addition to filling stomachs, the potato, which was easy to grow in northern climates, became an important source of vitamins (especially ascorbic acid) and minerals.

Maize from the Americas became a staple in the diet of many others, who, perhaps not enthusiastically, began substituting corn-meal cakes for the more expensive wheat bread. Maize and potatoes are staple crops that produce more calories per unit of land than any other (save cassava), and they certainly helped to sustain a growing urban proletariat. Perhaps, though, the greatest contribution to human health from maize was as animal feed. With more and more people forced from the land into cities, more space was available for domesticated animals. With hay and maize to sustain them, it became possible to carry greater numbers of animals over the winter. Thus another feature of the changing pattern of nutrition was a greater availability throughout the year of high-quality protein in the form of milk and cheese, and eggs as well as meat. Such protein would have helped people ward off many diseases more easily. A reliable supply of milk doubtless helped many more individuals to survive infancy and early childhood than had done so in the past. Improved transportation networks to deliver fresh foods more widely were also obviously vital in helping to improve nutrition.

A crossfire of debate continues over the importance of nutrition in the growth of the European population – and thus also over the importance of American crops in the European diet. It may be that answers are so entangled with and obscured by other complex forces that they cannot be teased out. Some light might be shed on the matter by examples from other parts of the world. In China, for reasons yet to be explained, there was a fall in the rate of mortality after the sixteenth-century introduction of maize and of sweet and white potatoes from the Americas. West and West Central Africa also experienced something of a population explosion after the introduction of cassava, maize, sweet potatoes, and peanuts. The irony is that the population was drained by a slave trade to the hemisphere that had provided the plants to begin with.

New Plagues – Yellow Fever and Cholera

As we have seen, Africa also sent deadly diseases westwards. By the end of the seventeenth century, yellow fever, in addition to haunting ports in the Caribbean, Central America, and Mexico, seemed to be ubiquitous along the eastern coasts of the continent. It struck Pernambuco in Brazil in 1685, killing thousands in Recife and Olinda and spread into Ceará before it burned out some 5 years later. To the north, the disease entered New York in 1668, Philadelphia and Charleston in 1690, and Boston in 1691.

In the eighteenth century, yellow fever extended its range to become a regular visitor to the ports of Colombia, Peru, and Ecuador in the Americas; and to Oporto, Lisbon, Barcelona, Malaga, and Cadiz in Europe. At the same time, it attacked the now-veteran Philadelphians with six epidemics. The disease also became decisive in Caribbean military campaigns. It thwarted Admiral Edward Vernon's 1741 assault on Cartagena in Colombia – half of his original landing force of 19,000 was lost to the virus; it helped in pruning 80,000 men from the British army in the West Indies during the years 1793–6; and it accounted for a sizable portion of the 40,000 French dead in their abortive attempt to regain San Domingue on the island of Hispaniola (now Haiti).

In the nineteenth century, yellow fever was especially prevalent in the port cities of southern USA, where, before the Civil War, it hammered Savannah with fifteen epidemics, Charleston with twenty-two, and New Orleans with at least thirty-three. After the war, it resumed this assault, which culminated in the 1878 epidemic. This moved inland up the Mississippi to leave countless dead in a swathe that cut from New Orleans to Memphis and beyond. Clearly, at least as far as the USA was concerned, yellow fever evened the score for participation in the African slave trade. Its losses to the disease far exceeded the number of slaves it imported.

Yellow fever also continued to slaughter Europeans in the Caribbean, most notably Spanish troops sent to put an end to Cuba's rebellion of 1868–78 (the Ten Years' War) and Frenchmen first sent to lay a railway across Panama and then to construct a canal. It also killed Europeans at home, invading numerous cities of Spain and Portugal as well as Gibraltar, and moving north to strike at the coasts of France and England.

Save for the 1821 epidemic in Barcelona and that of 1857 in Lisbon, however, yellow fever seemed a minor disease in Europe compared to the ravages of typhus and cholera. Typhus played a substantial role in turning the 1812 expedition of Napoleon to Russia into a catastrophe, and between 1816 and 1819 the disease ravaged Ireland. The revolutions of 1848 triggered typhus epidemics in eastern Europe, which then subsided until the First World War. During that war it killed a reported 2 million to 3 million soldiers and civilians. Afterwards, it continued to stalk the Russians and eastern Europeans by killing another 3 million or so.

Cholera, however, was easily the biggest epidemic news of the nineteenth century. Before that time (and thus before all the major advances in technology and transportation), the disease seems to have confined itself to India, where it had been observed and described by outsiders at least since the sixteenth century. From 1817, however, it appeared with increasing frequency outside India. By 1821, it had involved Java and China to the east and Persia to the west.

Disease and Imperialism

While cholera and some of the other 'old' diseases of civilization were being brought under control, civilization itself was spawning and spreading other infections. Medical advances opened Africa – previously known as the 'white man's grave' because of tropical fever – to European colonization as the nineteenth century drew to a close. The discovery of the cause of malaria and the establishment of a reliable supply of quinine (derived from the bark of the cinchona

Distribution of yellow fever in 1943

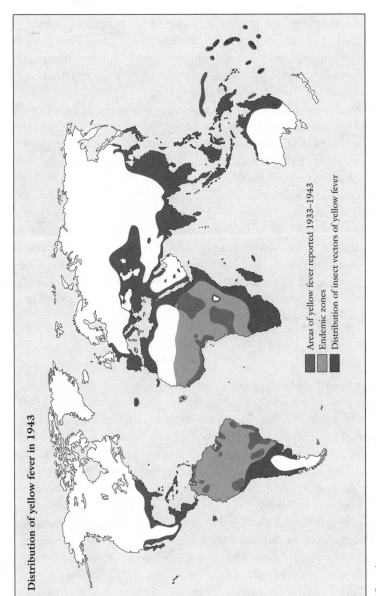

Areas of yellow fever reported 1933–1943
Endemic zones
Distribution of insect vectors of yellow fever

Map 4.

tree) to protect against it simultaneously provided a green light for imperial adventure.

Once established in Africa, however, Europeans sometimes seemed intent on turning it into a black man's grave. They forced Africans into mines to extract the continent's mineral resources; they seized fertile agricultural lands formerly occupied by tribal communities; they introduced alien breeds of cattle; they transformed barter economies into monetary economies; and they built railways and roads to link them.

In this proletarianization of Africa and in rearranging ecologies, the colonists unleashed massive epidemics of sleeping sickness and did much to extend the range of other illnesses. In addition, they brought tuberculosis to Africa. Highly mobile African labourers then spread it to all corners of sub-Saharan Africa, where it smouldered in the slums of an expanding urban poor. The nutritional status of Africans also fell sharply in the face of the implementation of cash-crop economies, which were often based on monoculture (such as cocoa in Ghana). And despite the efforts of missionaries, colonial medicine was mostly aimed at preserving the health of the oppressors, and seldom reached the oppressed.

Nutritional Diseases

Nutritional explanations of the waxing and waning of diseases are complicated by our lack of knowledge of what constitutes good nutrition. As we have seen, our hunter-gatherer forebears consumed an amazing variety of foodstuffs, whereas we, by contrast, consume relatively few. The archaeological record leaves no doubt that humans who surrendered their hunting and gathering ways for sedentary agriculture paid a stiff price in health. They became shorter and suffered considerably from anaemias as a result of an increasingly limited diet centred around a staple crop. At the same time, their young endured what appears to have been protein energy malnutrition after weaning, which doubtless contributed to soaring rates of child mortality.

Technological improvements in agriculture and plant breeding and the exchange of crops in the aftermath of Columbus's voyage of 1492, meant greater quantities of food to sustain more people.

But for those whose survival depended on a diet centred closely on a staple crop, it meant a tremendous sacrifice in nutritional quality. Hence the appearance of the classic deficiency diseases.

The poor in the American South, Africans, southern Europeans, and peoples in India, Egypt, and the Middle East who embraced maize cultivation frequently fell victim to pellagra, a disease characterized by diarrhoea, dermatitis, dementia, and ultimately death for as many as 70 per cent of its victims. The cause of the disease is complicated, but the major factor is a deficiency of niacin. It is not that maize lacks niacin. The trouble is that it has a chemical bond that does not release the niacin to the consumer unless that bond is broken with treatment by lime – a secret that native Americans knew but it did not get passed back to the Old World.

Beriberi is another disease linked to vitamin B deficiency, in this case thiamine. The affliction is normally associated with the rice cultures of Asia. Rice husks contain plenty of thiamine, but people have, over the ages, done their best to strip away the husk to make the grain more palatable, appealing, and amenable to storage. Traditional hand-milling of rice produced the neurological and cardiovascular symptoms of 'dry' and 'wet' beriberi for many people across the world and led to infantile beriberi, which was practically always fatal for nursing babies and toddlers with thiamine-deficient mothers. The problem became especially acute after the advent of steam-driven milling, and by the late 1950s beriberi had become a leading cause of death in parts of Asia, especially for infants.

Rice, however, has not been the only culprit in the aetiology of beriberi. The disease has also been caused by diets too closely centred on manioc meal and flour, and those confined to white bread before the adoption of enrichment procedures. Like pellagra, beriberi was particularly prevalent among institutionalized populations – for example, slaves on plantations, prisoners, children in orphanages, and inmates of ayslums – and those at sea for long periods of time.

The classic shipboard disease, however, was scurvy, triggered by a deficiency in vitamin C (ascorbic acid). Because humans do not synthesize their own vitamin C, scurvy is probably a very old disease. However, it takes some 30 weeks of vitamin-C deprivation for the classic symptoms of spongy, bleeding gums to appear, and even longer for old wounds to open and death to occur, so its appearance before the fifteenth century would have been relatively rare. But the desire for trade, exploration, and empire that accompanied the growing economic power of Europe sent ships to sea for periods long enough for the disease to develop; and it became the scourge of seamen for more than 300–400 years.

Scurvy also affected armies (especially during sieges), erupted in prisoner-of-war camps, dogged the heels of Arctic and Antarctic explorers, and tortured the Irish after the great failure of the potato crop in 1845–6, because potatoes contain vitamin C whereas the grains sent to relieve their plight did not.

In the middle of the eighteenth century it was repeatedly shown that citrus juice could prevent scurvy. It was not until the end of that century, however, that British sailors were regularly issued lime juice to combat the disease. By the close of the nineteenth century, with medicine in the grip of the germ theory, scurvy and the other nutritional diseases were often seen as the work of pathogens. It required the scientific knowledge generated in the twentieth century to get nutritional research back on track and to establish the concept of deficiency diseases.

All such deficiency diseases, at least when widespread, may be viewed as the consequence of nutritional problems caused by advances in civilization. The same is true for other ailments that, although not strictly deficiency diseases, are food-related. Ergotism, for example, is a disease caused by consuming cereal grains – especially rye – infected by the ergot fungus (*Claviceps purpurea*). Known since the time of Galen, it became prevalent in medieval Europe among poor people. Their bread, which constituted the bulk of the diet, was frequently made with spoiled rye, producing the 'convulsive' form when it affected the central nervous system and the 'gangrenous' form when it affected the blood supply to the extremities. The disease was often called St Anthony's fire. At least 130 epidemics occurred in Europe between 591 and 1789, and scores of thousands were killed. Outbreaks were reported from various parts of Europe as late as the 1920s.

A different kind of nutritional problem created by constricted diets is protein energy malnutrition (PEM), which, as we have seen earlier, is essentially a problem of the young and a problem that developed only as people settled into agriculture. Tell-tale evidence is seen on the teeth of early farmers, in the form of hypoplasias (growth-arrest lines) that indicate a real struggle for survival at about the time of weaning. In modern peoples, the evidence is plainly visible in the swollen bellies of kwashiorkor and the wasting away of marasmus, the two symptomatic poles of PEM.

The root cause of PEM is the weaning of a child from breast milk to a cereal pap that contains little or none of the whole protein that the child needs for its growth and development. Whereas hunter-gatherers were obliged to forage for their weaned youngsters, sedentary people concentrated on a staple cereal, which simplified the weaning process. Such simplicity, in turn, encouraged more pregnancies, so that one child was (and is) often abruptly weaned to make room for another. Thus the African word 'kwashiorkor' means the 'sickness of the deprived child'.

PEM often becomes full-blown when children acquire an infection and the latter, rather than the nutritional condition, gets the blame. Nonetheless, PEM is one of the world's great killers, especially in developing regions. It can retard the development and impair the health in later life of those that survive it as children.

Disease in the Modern World

Clearly, then, one result of the agricultural revolution – the concentration of diets on staple crops – was a mixed blessing of enabling more and more people to live but at significant costs to their health. The same might be said for the much more recent and ongoing industrial revolution, which, while creating the conditions for a further explosion in population, also produced general ill-health as well as some specific new diseases.

For example, black lung disease (coal workers' pneumoconiosis) cut life short for many coalminers; brown lung disease (byssinosis) became the curse of cotton textile workers; white lung disease (asbestosis) affected those engaged in working with asbestos; exposure to lead brought on lead poisoning; the 'phossy jaw' was an occupational risk of matchworkers who were exposed to phosphorus; and dust from stone, flint, and sand led to silicosis or 'grinders' disease'.

In 1775, London surgeon Percivall Pott pointed out that many males who had been chimney sweeps while boys later suffered from scrotal cancer. He linked this with irritation caused by soot, and thus identified the first cancer-causing occupation. Subsequently, ultraviolet light, X-rays, radioactive substances such as radium and uranium, and other irritants such as coal-tar derivatives were implicated in cancer.

Cancer, heart-related ailments, and probably Alzheimer's disease are ancient diseases of humankind. There is debate about why there seems to be a substantial increase in all three in the twentieth century, especially in the developed world. One possibility is that more people are living long enough to acquire them. Another explanation has to do with lifestyle – mass-produced and widely used tobacco products and distilled spirits, also products of the modern world, contribute considerably to at least two of these conditions.

It is probably the case, however, that a good number of other factors stemming from advances in civilization are also responsible. There may be more carbon in the atmosphere today because of forest clearance and cultivation than industrialization; but belching smokestacks and exhaust fumes from motor vehicles have put many other chemicals into the air we breathe, the foods we eat, and the water we drink. Moreover, many suspect that the incidence of skin cancers is increasing because of atmospheric pollution, which is increasing ultraviolet intensity. Heavy use of sodium has been implicated in both stomach cancer and hypertension. And foods and water are processed with chemicals that are under increasing scrutiny by both cancer and heart-disease researchers.

Greater longevity is certainly a factor in a greater frequency of some of the genetic diseases and genetic predisposition to other illnesses. In the past, a far smaller percentage of victims of these afflictions would have survived to reproduce and pass on the traits. As some geneticists have argued, in the developed world, at any rate, the principles of rigorous natural selection no longer apply. We have entered another stage – that of 'relaxed selection' – and we are having to pay for this with a greater frequency of diseases ranging from multiple sclerosis to mastoiditis.

Medicine has had the opportunity in the twentieth century to focus much of its research on genetic diseases and the chronic ailments – the new diseases of civilization – because of its triumphs over the old contagious diseases, culminating with the eradication of smallpox in the 1970s. But the collective self-confidence of the medical community has been shaken on several occasions during the past 100 years. This happened, for example, in 1918–19 when an influenza pandemic of unprecedented virulence swept the world, killing between 25 million and 50 million people. Hard on its heels came an epidemic of encephalitis lethargica (an inflammation of the brain and spinal cord) and another wave of killer influenza in 1920. How and why influenza suddenly became so deadly (especially to young adults) has never been satisfactorily explained – nor has its relationship with encephalitis lethargica.

The encounter of modern medicine with poliomyelitis, by contrast, has had a more satisfactory outcome. Poliomyelitis is an ancient viral disease of humankind but epidemics identified as polio became frequent only towards the end of the nineteenth century. This created the belief that it was a new disease, and the great New York epidemic of 1916 produced fears that polio was a modern-day plague – especially when what had been regarded as a children's disease began affecting adults. Such fears gradually subsided with the realization that, in the past, most children had been immunized early in life by the disease itself, which travels the oral-faecal route. Improved sanitation that in many cases had prevented this immunization was actually responsible for the upsurge of the disease. The introduction of vaccinations first by Jonas Edward Salk (1955) and then Albert Bruce Sabin (1960) has brought about a drastic decline in the disease in the developed world and much of the developing world as well. In 1994, the Americas were declared a polio-free zone after 2 years with no reported cases, and the World Health Organization hoped to eliminate the disease worldwide by the year 2000.

Medicine has, however, so far proved powerless against another disease. As was the case early on with polio, acquired immune deficiency syndrome (AIDS) has seemed to be a new disease. Unfortunately, the causative agent, the human immunodeficiency virus

(HIV), mutates even more rapidly than the viral agents of influenza, which has frustrated the development of both vaccines and effective antiviral drugs. Actually there seem to be two main types of the virus involved. HIV-1 was the first to be identified (1981), although in retrospect it would seem that the disease has been spreading silently for years. The principal means of transmission of most of its sub-types have been through homosexual contact and through blood and blood products. In 1985, HIV-2 was identified in West Africa; its pattern of transmission seems to be via heterosexual intercourse. HIV-1 and HIV-2 are now worldwide in their distribution, but both seem to have originated in sub-Saharan Africa where antibodies against HIV were discovered in stored blood dating from 1959, and where most of the world's cases (about two-thirds) were located as of 1995.

Because HIV impairs the immune system, patients often fall victim to illnesses such as pneumocystis pneumonia, tuberculosis, and other infections. Nonetheless, AIDS is a disease in itself, albeit one that can take a decade or longer after infection to manifest itself, with, what so far seem to be invariably fatal consequences. Such a hiatus, however, makes it difficult to calculate the spread of the disease, and thus projections must depend on estimates. Unhappily, even the most optimistic of these suggest that millions will die of AIDS. Some even predict that in terms of overall mortality the disease will take the lead as the biggest killer of humans in history.

Yet other deadly viral diseases have surfaced in Africa, among them Ebola, Lassa, Marburg, and Rift Valley fevers, and still others in South America such as Bolivian haemorrhagic fever and Argentine haemorrhagic fever. It is conceivable that, like AIDS, one or more of these could be unleashed on the wider world. In a sense they, too, are diseases of civilization – in this case of the developing world, where impoverished populations are swelling and chronic diseases of advancing age take second place to major infectious ailments.

Modern medicine has made it possible for increasing numbers of people to survive infancy and childhood in the developing world, but does little for them after that (except for notable campaigns such as those against smallpox or polio). However, in a world growing increasingly smaller as populations are knit ever more closely together, the question arises as to whether we can afford such neglect. Indeed, self-interest, if nothing else, may indicate the importance of cultivating health in the developing world, especially if that world continues to incubate diseases that reach out to kill in the developed countries.

2. The Rise of Medicine

Vivian Nutton

A round 1570, the Basle physician and medical professor
Theodor Zwinger traced the ancestry of the art of medicine
back to the ancient Greeks. Even if he, a good Protestant, could not
entirely believe that a pagan god like Apollo had created the healing
arts to benefit humanity, he accepted the half-god Asclepius as one
of the founders of medicine, and the mythical centaur Chiron, half
man and half horse, as the creator of pharmacology. But long before,
he believed, God had placed in the world healing substances for
the benefit of sick people, waiting to be discovered by subsequent
generations.

One may smile at Zwinger's historical fictions, yet his recourse
to legend conveys an essential truth; the evidence for healing and
medicine antedates any literary text or historical event. Archaeological excavations of sites thousands of years old have revealed bodies
that show signs of medical attention – broken limbs that have been
set, dislocations replaced, and wounds treated successfully. Some
skulls show signs of trepanation (holes drilled through the bone),
a procedure that demanded technical expertise and a rationale for
operating, although what that was is a matter for conjecture. We
may also suppose that various plants and other substances were also
used to treat those who felt ill, and that some individuals gained
a reputation for manual dexterity, herbal knowledge, or ability to
communicate with whatever force was causing the disease. In this
sense, medicine has always been with us, and to talk of the rise of
medicine is to labour the obvious.

The learned Zwinger was no fool, however, and his attempt to write a history of medicine was based on the secure belief that the medicine of his own day was the result of the progressive accumulation of learning over the centuries, and that those who possessed this knowledge, the doctors and surgeons, were the best (some would say the only) persons to be consulted when one fell ill. Self-medication might not be enough, while those who merely pretended to medical knowledge, frequently labelled quacks and charlatans, might kill as often as they cured. Medicine, in short, was being defined as something over and beyond mere healing, as the possession of a specific body of learning, theoretical and practical, that might be used to treat the sick. What this learning was, and how medicine came to supersede healing, are questions that this chapter will try to answer.

Ancient Healers of Babylonia and Egypt

Although Theodor Zwinger was right to place the origins of his tradition of medicine in Ancient Greece, the Greeks were not the only peoples of the eastern Mediterranean region who could claim to have invented medicine. Ancient Mesopotamia and Egypt had medical texts and traditions that long predated those of Greece. Those of India, China, and the Far East, although impinging scarcely at all on Western medicine until more modern times, have equal claim to antiquity.

The abundance of new discoveries from excavations in the Middle East, along with recent reinterpretations of fragmentary older texts, written on baked clay tablets, makes any characterization of Babylonian medicine extremely hazardous. Nonetheless, it is clear that acute observers noted down a large range of symptoms of disease, some of which can be readily identified with conditions such as epilepsy, scurvy, and bronchitis. As early as 1700 BC certain skin diseases were thought to be catching, and that direct, and even indirect, contact with a sufferer might be dangerous. But many conditions remained unknown, largely because they were associated, usually in head-to-toe order, with only one particular limb or organ.

A wide range of drugs was used, both internally and externally, and some drug lists were respected enough to be copied and commented on for hundreds of years. In several Babylonian tablets, a description of symptoms is linked to a diagnosis of the type of illness involved and, more frequently, to a statement of the likely outcome of the condition. A Babylonian medical text of about 650 BC gives a good description of some of the symptoms of epilepsy, as well as noting the more serious nature of convulsions occurring in sleep or recurring during an attack:

> If at the time of his possession, while he is sitting down, his left eye moves to the side, a lip puckers, saliva flows from his mouth, and his hand, leg and trunk on the left side jerk like a slaughtered sheep, it is *migtu*. If at the time of possession his mind is awake, the demon can be driven out; if at the time of his possession his mind is not so aware, the demon cannot be driven out.[1]

This emphasis on prediction fits in well with the Babylonians' expertise in astronomical forecasting, and in the casting of horoscopes through the examination of animal livers. Most striking of all is the frequent attribution of disease conditions to the hand of a god or a spirit, often accompanied by a prognosis of death.

It is not surprising, then, to find two types of healer mentioned in the Babylonian texts, one working largely with drugs, potions, bandages, and the like, the other akin to an exorcist in using incantations and healing rituals. Whether these groups were in conflict or complemented one another – or, indeed, whether one person could perform both types of healing – is controversial, but there is ample evidence for both being officially recognized. The law code of Hammurabi (reigned 1792–1750/1743 BC) specifies the fees to be paid to a healer for a particular operation on a sliding scale, depending on the status of the patient (or animal), as well as draconian penalties for failure, akin to those to be imposed on incompetent architects or shipwrights.

In spite of these potential hazards of failure, it is clear that many minor surgical procedures were carried out (one text discusses a case of nosebleed incompetently treated by bandaging), and there are even records of attempted caesarian section. In short, we are far from the situation alleged for Babylonia in the fifth century BC by the contemporary Greek historian Herodotus, of a land without doctors, in which the sick were brought into the marketplace and had their cases diagnosed and treated by passers-by who had had, or who knew of others with, a similar condition.

Herodotus may simply have misunderstood the common Middle Eastern custom where the sick are placed outside the house for friends and neighbours to talk to and advise. In his comments on Egyptian medicine, however, he was better informed, and far more enthusiastic. He noted a multitude of specialists, one for each disease, and claimed that the whole country was filled with doctors, of the head, the teeth, the belly, and of more obscure diseases. He was not alone in his high regard for Egyptian healers. The king of Persia had Egyptian court doctors, and about 500 BC had sent an Egyptian physician, Udjohorresne, back to Egypt to restore the 'house of life' (a medical institution), 'because he knew the virtues of that art'.[2] Some 750 years earlier, the King of the Hittites (Central Turkey) had asked Rameses II of Egypt for a physician and an incantation-priest to attend his sister, and Egyptian physicians appear in other early diplomatic documents.

The high reputation of Egyptian doctors was owed to their skills as diagnosticians and as surgeons; in the Edwin Smith papyrus of surgery, forty-two out of fifty-eight examinations led to recommendations for treatment. In spite of the presence of incantations, magic, and religious cures, the medical treatises are generally careful to distinguish between them and leave these to other healers. Touching, seeing, and smelling the patient (even taking the pulse) gave the physician an insight into the workings of the body, whose pathological changes were frequently ascribed to the results of putrefying residues collecting within it; heat from the anus, for example, might cause weakness of the heart. Hence the need to pay special attention to stopping the production of pus and to cleaning the body, with purges and enemas as well as washings and perfumings.

Such procedures were also followed in mummification, by which a corpse was preserved. It is open to debate whether the removal of the organs in mummification amounts to anatomy, and whether the knowledge of the mummifiers was passed onto the physicians, but certainly there was not in Egypt the same taboo on handling a corpse that is found in many other societies.

Above all, the Egyptians were famous for their drugs. They ranged widely, from the humble leek, to the fat of the hippopotamus, and from pomegranate to fried mice and lapis lazuli. 'Bring me honey for my eyes and some fat ... and real eye paint, as soon as possible', wrote the painter Poi to his son Pe-Rahotep around 1220 BC. 'I am weak. I want to have my eyes and they are missing.'[3] The drugs came from the Eastern Mediterranean, Africa, and Asia. To us now, the combination of identifiable ingredients and strange semi-magical substances is less important than the vast range of sources they imply.

Greek Medicine

Both Egyptian and Babylonian medicine show evidence of accurate observation, as well as hierarchies of practitioners. What their writings do not yet reveal is the questioning, argumentative, and speculative discussions that mark early Greek medicine, as found in the *Hippocratic Corpus*, the collection of some sixty tracts ascribed to Hippocrates (active about 410 BC). Hence, scholars have often asserted the independence of Greek medicine from that of neighbouring civilizations, a claim more likely to be true of Greek theory than of actual therapeutic practice.

The variety of treatises in the *Hippocratic Corpus* is typical of a period when the practice of medicine was evolving in Greece from a family system, exemplified in the legends of Asclepius and his descendants, one of whom was said to be Hippocrates himself. The famous Hippocratic Oath represents a half-way stage, setting the teacher as a quasi–father figure to the student, but other evidence shows a multiplicity of competing healers – rootcutters, physicians, obstetricians, incantatory priests, exorcists, bone-setters, surgeons, to say nothing of interested laymen and laywomen, self-medication, and divine intervention. Medicine was an open art, and the speculations of philosophers such as Empedocles and Plato in the fifth and fourth centuries BC were as important in influencing and spreading medical ideas as those of more practical medical men.

In this medical marketplace, each seller could tout his or her wares, in opposition to or in cooperation with others, and the choice was left to individual patients. In such a situation, laying down rules for good practice served as both medical ethic and advertising, not only emphasizing the effective contributions of one healer but distinguishing them from the dubious or useless practices of another.

Religious healing was an ever-present alternative that was sought particularly in chronic cases. Few doctors rejected divine intervention, and most believed in a divinely ordered world, yet they were also convinced that their treatments were effective without the guidance of the gods, and could not be accused of being magical. Others might disagree. The onset of an epidemic often resulted in attempts at religious cures, by public ceremonies or by the introduction of new gods thought capable of ending the mass disease. Thus the mysterious epidemic that affected Athens and other parts of Greece in 430–427 BC helped to spread the worship of Asclepius, who superseded Apollo as the pre-eminent Greek healing god (although almost any deity could cure, and there were many local healing cults).

At shrines of Asclepius, especially at major temples in Tricca (N. Greece), Epidaurus (S. Greece), Lebena (Crete), Cos, and, later, Pergamum (now Turkey), sufferers would stay overnight (incubate) within the temple. If fortunate, they would receive healing in a dream, either directly from Asclepius or in the form of instructions interpreted by his priest and often compatible with the recipes and advice of secular physicians. Such healing was perhaps cheaper and more accessible than the services of a physician.

Numbers of healers are impossible to determine. Few towns had more than 2,000 inhabitants, and full-time healers could have existed only in Athens and other big cities or by travelling around a region. Many doctors clearly combined income from medicine with farming and other pursuits – blacksmiths with a sideline in bone-setting are not unusual even in the Middle Ages. Some went to larger towns to study as apprentices; others, especially on the island of Cos, were taught within their families; still others relied entirely on their own skills and what they could pick up by observing or listening to medical debates in the marketplace.

Some big towns, especially Athens from about 500 BC, tried to secure the services of a resident doctor by paying a retaining fee (incidentally also attesting a hoped-for competence). However, the state did not intervene in the relationship between doctor and patient, and although such civic doctors might voluntarily treat citizens for nothing, non-citizens (who were especially numerous in Athens) had to pay in full.

The medicine that these doctors practised was based primarily on dietetics – that is, regulating the whole lifestyle. Drugs were used (those from Egypt had a great reputation), but surgery was very much a treatment of last resort. Swabbing with wine reduced sepsis in hernia operations. Recommendations for the treatment of fractures, dislocations, headwounds, and uterine prolapse sound very modern, but detailed knowledge of the internal organs and arrangement of the body was lacking. Comparisons with animals or everyday objects took the place of careful observation. The internal economy of a woman, for instance, was imagined as a tube, in which the womb wandered from its normal position, to which it might be attracted back by sweet, or repelled by foul, substances introduced into the vulva or the nose.

Anatomical knowledge changed at the end of the fourth century BC. The philosopher-scientist Aristotle and his followers embarked on a massive programme of zoological and biological investigation, and his contemporary Diocles of Carystos is credited with the first book on dissection (but of animals). The breakthrough into human anatomy came outside Greece, in the newly founded city of Alexandria at the mouth of the Nile in Egypt. The conquests of Alexander the Great (reigned 336–323 BC) had brought Greek civilization out of the Aegean basin (and Sicily) to cover the whole of the Middle East, from Libya to the Punjab. Although his empire fragmented at his death, his successors maintained their Greek (Hellenistic) culture. Chief among them was Ptolemy, who ruled in Egypt from 323 to 282 BC and who created in Alexandria a major culture centre with a famous library and 'Hall of the Muses'.

Here, perhaps freed from some of the constraints on mutilating a corpse known in Greece, two Greek physician-scientists almost simultaneously around 280 BC began to investigate the internal body. Herophilus examined carefully the layout and organs of the body, giving names to the duodenum and other anatomical structures. He dissected the eye, and, following his master Praxagoras of Cos, studied the pulse as a guide to illness. His contemporary, Erasistratus of Ceos, was far more radical in his claims.

Erasistratus dissected the brain, trying to establish how movement and sensation were produced, and, using analogies from Alexandrian science, described the body and its processes in mechanical terms. He challenged many of the doctrines associated with Hippocrates. He had little time for humours, and thought that the arteries contained only air, *pneuma*, a form of refined air produced in the heart. He explained the presence of blood in the arteries as resulting from seepage or from attraction following the escape of *pneuma* and the temporary creation of a vacuum. He rejected equally strongly the view of Plato and Aristotle that everything was created for a purpose (teleology), favouring a mechanical development.

Although later scholars praised Erasistratus's anatomical discoveries, especially in the brain, most doctors found them largely irrelevant. Indeed, one influential group, or sect, the Empiricists, rejected all anatomical investigation and theoretical speculation, in favour of treatments based on comparisons with what had succeeded in the past in similar cases.

The Greek world from 250 BC onwards fell more and more under the military power of Rome, which extended its control over Italy, southern France, and Spain, and, by AD 100, ruled from southern Scotland, the Rhine and Danube, to the Sahara, Israel, and the borders of modern Iraq. However much Roman chauvinist politicians might have deplored the arrival of Greek medicine and its new-fangled theories, along with luxurious furniture and silk dresses, by 80 BC Greek doctors and Greek ideas were common in Italy, especially in Rome. There even grew up a new medical sect, the Methodists, who from around AD 60 were dominant in Latin medicine. They combined a view of the body made up of atoms and pores, and of illness as an imbalance between them, with propaganda stressing the simplicity and effectiveness of their diagnoses and cures. In this they were repeating the slogans of an earlier Greek immigrant, Asclepiades, around 92 BC, who had gained a wealthy clientele by his claim to cure 'swiftly, surely, pleasantly'.

Roman practicality was shown in their public works, sewers, and aqueducts (these were also features of Greek towns by 50 BC) and in their provision of 'hospitals'. These catered for two social groups, domestic slaves (100 BC–AD 70), and soldiers in permanent forts in newly conquered territory (9 BC–AD 220). Large fortress hospitals, as at Chester (England) or Inchtuthil (Scotland), were for legionaries (not locals), and were designed on a plan of rooms opening off a square corridor. Situated usually many miles behind the frontier, they catered for the sick rather than those seriously wounded in battle. A few small forts housing non-citizen soldiers – at, for example, Fendoch in Scotland – had hospitals on a reduced scale, but a change in military strategy around 220 to reliance on a mobile fieldforce put an end to these permanent hospitals.

If in the Latin-speaking Western half of the Roman Empire, medicine was generally carried out by relatively humble immigrants, the Greek doctors who lived in the Eastern half flourished intellectually and socially. Many were among the elite of their towns, acting as magistrates or officials and serving also as civic physicians – practitioners distinguished, so lawyers declared, for 'their morals and medical experience', and also for their tax privileges. Latin medicine, even in Celsus's *On Medicine* (AD 40), an elegant handbook for laymen based on Greek sources, does not begin to compare with the Greek investigations into drugs of Dioscorides nor the therapeutic insights at the bedside of Rufus of Ephesus or the Methodist writer on gynaecology, Soranus of Ephesus (both around AD 110). These were in turn overshadowed by Galen of Pergamum.

Within 30 years at most, Galen's books were being studied in Egypt and somewhere near Carthage in modern Tunisia also by the Latin writer Gargilius Martialis, author of a book on garden vegetables, fruits, and herbs. Galen set a new agenda for medicine in the Greek-speaking world, from which alternative views to his were gradually extruded. As the comforting certainties of Greek city life gradually disappeared under political chaos and invasions of barbarians, Galen's apparent mastery of the medical literature of the past, as well as his achievements in anatomy and all other branches of medicine, were viewed as impossible to emulate. Medical writers continued to add their own discoveries, but more often they produced large encyclopedias of past learning or elegant restatements of standard doctrine. Oribasius, for example, in the fourth century produced at least four separate *Synopses*.

The preservation of sound learning in an increasingly impoverished age, when medical texts had to be copied laboriously by hand

and drugs and surgical instruments were hard to find, is praiseworthy. More controversial but harder to pin down are three related developments.

Between AD 200 and 600 there was formed in medicine, as in literature and philosophy, a canon of works of Galen and Hippocrates that was accorded a special place in teaching, certainly at Alexandria and perhaps elsewhere. Medicine was now becoming defined in terms of specific book-learning, and could be tested as a series of responses to questions on books. The second development was a growing split between medical theory and practice, with the former being treated with somewhat greater respect. Finally, Galen's demands for the philosopher-doctor were interpreted to mean that a doctor must first study philosophy (that is, logic and some of Plato's and Aristotle's theories of matter and the universe). This erudite paragon, found in Alexandria, Athens, or the new capital of Constantinople (now Istanbul) was far removed from, and perhaps less familiar than, the backwoods jacks-of-all-trades, who offered their services to the sick – the magical healer, the peasant farmer-cum-bone-setter, the diviner, the travelling drug salesman or oculist, the amulet maker, the barmaid-cum-midwife, the teacher turned recipe writer, or the wise woman with a wonder-working hyena skin. The theoreticians became accepted as the true physicians, even though their opponents might allege, sometimes with justice, that their intellectual expertise was confined to words and not to therapy.

The Christian View of the Sick

More significant than any of these internal changes within medicine was the recognition, from 313 onwards, of Christianity as an (later the) official religion of the Roman Empire. Like Judaism, from which it took much, Christianity had an ambiguous attitude towards medicine. Some preachers, expounding the healing miracles in the Gospels, emphasized the power of faith to cure disease (although few went so far as to claim that that was sufficient), and, especially from 370 onwards, the shrines of saints and martyrs became places of pilgrimage for the sick, vying with, and ultimately replacing, the pagan temples of Asclepius.

Both Christianity and Judaism also believed in the notion of a whole community bound together by religion, in which everything, including medicine, had its place, and where religious doctrines and religious authority might rightly intervene in what had earlier been purely secular affairs. It was, for example, important to prepare the patient for a good death, leading to an eternal life in heaven, and hence to involve a priest at the bedside as well as a doctor.

Irksome though this intervention might occasionally appear, the church viewed medicine positively on the whole. True, some of its most eminent practitioners in the fifth and sixth centuries were unrepentant pagans, but Galenic medicine, with its appeal to a monotheist creator, could easily be assimilated, and the workings of drugs and the skills of the surgeon held up as prime examples of the bounty of God towards humanity. Although church institutions offered a potential source of conflict with medicine, this was outweighed by the ways in which, increasingly, the church acted as the preserver of learning, including medicine.

Nowhere was this more evident than in a new institution, the hospital, the product of Jewish and Christian ideas on charity. Ancient charity had been narrowly defined, limited to particular groups, usually of male citizens. The Jews and Christians broadened this to include their fellow-believers and, in the case of Christians, all who might be in need, for all were potential Christians. By AD 60 the Jews had built hostels for those on pilgrimage to the Temple at Jerusalem, in at least one of which medical assistance was available. Christianity extended these hostels geographically. By 400 they were common in Asia Minor (modern Turkey) and the Holy Land, and by 450 had spread to Italy, North Africa, and southern France. At the same time, church laws throughout the Middle East specified that each community should set aside a room for looking after those in need.

Most 'hospitals' were small, but in Constantinople or Jerusalem some had 200 or more beds. As the variety of names used for them shows, they catered for many different groups – the sick, the old, the poor, and the stranger; sometimes together, sometimes not. Some institutions specifically excluded the maimed and sick, others treated them in separate wards. Increasing size brought administrative specialization, into wards, by sex, and, by 600 in one hospital at Constantinople, by illness. Medical assistance was available in the biggest hospitals, but most provided only care (food, warmth, and shelter), although this should not be despised as an important component of the process of cure. Some hospitals were run almost as family businesses, others as extensions of a bishop's role as father of his flock. They were all examples of Christian charity in action.

From the fourth century onwards, doctrinal splits within the Christian church contributed towards the very gradual political and military disintegration of the Roman Empire. The Western half, Latin-speaking and centred on Rome, had by 570 become an amalgam of barbarian states. In the East, the central government of Constantinople continued to exercise control over the eastern Mediterranean until the Arab conquests of the seventh century restricted it largely to the Aegean basin and Asia Minor.

In a region stretching from Egypt through Syria to Persia, a local language, Syriac (akin to Hebrew), competed with Greek, as the language first of the church and then of advanced culture. By 531 the texts of Galen that formed the basis for the Alexandrian medical curriculum had been translated into Syriac, and medical compendia were being written in Syriac of a standard comparable with those in Greek. The ready availability of Syriac translations of Aristotle helped to confirm the authority of Galen, so often an Aristotelian in his ideas and prejudices. Once again Greek medicine was transplanted into another linguistic society.

The Arab Influence

The Arab conquests of the seventh century grafted a new political order onto a basically Christian, Syriac-speaking society. Although the Arabs had their own medicine, based on herbs and chants, they were not numerous enough to impose it on their new subjects. Besides, the Koran and the traditions that soon grew up around the figure of the prophet Mohammed said very little about medicine; and the little there was could easily be reconciled with Galen's teleological monotheism and, at least at first, impinged little on a conquered Christian population. Here, the practice of medicine long continued as a non-Muslim speciality, families of Christian or Jewish physicians attending the ruling families for centuries. A specifically

Islamic medicine, the so-called 'Medicine of the Prophet', does not appear important until the tenth century.

Of medicine under the early Caliphate, we know little. Only with the transfer of power from Damascus to Baghdad in 762, and under such rulers as the Caliph Harun ar-Rashid (reigned 786–809), does light return again. This period saw in the Middle East a conflict between Islam and those who believed in Manichaeanism, a religion with many adherents in Iraq and Iran. Manichaeanism had long been attacked by Christianity as a dangerous heresy, and Islamic authorities turned to their Christian subjects for assistance against a common enemy. This is the background to a massive takeover of Greek philosophy and science, whose Aristotelian insistence on the purposefulness of the divine creator struck at the Manichaean notion of a world divided between good and evil. Texts on logic and philosophy were translated into Arabic, and were followed by medicine, often at the behest of government officials and with government support.

The major ninth-century medical figure in Baghdad was a Christian Arab, Hunain ibn Ishaq, an amazingly accurate and productive scholar, who travelled to the Greek Byzantine empire in search of rare Galenic treatises. In all, he, his pupils, and a few contemporaries translated 129 works of Galen into Arabic, often making a translation first into Syriac. His labours provided the Arabic world with more Galenic texts than survive today in their original Greek, and with versions that are both technically accurate and stylistically elegant.

In an eventful life (he was once imprisoned by his royal master), Ibn Ishaq also wrote a major tract on eye diseases and a summary of Galenic medicine in the form of *Questions and Answers* (c. 850). The group of Christian doctors to the Caliph (including for four centuries members of the Bakhtishu'a family) all engaged in similar tasks of translation or reinterpretating their Galenic heritage for Arab patients and patrons.

This successful transfer of classical knowledge into yet another language (there are contemporary translations also into Armenian and Hebrew) led in the tenth to thirteenth centuries to a massive expansion of medical writing in Arabic. Ar-Razi, or in Latin Rhazes, described smallpox and measles accurately, as well as his chemical experiments; al-Biruni wrote at length on the plants and herbs he had seen in his travels in Afghanistan and India; and the Syrian physician Ibn an-Nafis argued strongly against Galen for some form of circulation of the blood (Galen had argued that blood produced in the liver was all used up as nutriment and its residues excreted). But these new discoveries, however impressive they might now seem, were unusual (and Ibn an-Nafis reached his conclusion by logic, not experimentation).

More typical were attempts to develop and systematize Galenic ideas. Galen had once suggested ranking drugs according to their degrees (or grades) of action, but he himself had suggested grades for only a third of the medicinal substances he discussed. Arabic pharmacologists extended his system to a wider range of substances, which they then combined in complex mixtures designed for the individual patient. Elsewhere, as with Galen's ideas of the eye or on urines, his opinions were scattered throughout his enormous works, and it was Arabic authors who brought them easily together. Finally, there were compendia, of all sizes, expanding what Galen had hinted at and amalgamating a variety of diffuse observations into a coherent whole. Thus it was Arabic authors who first wrote about the three spirits ruling the body (Galen had accepted the psychic spirit in the brain and nerves, and possibly the vital spirit in the heart and arteries, but his reference to a natural spirit in the liver and veins was at best muted), and who developed his ideas of a physicalist psychology.

The most important of such compendia were those by ar-Razi, al-Majusi (Haly Abbas), and Ibn Sina (Avicenna). Ibn Sina's *Canon of Medicine*, which still retains its primacy within this tradition as it is taught today in the Muslim world, displays a wondrous appreciation of all Galen's medical writing, and is tightly structured by Aristotelian logic. It is no coincidence that Ibn Sina, like Ibn Rushd (Averroës) and the Jewish physician Moses ben Maimon (Maimonides), active in twelfth-century Muslim Spain, North Africa, and Cairo, was famous as a philosopher as well as a physician, for Galen had encouraged the study of philosophy and logic, and his method of argumentation invited philosophical enquiry just as it did experimentation. Others took Galen's insistence on book-learning almost to excess: the wife of Ali ibn Ridwan at his death in 1068 is said to have dumped all his huge Galenic library into the fishpond, as she did not wish any longer to share the house with her late husband's great love.

This bookishness, possible only in a wealthy and learned society like that of medieval Islam, may have helped to downgrade manual skills such as surgery; the best doctor was the one who could diagnose correctly without even seeing the patient. But that did not prevent some writers – for example, al-Zahrawi (Albucasis) – from producing excellent surgical textbooks, in which they reported details of complicated abdominal operations. New techniques were invented for the treatment of cataract and other eye complaints, just as other scholars promoted new theories about the mechanics of vision. But the sheer danger of surgery may have been the greatest handicap to its further development.

How far the Islamic world took over the medical institutions of the Greek world is an open question. Certainly, by the eleventh century, there were large hospitals in every major Muslim town (and with a Muslim religious bias to match that of a Christian hospital). Medicine was also being formally taught within the hospital setting, with certificates granted for attendance. Theoretical treatises on the duties of the 'Market-superintendent' imply that this official had to examine candidates in medicine and surgery before they could practise, but evidence for theory translated into action is hard to find.

More plausible is a picture of a variety of overlapping types of healing, in which the learned Galenic tradition was but one part, alongside the medicine of the prophet, astrological and magical healing, and, by the eleventh century, healing at the shrine of famous Muslim 'saints'. In spite of the traditional picture of a unified Islam, Jews, Christians, and other groups still continued to offer their own forms of healing, within and without their own communities.

The Mongol invasions of the early thirteenth century devastated the eastern half of the Islamic world, and civil war, and the increasing success of the Christians, pressed hard on the Islamic communities of Spain and North Africa. The openness to Hellenism of ninth-century Baghdad was replaced by a more fundamentalist Islam, in which adherence to tradition, both religious and medical, was enjoined on the community of the faithful. Even so, medicine in thirteenth-century Cordoba or Cairo had arguably reached a higher level of sophistication and effectiveness than anywhere in the Western world, with the possible exception of Constantinople.

Medicine in the Byzantine World

In Constantinople, as the Byzantium Empire shrank to become little more than the area around the capital, professors argued, taught, and perhaps even demonstrated in the Galenic tradition of learned medicine. There were hospitals, like the Pantokrator, a royal foundation in 1136, whose fifty or so patients (and outpatients) were, according to the charter, to be provided with a more than adequate diet and treated by a trained medical staff with a wide range of drugs and therapies. But, even if the demands of the charter were fulfilled, the hospital itself could have made only a tiny contribution to the health of the city, its population then numbering some 300,000. Outside Constantinople, there was much less provision for the sick. In 1185, Thessalonica, the second city of the Empire, had only one hospital.

For all its failings, however, the medical services of the Byzantine Empire were far superior to those of the contemporary West, and the capture of Constantinople by the Crusaders in 1204 may have led to the copying in Western Europe of some Byzantine medical institutions. For example, from 1250 in some towns in France and northern Italy hospitals had up to 200 beds and a large medical staff, and became the focus of community care for the sick.

Medicine in the Dark Ages

The situation in Western Europe in the preceding centuries – during the so-called Dark Ages (roughly 500–1050) – was very different. Here the crumbling of Roman imperial power brought about a catastrophic downturn in economic prosperity, most noticeably as expressed in the life of towns. Although doctors continued to practise medicine in some of the more important towns, there is evidence for a massive decline in the number, and quality, of medical writings available. Short handbooks replaced learned disquisitions, digests their original tracts, drug lists academic pharmacopeias. Although law texts continued to repeat rules for civic physicians and the costs of slave physicians, they were legislating for the past, not present reality.

Two features stand out in this decline. The first is the preminence of 'do-it-yourself' handbooks, primarily of dietetic medicine, which presented a small amount of basic theory with a concise exposition of a few diagnoses and treatments. By contrast, only a handful of Hippocratic and Galenic texts were available in translations made in northern Italy around 550, and even Latin Methodist medicine was poorly represented. The second feature is the ecclesiastical takeover of medical learning – and learning in general, for few outside the ecclesiastical community could read.

Probably only within monasteries or, from the ninth century, the schools that grew up around certain major cathedrals, such as Laon and Chartres in France, were medical texts in Latin being copied and studied. Only about 150 manuscripts of medicine survive today from the period 800–1000, and in the latter year there may have been no more than 1,000 in all Europe, and these were confined to a small number of centres. Yet there was some preservation of classical learning. Medicine in Anglo-Saxon England, almost unique in being written in a vernacular language, shows traces of Greek learning and uses some drugs and drug recipes from the eastern Mediterranean.

This relatively learned medicine was supplemented by the healing offered at shrines and by holy men. Tales abound of so-called miraculous cures, and, by 1000, shrines were competing among themselves in the number of their cures. Some saints were almost specialists – St Dymphna was favoured for mental diseases, St Roch for plague, St Hubert for rabies sufferers, and St Blaise for throat complaints. Others serviced a locality – for example, the shrine of St Godric at Finchale (County Durham) was mainly visited by sufferers from northeastern England. Only a few shrines, like that of Roquemadour (southern France), drew pilgrims from all over Europe. Nor were the cults necessarily directed against secular healers. They might advise patients to rely on God and the saints, and, in turn, St John of Beverley or some other saint knew which diseases could be treated by secular means and by secular healers. Besides, in an age when secular healers were few, the sick needed to rely on a variety of resources.

The change from Dark Age medicine is generally located around 1050 in the region of Salerno, southern Italy. Here was a thriving medical community in touch with the Greek and Arab worlds, as well as the wealthiest and intellectually most advanced abbey of Europe, Monte Cassino. From 1080 or so, the Salernitan masters reintroduced theoretical speculation into medical teaching. Aided by contacts with Constantinople, and, from 1200 onwards, by Latin translations of some Arabic texts by Constantine the African, they re-established Galenic academic learning, combining commentary on a few set texts with philosophical discussion of wider issues and, by 1250, with practical demonstrations of animal anatomy. Galenism was reintroduced in Arabic form, in particular via the medical compendia of al-Majusi and the so-called *Introduction of Johannitius* (an abbreviated version of Hunain ibn Ishaq's *Questions and Answers*). The *Rule of Salerno* (*c.* 1300), a Latin poem, translated later into many languages, helped to spread a knowledge of classical dietetics throughout Europe.

The Arabic basis of Latin medicine was further strengthened by a series of translations made in Spain by Gerard of Cremona and others of such texts as Ibn Sina's *Canon*, and *On the Grades of Drug Action* by al-Kindi. By 1190 many texts of Galen had been translated, largely from the Arabic, along with most of the major Arabic works of medicine: by 1350, thanks to the South Italian Greek Niccolò da Reggio, many minor Galenic works became available in Latin, although few bothered to read them. There were three consequences of this translation movement. First, the amount of learned medical material suddenly burgeoned beyond all recognition. Second, the language of medicine was heavily arabized (for example, *siphac* for peritoneum), and its therapeutics depended heavily on Arabic sources, especially in pharmacology and surgery. Third, there was now a heavy philosophical component, based on Aristotle, whose Latin revival, also from Spain, helped and in part determined the character of medieval learned medicine. Nobody could properly understand the new medicine without some knowledge of the technicalities of Aristotelian science (or natural philosophy).

Development of University Medicine

Translation accompanied the development of university medicine, first in northern Italy, in the wealthy towns of Bologna and Padua, and then in France (Paris and Montpellier), and in England (Oxford). Germany lagged behind, but by 1400 many areas of Western Europe had their own institutions of higher learning. Medicine came late into the universities. Professional associations of medical teachers, as at Salerno, joined universities only when they saw the advantages of the new institutions' ability to secure their own rights and privileges in law and theology, and many universities, especially in France, never had a medical faculty.

Once in the universities, the doctors readily adopted university procedures – lectures on set texts, such as *The Introduction of Johannitius*, Ibn Sina's *Canon*, and some Galen, debates on medical questions, and a theoretical (heavily Aristotelian) bias – and university prejudices. Because their medicine was based on texts, they increasingly argued that proper medicine depended on such knowledge, and that they, as university graduates, alone had the right to decide who should or should not practise medicine – a textual examination supplemented, and at times replaced, practical instruction by apprenticeship.

The numbers of medical students were tiny (not surprisingly, since a medical degree took at least 7 years of study, including a full course in the arts): most universities, except for Bologna and Padua, saw only one or two medical graduates a decade. But by appealing to an increasingly university-educated elite of administrators, they often succeeded in imposing themselves and their own qualifications on the medical community. A popular saying on the prospects of university doctors and lawyers in about 1250 was 'Galen gives riches, Justinian offices'. The view was held that if only graduates could practise, there was legally no place for Jews and women (who might even perform surgery and often attended male patients), and a potential source of conflict with other organizations, especially medical guilds or colleges, who took a more realistic view of medical competence.

Medieval university medicine is indeed often speculative and highly theoretical. Yet its claim that a proper understanding of

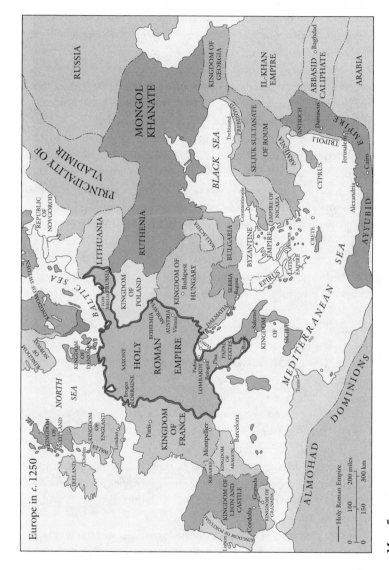

Europe in c. 1250

RUSSIA

MONGOL KHANATE

KINGDOM OF GEORGIA

IL-KHAN EMPIRE

ABBASID CALIPHATE ○ Baghdad

ARABIA

PRINCIPALITY OF VLADIMIR

BLACK SEA

SELJUK SULTANATE OF ROUM

○ Trebizond

ARMENIA

○ ANTIOCH
Damascus ○
TRIPOLI
Jerusalem ○
Cairo ○

EMPIRE

REPUBLIC OF NOVGOROD

LITHUANIA

RUTHENIA

MOLDAVIA

BULGARIA

BYZANTINE EMPIRE

EMPIRE OF NICAEA

CYPRUS

CRETE

Alexandria

AYYUBID

KINGDOM OF SWEDEN

BALTIC SEA

KINGDOM OF POLAND

KINGDOM OF HUNGARY

○ Budapest

SERBIA

Ragusa

Constantinople

Athens ○

LATIN EMPIRE

EPIRUS

MEDITERRANEAN SEA

DOMINIONS

KINGDOM OF DENMARK

Pom BRULY PRUSSIA

SAXONY

BOHEMIA

AUSTRIA
Vienna ○

DALMATIA

HOLY ROMAN EMPIRE

LORRAINE
Bruges ○

Padua ○
Bologna ○
Pisa ○
LOMBARDY

Genoa

PAPAL STATES

Rome ○

Salerno ○

KINGDOM OF SICILY

Tunis ○

NORTH SEA

KINGDOM OF SCOTLAND

KINGDOM OF ENGLAND

IRELAND
WALES
Dublin ○
London ○

Paris ○

KINGDOM OF FRANCE

Montpellier ○

NAVARRE

KINGDOM OF ARAGON

Barcelona ○

KINGDOM OF LEON AND CASTILE

KINGDOM OF PORTUGAL

Lisbon ○

Cordoba ○
Granada ○

KINGDOM OF GRANADA

ALMOHAD

——— Holy Roman Empire

| 0 | 100 | 200 miles |
| 0 | 150 | 300 km |

Map 5.

health and disease required an understanding of the fundamental structures of the body is not foolish, neither is its attempt to relate questions of medicine to wider 'scientific'. In the thirteenth century, teachers such as Taddeo Alderotti at Bologna and Arnald of Villanova at Montpellier were expert physicians as well as expositors, and could call on a formidable range of learning. Their fifteenth-century successors went further in emphasizing the practical basis of therapeutics, and in linking the medicine of the classroom to that of the bedside. Many university statutes, especially in Germany, demanded a period of supervised practice before granting a degree; whether they were enforced is another matter.

Below the university doctor in the medieval medical hierarchy stood the surgeon. In Italy and Germany, he might have been trained in part at a university, although a guild-apprenticeship was more common, and, even in London, the surgical elite had more in common with physicians than with their lower competitors, especially barber-surgeons. They had their own books, and some of their successful treatments – of abdominal injuries, anal fistulae, bladder stones, and cataracts – are impressive, and are far more than mere burning and bleeding. There were innovations, such as in the treatment of inguinal hernia, and in some artificial limbs, and even university men might have been forced to acknowledge the expertise of itinerant bone-setters or tooth-extractors. Bleeding, a favoured remedy and prophylactic was often carried out, especially in spring, by a local barber, who might also attend to cuts, bruises, and the ubiquitous ulcerations.

Others also offered their services. Although excluded as non-Christians from universities, Jews were often favoured as practitioners, especially among the aristocracy. The drug trade was in the hands of apothecaries and spicers, importers of drugs from far afield, who might also offer medical advice to their clients. Women were often attended by female healers or midwives, but it would be wrong to imagine that women's diseases were left entirely to women, or that women with healing skills confined themselves only to women and children. Although regulations might endeavour to restrict them in this way, they were never universally enforced.

This situation reflects the multiplicity of institutions and organizations with pretensions to authority over medicine – the church, guilds, medical colleges (usually, but not always, of medical graduates), town councils (increasingly involved from 1200 or so in selecting a public doctor), and magnates of all descriptions. Sometimes authority was mediated through an individual (for example, a royal physician), sometimes through a committee. In fifteenth-century Brussels, midwives were licensed by a board of ecclesiastics, doctors, and midwives themselves; in Bruges in 1486, the town council had authority over them. 'On 24 March, paid by order of the council to Mary, widow of Henry Craps, and two other midwives, for having at the council's request questioned and examined a woman seeking to show knowledge in that field . . . twelve gros and three solidi each.' The conflicts, common in the sources, between doctors and surgeons, or medical men and lay administrators, are typical of this fragmentation of authority in Europe. Effective resolution of these conflicts reflects far more the growing effectiveness of the state than any public consensus about the suitability of types of healing.

The growing state involvement is shown by the Health Boards, which were first developed when the Black Death arrived in Europe in 1348. Originally temporary creations, even in small communities, to face the plague, they had become permanent in most major towns of Italy by 1500. Composed of laymen, with medical advisers and often large staffs, they could impose quarantine (first at Dubrovnik in 1377), remove the sick to isolation hospitals, ban goods from entering or leaving, clean the streets, unblock waterways, and compile lists of the dead. Their information networks sometimes stretched far, and their powers of punishment were draconian. In effect, the sophisticated northern Italian towns faced the great challenge to their lives by effective administrative measures, in which a directly medical response formed only one part.

The Black Death – perhaps bubonic plague with complications – first noted in Asia in 1346, was the greatest medical disaster of the Middle Ages, killing in its first wave, from 1347 to 1350, perhaps 25 per cent of Europe's population. It also became endemic, with possibly even graver consequences. Between 1350 and 1400 the average European lifespan may have shrunk from 30 to a mere 20 years, and Florence lost almost three-quarters of its population between 1338 and 1447. (Reasonably accurate figures for population and mortality begin in Italy around 1350, but are absent from much of northern Europe for two centuries more.)

The Black Death differed from earlier epidemics in its extent and in its ubiquity. Leprosy, which was widely feared in the twelfth and thirteenth centuries and which was explained in the same way as plague, affected fewer individuals, who could be easily segregated from the community in a leper house in a form of living death. But plague struck both more extensively and with harsher results. Death might be swift, and the imposition of rule by a Health Board might bring financial ruin.

How healthy was medieval society? In a crowded Italian city in 1480, the poor rarely lived beyond thirty, and even in the countryside few attained the age of forty. Diarrhoeas, smallpox, tuberculosis, typhus, measles, and meningitis were common, colics and the ubiquitous 'fever' frequent, and winter chills carried off many of the old and malnourished. Accidents, drownings, and burnings were often recorded, as were malarial fevers, kidney and bladder stones, and intestinal disorders. Degenerative diseases, such as cancer, were less common, because the population died at a relatively young age. The evidence of skeletons shows that few, even among the young, escaped without some debilitating disease.

The process of childbirth was particularly hazardous. Medical texts, largely based on Greek ideas, emphasized that woman was a weaker (and wetter) version of man, and hence more prone to disease, never more so than in pregnancy. The delivery itself was made without forceps or effective anaesthetics (although some opium-based drinks might have reduced pain a little). Although caesarian section is mentioned, evidence for its use is disputed. All that could be done was to ensure, as far as possible, that the child in the womb lay in the best position for an easy birth – a recommendation far from simple to achieve. There are agonizing stories of women dying in labour, or from later complications, and although many of the recommendations for the care of the newborn are eminently sensible, the *Books of the Dead* reveal a veritable massacre of the innocents.

Mental diseases were treated in a variety of ways. Doctors generally believed in a strong link between physical and mental well-being, and paid attention, even in fevers, to the general psychological state of the patient. For some sufferers from mental diseases, physical remedies might be suggested – good food, healthy walks, and very occasionally drugs to change the overall humoral balance. Others sought a cure from God or the saints, by pilgrimage to a shrine or a holy dance, or indeed saw some conditions as 'holy folly', a special mark of grace, far beyond the love-madness sung by the medieval troubadour. Although we hear of the mad locked up in chains – in fifteenth-century Nuremberg (Germany) one could hire a cell in the town gaol – they were mainly looked after at home, within their own community and frequently given tasks that would integrate them with society and reduce the frightening aspect of their disorder.

The borderline between madness and divine inspiration is narrow and it is hard for modern scholars to interpret the narrative of a mystic or madwoman like Margery Kempe without using anachronistic categories. Yet it is fair to note that she lived in the world, bore fourteen children, travelled to the Holy Land and Germany, and was certainly aware of the different types of psychological experiences that she felt over many decades.

Margery Kempe, who was born in England in 1393, was a wealthy woman, familiar with practical medicine. After a period of insanity, she made pilgrimages to Jerusalem, Rome, Germany, and Spain and described them and her spiritual experiences in *The Book of Margery Kempe* (*c.* 1423). This narrative, which is one of the earliest autobiographies in English literature, reveals the interaction between medicine and late-medieval society. It describes a learned medicine with roots in the Greek past but not unintelligible to the lay person: the good housewife might be more effective in providing healthy remedies than many an expensive physician or surgeon.

To some of her companions she was a sick woman, a nuisance with her interminable wailings; to others, she had been chosen as a mouthpiece of God. Her account describes her relationship with others in society, and gives an insight into how her condition was viewed by others at the time.

Many said there was never saint in heaven that cried as she did, and from that they concluded she had a devil within her which caused that crying. And this they said openly, and much more evil talk. She took everything patiently for our Lord's love, for she knew very well that the Jews said much worse of his own person than people did of her, and therefore she took it the more meekly.[4]

Margery lived to a ripe old age, and cared for her husband when he, too, was senile.

The picture that Margery Kempe portrays is very different from that of modern medicine. It is not that many diseases were hard, if not impossible, to cure – although medieval drugs may have worked more often than we think, and they certainly would have wrought little harm – but the whole context of medicine has changed. The Galenic–Arabic tradition stressed a holistic form of medicine, and, whether we are dealing with Islam, Christianity, or the scattered Jewish communities of medieval Europe, there was a social involvement that is often lacking today. Birth was a process attended by the women of the village; cleaning the streets might be a task imposed on all citizens; and death was an occasion for an assertion of communal values as well as private grief.

Yet medicine, and medical institutions, were also challenging some of the older ways. A new vocabulary of medicine, the growth of medical inquests and autopsies, Health Boards, Death Books, public physicians (and official pharmacopoeias), and the isolation of lepers and plague victims, all gradually contributed to a move away from a communal consensus within medicine. Some might argue that this was a move towards a more effective system of health care; others that in 1500 this was centuries in the future; and others that an important part of the healing process, the interaction of patient and therapist, was being subverted to a medical monopoly.

Whichever point of view is adopted, medieval medicine was far from being static, unchanging, or entirely given over to the contemplation of past authorities. It was, in fact, capable of responding effectively to the challenge of disease within its own terms, and by invoking communal and religious responses, by involving caring and curing, it may have done as much as was possible until the therapeutic revolution of the late nineteenth and twentieth centuries to maintain health.

3. What Is Disease?

Roy Porter

Understanding the history of medicine presents many challenges. Not only has medicine itself undergone profound change in its encounters with disease and death, but the very conception of illness – its nature, causes, and meaning – is complex and enigmatic. Perceptions of sickness have varied greatly over time and place, shaped by diverse circumstances. Different social groups conceptualize illnesses disparately. In Shakespeare's time, melancholy was called the 'courtier's coat of arms' and regarded as an eligible, fashionable disorder of the elite; but a poor person suffering similar symptoms – what we might call depression – was considered 'mopish' and rebuked for being sullen. Gender has counted too: the condition that in 1800 would have been called 'hysteria' in a woman might have been diagnosed as 'hypochondria' in a man. Not least, illness may be regarded differently by patients and practitioners. Sufferers experience the personal side of being sick; doctors, especially those with scientific pretensions, are more likely to emphasize its objective aspects, the facts underpinning diagnoses and prognoses.

Disease and Illness

Chapter 1 dealt with 'disease' as a biological force in the economy of Nature, showing humans and microbes locked in a Darwinian struggle for survival; this chapter looks at 'illness'. The terms are often used interchangeably: 'he's got a disease', we say, or 'he's suffering from an illness'. Yet they may also be differentiated. After all, it makes perfect sense to say of somebody with a tumour: 'he's got cancer, but he's not feeling ill'. 'He's sick' is said of someone with a hangover, without generally implying that any 'disease' is involved – although we might think he was also suffering from alcoholism, a rather particular species of disease.

In modern English parlance, disease is normally an objective thing, often triggered by a pathogen, such as a bacillus or a virus, and marked by telltale symptoms – a rash or a raised temperature. Illness, on the other hand, denotes something subjective, feelings of malaise or pain. They may be two sides of the same coin, but not always. This may seem semantic quibbling, but words are often revealing symptoms of underlying realities. And our habit of distinguishing between disease and illness itself betrays historical transformations. For the term 'disease' has developed from 'dis-ease'; similarly, malaise from 'mal-aise' (ill at ease, a state of discomfort). Thus, within the modern, scientific concept of disease lurk softer, more subjective, and historically antecedent connotations. The emergence of the neutral, scientific concept of 'disease' from earlier ideas of 'dis-ease' (akin to our 'illness') offers an insight into different cultural perceptions and changes over time.

Healing and Holiness

First, it is worth glancing, for contrast and comparison, at conceptions of sickness in what might be called traditional societies; groups without an indigenous written culture, ones in which medical skills are orally transmitted. It would be entirely wrong nowadays to accept the derogatory Victorian verdict on the medical beliefs of such societies, condemning them as primitive, superstitious, and irrational. We feel confident that we have 'progressed', and science certainly furnishes Western healing with powers that the medicine-man or witchdoctor lacks. But tribal medicine 'makes sense' no less – and, in some ways, far more – than Western medicine.

It is easy to spot similarities between the traditional medicine of Africans or Australian Aborigines today and the religious framework that cradled illness and healing in medieval Europe. Medical magic was then explicit within folklore, the Church, and learned medicine alike. Religion and medicine shared a common orientation in the Middle Ages – that of making whole. Etymologically, 'holiness' and 'healing' stem from a common root (the idea of wholeness), as do salvation and salubrity, and also cure, care, and charity (from the Latin, *caritas*). But our culture (being literate and analytical) has also developed demarcations between the body on the one hand and, on the other, the soul, mind, or spirit. Such dualisms have fostered a differentiation of medicine from faith, and of doctor from priest, the one attending the cure of bodies, the other the 'cure of souls'. Such distinctions have been contested, and physic and faith have continually crisscrossed or collided, engaging in border disputes. Although often complementary, there remains potential for conflict; while separate, there remains scope for unification.

Not least, Western medicine developed within dominant value-systems established by the Church (until quite recently, medicine remained a junior, subaltern profession, less prestigious than the cloth). Like other great faiths, Judaeo-Christianity proclaims a dualistic cosmology that ennobles the soul or mind while disparaging the body, which is often viewed as the soul's prison house. Spirit is immortal; the flesh, by contrast, is weak and corruptible, and, thanks to Original Sin, theologically depraved. It was Adam and Eve's disobedience in the Garden of Eden at the Fall that created vile bodies and brought sin, suffering, and death into the world.

Anxieties about the corruptions of the flesh are registered in the strict body regulation demanded of the Chosen People in the Pentateuch and upheld ever since within Judaism's elaborate rituals concerning hygiene, diet, and sex. Cleanliness had to be defended against such defiling pollutions as the blood of a menstruating woman. It was a Talmudic requirement that Jews should not live in a city without a physician. Mistrusting the fallen body, early Christians responded with defences of their own. Drawing on traditions of Eastern asceticism, the Desert Fathers mortified the flesh and exalted continence. The lusts of the flesh had to be tamed to free the spirit. In the Middle Ages, chastity, fasting, and self-flagellation became hallmarks of holiness.

The disciplining of the flesh has been a key element in many faiths. Christianity, however, encodes especially complex attitudes towards the body. It personalizes the Deity (God the Father), and weaves Him into the plot of the terrestrial world. God has an only son, who is born in the flesh, before being crucified in bodily agony.

Incarnation and sacrifice are in turn commemorated in the Eucharist, whereby, for Roman Catholics, sacramental bread and wine are literally transubstantiated into the Saviour's body and blood. Through divine propitiation, believers are promised bodily resurrection at the Last Judgment. While abhorring the flesh because tainted by sin, Christianity, in short, also emphasized a certain sanctity immanent within it. While asceticism was prized, mortification was never to be pursued to the point of self-destruction. Suicide was a mortal sin: being God's creature, how could man be free to dispose of his own body?

Christianity, Pain, and Suffering

To modern medicine, pain is an alarm bell, part of a system that warns of trouble within; it is thus a necessary evil. To some churchmen, it has been a positive sanctification: it was not unusual for evangelists to follow St Paul and commend the 'thorn in the flesh'. The great Victorian Baptist preacher, Charles Haddon Spurgeon, was convinced that 'the greatest earthly blessing that God can give to any of us is health, with the exception of sickness ... A sick wife, a newly made grave, poverty, slander, sinking of spirit, might teach us lessons nowhere else to be learned so well'.[1]

The man in the street has been less enthusiastic about pain – Christian zealotry may seem to verge on masochism – and philosophers have felt obliged to confront the problem of pain. What is it for? Should it be enjoyed or endured? If shunned, how? A prime aim, for example, of the Epicureans (followers of the Greek philosopher, Epicurus) lay in devising damage limitation, designed to curb self-inflicted exposure to agonies: the simple life would avoid giving hostages to fortune. Stoicism similarly recommended soaring above worldly passions, for they brought disappointment not pleasure.

Christianity taught that pain and sickness were not original to God's design. Agony had entered the world through Original Sin, through which man was condemned to labour by the sweat of his brow and woman to bring forth in pain; after the Fall mankind would thereafter suffer disease and death. Thus the Bible construed pain as the penalty for disobedience – a notion reinforced by etymology, the word pain being derived from *poena* (the Latin for punishment).

Scripture further showed God visiting woe upon the wicked through pestilence, while chosen individuals were devoutly to rejoice in the Cross of illness. As Job's trials showed, the pious response to divine affliction was to be long-suffering. Martyrdom to disease in this vale of tears might be as glorious as martyrdom to the infidel. Especially within Catholicism, expiatory mortification of the flesh, with goads, hair-shirts, and fasting, struck a blow for holiness.

Yet caution was always urged upon Christians, lest they fetishized pain, glamourizing the man of sorrows. And charity also required succour for the sick and relief of distress. Thus Christian doctrine regarding welfare, philanthropy, and medicine grew extremely complex. Suffering was a blessing, yet it was also to be alleviated by medicine and charity. Ambiguities similar to these are also mirrored in the casuistry of the Churches' teachings towards war: Christians should turn the other cheek, but just wars may be holy.

Medicine within Christendom

Over the centuries, certain fundamentalist Christian sects have condemned medicine as more or less impious. Some Calvinists in Britain and North America rejected smallpox inoculation and vaccination on the grounds that implantation of diseased material into a healthy person risked breaking the Sixth Commandment. Jehovah's Witnesses originally denied the germ theory, and still refuse blood transfusions, convinced that they contravene Scripture (Genesis 9:4) – although, somewhat eccentrically, they today accept organ transplants. Nevertheless, the main Christian churches have routinely accepted that medicine has a valid role. Was not the Evangelist Luke 'the beloved physician'? And did not Christ himself, while instructing physicians to heal themselves, give proofs of his divine powers by some thirty-five such curative miracles? The apostles exercised healing as 'a gift of the spirit' (1 Cor. 12:9). From the start, Christianity was a healing faith.

Christianity's vision of the body – fallen, yet God's instrument – suggested a division of labour between the churches and the medical profession. Priests were to tend the salvation of the soul, while the ailments of the body became the physicians' prerogative. The Fourth Lateran Council (1215) in Rome forebade clerics to shed blood through the practice of surgery, and warned against immoderate involvement of clerics in treating physical complaints. Doctors and priests thus mapped out 'separate spheres' – in principle, a mutually acceptable *modus vivendi*. Matters pertaining to the soul were rendered unto the Church; and the body was rendered unto the 'Caesar' of the doctors. Peaceful coexistence was the norm but border flare-ups were inevitable.

For one thing, Catholicism energetically involved itself in healing rituals, championing recourse to relics, offerings made in fulfilment of vows, pilgrimages, holy waters, and, above all, shrines and cults. Saints won reputations for special healing powers: for example, to cure toothache, you prayed to St Apollonia (d. 249), who had been martyred by having her teeth yanked out. Some other examples are noted in Chapters 2 and 8.

Down the centuries, holy people have claimed healing gifts. In Restoration England, the Irish gentleman Valentine Greatrakes healed by prayer and laying on of hands; a century later, Bridget Bostock from Cheshire cured with holy spittle; in mid-nineteenth-century France, the visions of Bernadette Soubirous, the miller's daughter, led to Lourdes becoming a leading healing shrine, today visited by around 3 million pilgrims a year. 'Miracle' healing has commanded a mass appeal, and the less the medical profession and even churches countenance marvellous cures, the more faith-healing falls into the hands of hucksters.

Epidemics often excited confrontations between the Church and the medical profession, public authorities and the people, as to the meaning of diseases and the measures required. Plague above all provoked such problems, for bubonic plague was lethal, rapidly fatal, and spread like wildfire, imperilling whole communities. Laden like leprosy with Scriptural associations and moral metaphors, plague was typically interpreted as a visitation, requiring public atonement. In the fourteenth century, the Black Death led to expiatory flagellant movements and anti-Semitic pogroms. Faced with plague, Church authorities in Renaissance Italy proclaimed mass intercessions and propitiatory prayers. The municipalities, for their part, counterordered quarantine and isolation, sometimes banning religious processions. This prompted tests of strength, the populace typically siding with the priests (for public-health decrees like quarantine were commercially ruinous). On one occasion the entire Florentine Health Board was excommunicated.

In Tudor and Stuart times, plague led to tussles in England between royal health policy and protesting Puritans. The Crown and city corporations responded to epidemics by containment, bolting city gates, banning markets, and quarantining sufferers and suspects. Preachers condemned such measures as misguided, medically worthless, and (because they seemed to fly in the face of Providence) impious. 'It is not the clean keeping and sweeping of our houses and streets that can drive away this fearful messenger of God's wrath', wailed the Puritan pastor, Laurence Chaderton, 'but the purging and sweeping of our consciences from . . . sin.'[2] True Christian fellowship demanded not hygiene but holiness, not sequestration but trust in God.

Witchcraft became a prime bone of contention between the medical and religious outlooks. The baselines were well established. Almost all agreed (here pre-industrial Europe mirrors modern tribal societies) that the Devil and his minions could wreak bodily evil: sickness and death were indices of such diabolical power. When someone fell ill without obvious cause, accusations of *maleficium* (malice) might follow. But could one be sure that the victim was bewitched? Faced with such symptoms as fits, vomiting, confused speech, or delirium, there seemed three possible explanations: disease, fraud, or demonic possession. Doctors developed examination procedures to decide the matter. Were there unambiguous wounds or ulcers? Could the Devil's stigma (*stigmata diaboli*) be discerned? Priests had trials of their own: how did the victim respond to prayer, to display of the Cross?

In most instances, religious and medical experts concurred. But not always. In 1602, Mary Glover fell sick with fits and Elizabeth Jackson, a London charwoman, was accused of bewitching her. Testifying in court, the physician, Edward Jorden, contended that her disorder was organic. Puritan counterwitnesses protested that this was a case of demonism, a view upheld by the judge, Sir Edmund Anderson, a noted hammer of witches. Overruled, the angry Jorden published a book called *The Suffocation of the Mother* (1603),

arguing that the accepted signs of witchcraft were generally produced by a somatic disease that he called 'the Mother', an old term
for hysteria.

Jorden did not deny the reality of diabolism in general, he merely
claimed that it did not apply to Glover. Nor did the case produce a clear line-up of physicians versus priests. Leading Anglican ecclesiastics supported Jorden, for the bishops wanted to put a
damper on witchcraft accusations, which they saw as being exploited
by Roman Catholics and Puritans alike in their battles against
the Church of England. Although to us it might seem paradoxical, Anglican bishops were eager to wash their hands of devil-
dabbling, and were happy to consign cases of 'possession' to the
doctors.

In the long run, governments, church establishments, and ruling
elites throughout Europe, terrified by the anarchy of the witchcraze,
'medicalized' demonism. Indeed, in the eighteenth century, in the
rationalist atmosphere of the Enlightenment, belief in diabolism,
once so orthodox, became condemned as bigoted or even psychopathological, a mark of the lunatic fringe. This in turn spot-
lighted a new malady, religious insanity (see Chapter 8).

The Medical View of Illness

Alongside Christian beliefs about sickness, suffering, and healing –
with their transcendental visions of providence and punishment,
trial, and tribulation – medicine was all the time offering its own
theories of the nature and meaning of sickness. The medicine of the
Greeks and Romans bequeathed a complex message. On the one
hand, the Hippocratic tradition, laid down in writings thought to
be by Hippocrates of Cos, insisted that sickness was of the body, and
that the body formed part of the comprehensive economy of Nature
(*physis*): hence, physicians should study physis. Hippocrates – or,
more accurately, one of the anonymous authors of the *Hippocratic
Corpus* – poured scorn on the superstitious view that sickness was a
supernatural visitation.

Behind this Hippocratic onslaught was a push towards the creation of a more coherent professional identity. In early Greece, there
were no state privileges or legal safeguards for the medical art, and

anybody was free to jockey for trade in the medical marketplace. In such circumstances, the Hippocratic doctors strove in various ways – witness the celebrated Hippocratic Oath – to elevate themselves above other healers. Imposters and disreputable healers 'who first attributed a sacred character to this malady', a Hippocratic author complained, 'were like the magicians, purifiers, charlatans and quacks of our own day, men who claim great piety and superior knowledge. Being at a loss, and having no treatment which would help, they concealed and sheltered themselves behind superstition, and called this illness sacred, in order that their utter ignorance might not be manifest'.[3]

Naturally, the Hippocratics also thought they knew more than other people; but their claim to unique expertise lay in appropriating the organic. As pioneered by the Hippocratics and passed down through the great Galen, medicine was expertise in the body. Greek medical theory thus plucked sickness from the heavens and brought it down to earth. Historians have regarded the Hippocratic programme as, symbolically at least, constituting the foundation of scientific medicine, through denial of a supernatural causation of disease and concentration on the body.

Yet, as emphasized in Chapter 2, if Graeco-Roman medicine was secular and naturalistic, it was also holistic. It focused upon what it called the humours, those fluids whose equilibrium was vital for life: the body must not become too hot or too cold, too wet or too dry. It emphasized 'animal spirits', superfine fluids mediating between the body and the mind. And it postulated various 'souls' that governed bodily functions – a 'vegetable soul', directing nourishment and growth (that is, autonomic processes and metabolic regulation); an 'animal soul', governing sense, feeling, and motion (similar, in our terms, to the sensory/motor system); and an 'intellectual soul', regulating the mental powers (that is, what Renaissance theorists of human nature later designated as reason, will, memory, imagination, and judgment). In short, the human animal was presented as a complex, differentiated integrated whole. The humours formed one facet, and their balance was reflected in the 'complexion' (or outward appearance) and the 'temperament' – or, as we might say, personality type. Humours, complexion, and temperament constituted an interactive system.

Greek medicine was thus 'holistic' or 'whole person' in two crucial ways. First, it assumed that health and illness were 'organic' or 'constitutional' in the sense of deriving from inner processes. It did not see illness as typically caused by invasive pathogens: the cause of sickness was largely internal. Second, all aspects of the person were interlinked. The body affected the mind, as with fever causing delirium. Equally, however, passions and emotions influenced the body, producing what we would call psychosomatic complaints.

Thus Greek medicine – and by extension the learned medicine espoused by bookish physicians through the Middle Ages and the Renaissance – adopted a constitutional or 'physiological' doctrine of sickness. It was the product of physical processes, not of spirit possession or sorcery. It was an expression of changes, abnormalities, or weaknesses in the whole person; peculiar to the individual, it was 'dis-ease' rather than disease. Such a person-centred view could underwrite a certain therapeutic optimism: relief was in the hands of the 'whole person'. Classical medicine taught that the right frame of mind, composure, control of the passions, and suitable lifestyle, could surmount sickness – indeed, prevent it in the first place: healthy minds would promote healthy bodies.

Mechanical Science

Medical thinking took its cue from the Ancients for a long time: Galen of Pergamum, in particular, was deified throughout the Middle Ages. But the tradition was to be challenged by the Scientific Revolution, especially its onslaught on the person-centred and vitalistic views ingrained in Greek, and especially Aristotelian, science. Champions of the 'new science', such as the seventeenth-century philosophers René Descartes and Thomas Hobbes, denounced Aristotle for falsely endowing Nature with vitality, proclivities, appetites, will, consciousness, and purposes ('final causes'). In reality, they argued, Nature was made up of particles or corpuscles of inert matter. The motions of planets, or of balls falling from the Tower of Pisa, were not to be explained in terms of any 'desires' but through the laws of mechanics, of matter in motion, which found ideal expression in the language of geometry and number. Nature was in truth a machine.

This view of Nature – seen as particulate matter uniformly moved by immutable, universal laws (Hooke's Law, Boyle's Law, and such like) – had momentous implications not just for understanding the Solar System or the trajectories of cannon but also for the conceptualization of living beings. Were animals machines? Were humans machines? These were tempting if perilous possibilities pondered on by the fashionable members of London's Royal Society and its equivalents in Paris and Florence. During the seventeenth century, scorn was poured on the 'humours' – they were dismissed as empty verbiage. Thanks to dissection techniques rendered prestigious by the Flemish anatomist Andreas Vesalius, attention was refocused on the solid body parts. Arguing for the circulation of the blood, the London physician William Harvey depicted the heart as a pump. Dissection and experimentation spurred inspection of muscles, cartilage, fibres, vessels, and interpretation of their operation by analogy with levers and springs, pulleys and pipes in man-made mechanisms like mills and clocks.

Analysis of the transformations in anatomy and physiology arising from the Scientific Revolution is provided in Chapter 5. They had the profoundest implications for conceptions of health and disease: wellbeing became compared to the running of a well-tuned, well-oiled machine, and sickness was depicted as a mechanical breakdown, due perhaps to a blockage, fuel shortage, or excessive friction.

The mechanical outlook's appeal was enhanced by the new dualistic philosophies associated above all with Descartes. He postulated two radically different entities, extension (material) and mind (immaterial). Only the human soul or mind possessed consciousness. Literally everything else in Nature, including the human body and all aspects whatsoever of all other living beings, formed part of the realm of what Descartes called 'extension' (obeying the laws of mechanics). 'Extension', which included all other living creatures, was a legitimate terrain for scientific investigation. By Descartes' deft manoeuvre, mind had, so to speak, been mystified, while the body was laid bare.

Such a demarcation clearly had attractions for medicine. If the body's workings were purely 'mechanical', its territory must be the exclusive property of medical science. A huge KEEP OUT notice had, as it were, been pinned to the body, excluding theologians, moralists, and any one else considering fishing in medicine's pond. Moreover, if the flesh truly were a machine – no more, no less – it should prove as comprehensible as the workings of a clock. Reductionism now, for the first time, loomed large in medicine's agenda: explaining the whole in terms of its parts, the complex in terms of the simple, the biological in terms of the physical or chemical.

The mechanical world-view with its attendant mind-body dualism unleashed an extraordinarily productive programme of anatomical and physiological research that bore exceptional fruit, in the nineteenth century, with experimental physiology and cell biology and, in the twentieth, with molecular biology. Nineteenth-century medical scientists felt increasingly certain that for each sickness they would find, under the skin, tangible localized lesions: an inflamed organ, an obstruction, a tumour, or pathogens and parasites. Material interventions – drugs and surgery – would relieve or cure. Confident professional articles of faith proclaimed the autonomy and authority of biomedical science. Such developments imparted a new scientific aura to nineteenth-century professional medicine. Biomedicine claimed an explanatory monopoly over the body, its exploration, and its treatment. Proponents of scientific medicine, such as the German bacteriologist Robert Koch, discoverer of the cholera bacillus, believed they had cracked the secret of disease.

So the core medical project over the past two centuries has lain in exploring the workings and the malfunctions of bodily tissues and cells. Chapter 5 examines the role in this of the laboratory and the medical specialisms it has sustained. For example, thanks to the microscope and the rise of cytology, cancer and other cellular diseases could be investigated for the first time. On the microscope slide were exhibited the bacteria and viruses responsible for infections: disease organisms became visible. Furthermore, biochemistry has examined deficiency and digestive diseases, endocrinology has explained hormonal imbalances, neurology has revealed the basis of behavioural disturbances in the central nervous system, and modern genetics is cracking inherited conditions such as Huntington's chorea.

Alongside the laboratory, the hospital played a major part in establishing disease as objective ('ontological'). As the French thinker Michel Foucault emphasized in his study *The Birth of the Clinic* (1963), the vast nineteenth-century expansion of hospitals created disease showcases. The presence under a single roof of scores of cases of tuberculosis or typhus switched attention from the individual to the type. What seemed significant in the hospital was not the slightly diverse symptoms of this or that patient but the fact that diseases routinely followed essentially the same course in case after case, and that clinical regularities could then be confirmed in the morgue through postmortem pathological examination. Nicholas Jewson, a British medical sociologist, has spoken perceptively of the 'disappearance of the sick man' in the nineteenth century: doctors directed their gaze not on the individual sick person but on the disease of which his or her body was the bearer.[4]

Hospitals also became sites for surgery; and the progress of surgery – especially after anaesthetics and antiseptics made abdominal surgery feasible and safe (see Chapter 6) – proved the capstone and ultimate vindication of the programme of medical research and thinking espoused from the seventeenth century. For surgery was human engineering; as with car maintenance, one peered under the bonnet and repaired faulty parts. Nowadays, transplant surgery permits, for the first time, replacement of parts that are beyond repair. Mechanical and reductionist approaches found their culmination in spare-part surgery.

Body and Gut

The laboratory and the hospital created and confirmed a viewpoint disposed to think of disease as an objective, physical entity, and so contributed to a shift from 'dis-ease' to diseases, or from 'physiological' to 'ontological' conceptions of disease. So, too, the emphasis changed in general practice and bedside medicine. In premodern medical consultations, the doctor's job was mainly to manage the patient's condition – generally with some pretty ineffectual drugs washed down with a hefty gulp of the placebo effect. With the advent of scientific medicine, it was transformed to attacking the disease. The mark of this shift was the emergence of physical examination and its accompanying diagnostic technology – a topic fully examined in Chapter 4.

Before the turn of the nineteenth century, when a patient saw a doctor, the physician first had to be put in the picture. This was achieved through the sick person relating his 'history': when and how the complaint had started, what might have precipitated it, the characteristic pains and symptoms, and whether it was new or recurrent. The patient would also recite the main features of his lifestyle – eating and sleeping habits, bowel motions, details of emotional upsets, and so forth.

The practitioner would appraise this history in the light of prior experience. He would also conduct some kind of physical scrutiny of the body, but, by today's standards, this was cursory. It would be conducted by the eye, not by touch, paying attention to such features as skin colour and lesions (rashes or spots), swelling, and inflammation. Doctors would commonly feel the pulse with the finger, making a qualitative assessment (was it languid or racing, regular or erratic?), look at the tongue, listen to coughs, and sniff bad odours.

Physical examination was perfunctory. For one thing, too much touching or exposure of the patient's body was liable to be thought indelicate. Groping beneath the clothes was undignified to a genteel physician. For another, traditional medicine had no diagnostic instruments to augment the senses. Stethoscopes, ophthalmoscopes, and other gadgetry were not introduced till after 1800, and even then they met resistance from patients and practitioners alike. To the end of her days, Queen Victoria was noted for her 'great aversion' to the stethoscope. In all the 20 years he attended her, remembered the Queen's last physician, Sir James Reid, 'the first time I had ever seen the Queen . . . in bed' was when she was actually dying, and it was only after her death that he discovered that she had a 'ventral hernia, and a prolapse of the uterus' – proof that he had never given her a full physical examination.[5]

In traditional medical consultations, the physician was reliant on what the sick person said and his skill in interpreting the patients' words. This did not leave him in too parlous a state, because lay people, both educated and illiterate, had entrenched notions of their own about their systems and what made them ill. Letters and autobiographies from earlier centuries reveal deep preoccupation with matters of health and with attempts to plumb the sources of sickness.

Samuel Pepys, for example, still subscribed to a humoral theory of illness, stressing 'cold' and therefore the role of phlegm. Cold was dangerous because it 'clogged the pores' and thus impeded healthy expulsion of 'peccant humours'. For commonsense humoral thinking, the key to health lay in the body functioning as an efficient throughput system. Abundant food and drink were necessary to stoke the vital fires (the 'flame of life' was a popular metaphor). But regular evacuation was equally needed to prevent blockages. Hence people set great store by taking vomits, letting blood (venesection or phlebotomy), undergoing 'sweats', and, above all, in purging themselves (see Chapter 4). Regular and energetic evacuations helped maintain good 'flow'.

The situation was to change, and the development of physical examination was an important factor and marker. Emerging during the nineteenth century, it revolved round a sequence of highly stylized acts performed by the doctor – feeling the pulse, sounding the chest, taking blood pressure, inspecting the throat, taking the temperature, and so forth. The patient would commonly be made to lie on a couch and loosen or remove clothing. Many procedures involved touching body zones not normally exposed or handled. From the stethoscope through the X-ray to the biopsy and the CAT- or PET-scanner, mechanical means have successively permitted scientific medicine to peer right through the body, and see disease independently of the individual who happens to be its carrier.

Through such means, physical and symbolic, the medical profession has radically transformed its viewpoint. With its costly technology, its research and laboratory programmes, modern medicine promotes its claim to be scientific, and hence to be as attentive to the objective laws of disease as, say, physics is to particles. This minute concern with cells and pathogens has, of course, risked the wrath of uncomprehending critics, asking: *cui bono?* Two centuries ago, Samuel Coleridge damned doctors for such debasing and blinkered somatism: 'They are *shallow* animals', judged the poet, 'having always employed their minds about Body and Gut, they imagine that in the whole system of things there is nothing but Gut and Body.'[6] Yet clutching the coat-tails of science has also lent medicine immense authority and prestige – as well as greatly advancing medical knowledge and its capacity to vanquish disease. Many now have cause to be grateful that medicine knows so much about the gut.

Science and Stigma

This tale of the rise of medical science is, however, only one side of the story. For one thing, the science of disease long remained and still remains in key respects less an accomplished reality than a programme. There has always been rivalry over concepts of scientificity and contention concerning models of causation. As is explored in Chapter 5, experimentalists, epidemiologists, public-health experts, and clinicians have been at loggerheads regarding the classification and causation of individual diseases and of whole divisions of disorders.

In the eighteenth century, controversy raged over the value of disease classification, or nosology: were there truly different species and varieties of disease that could be classified taxonomically? Or, as the radical Scottish doctor John Brown and his followers (called Brunonians) claimed, was there but one disease that struck at different levels of intensity in different ways? Disputes about the part played by 'nature' and 'nurture' and 'seed' and 'seed-bed' were to the fore in the late nineteenth and early twentieth centuries – controversies given greater edge by the founding of movements aiming to curtail the fertility of alleged hereditary 'degenerates'.

Tuberculosis was the scourge of early industrial society. Was it a hereditary malady? Was it a self-inflicted condition that the indigent brought on themselves by their squalid habits? Or was it the consequence of the wretched urban environment in which the labouring poor were forced to live? Competing theories were fiercely debated through the Victorian era in Europe and North America. All were wrong: tuberculosis proved to be caused by a bacillus, discovered in 1882 by Robert Koch.

Thus the pretensions of medical science to penetrate the causes of disease – and hence to direct preventive and remedial action – have often run ahead of copper-bottomed knowledge. And it would be simple-minded to believe that discovery of the presence of harmful bacteria finally settled all issues. For tricky questions remained as to why the tubercle bacillus precipitated the disease in some people, yet not in others. Medicine still seemed different from physics, for evidently bacteria did not cause disease in precisely the way that lightning caused thunder. The same debate now rages about the human immunodeficiency virus, HIV. From 1984, the official line has been that HIV was the 'cause' of AIDS, but some medical researchers now believe that this is far too simple a model for understanding AIDS, and think that 'co-factors' are equally important. Some – a minority – even claim that the presence of HIV is no certain indication that a person will develop AIDS.

The cause of epidemics led to the keenest debate from the Renaissance into the bacteriological era. Why did certain fevers ravage communities? And why did some individuals succumb to infections while others escaped? Stressing internal balance, Greek humoralism was effective at explaining why an individual fell sick, but theories seeing sickness as principally constitutional only went so far. They hardly explained Black Death or smallpox – or the seemingly 'new' diseases on the march, such as syphilis which appeared at the close of the fifteenth century. Some said it was brought back from the New World; others that it spread from Italy or from France (the 'French disease'). Whichever, rotting genitals bore tell-tale marks of a disease communicated by direct and intimate contact, and speculations abounded. In the sixteenth century, an Italian physician, Girolamo Fracastoro, advanced the first influential 'contagionist' theory of disease: syphilis, he contended in *Syphilis, Sive Morbus Gallicus* (1530), was spread by 'seeds' sown by human contact.

Thus sexually transmitted diseases and 'contagionism' arose at the same time and became melded in the mind. Certain consequences followed. If disease was contagious, could not its spread be halted by taking sufferers and suspects out of circulation? Renaissance Italy accordingly developed quarantine systems; not least, the hospitalization of those new moral lepers, syphilitic prostitutes.

The notion of contagion became familiar, fearsome, but contentious in the early modern world, because of its weighty moral as well as medical overtones. For it was already powerfully associated with infection by the Devil and with magic's invisible arrows. Everyone knew that diabolical *maleficium* was transferred from person to person: what else was 'possession'? Witchcraft could similarly involve the power of charms or the evil eye. In other words, the notion of a 'contagious disease' was, from the start, connected in the popular mind with magic and diabolism.

Residual associations between contagion, astrology, magic, and the occult explain the appeal of a counter-theory of epidemics that rose to prominence in the eighteenth century – the notion of 'miasma'. 'Miasmata' were atmospheric exhalations given off by stagnant ponds, rotting vegetable and animal matter, human waste, and all that was filthy and putrescent. Miasmatism seemed to explain why it was slum districts and the poor who were most severely stricken in times of epidemic. Moreover, with its palpable linking of soil, environment, atmosphere, and sickness, 'miasmatism' seemed scientific, open to empirical investigation.

Faced with the raging epidemics of early industrial cities, vehement struggles ensued between contagionists, miasmatists, and many other '-ists'. Arguments were medical; but they were also implicitly or explicitly political, economic, and moral. Insofar as the contagionist position was linked with calls for quarantine, for example, it roused the wrath of commercial interests fearful of the interruption of trade. Alternatively, insofar as the wretched habitations of the poor were thought to breed disease-bearing miasmata, miasmatism could become a fatalistic doctrine (the destitute created unhealthy environments) or a call for change (slum clearance and public-health measures would reduce sickness).

If bacteriology finally settled those debates, questions of the origin and nature of disease still arise. Even today, major, widespread, and often lethal diseases still elude full scientific elucidation. Most cancers fall within this category. The involvement of hereditary factors, environmental elements, and viruses in carcinomata remains deeply contested amongst cancer specialists. We await full elucidation of many degenerative diseases, from arthritis to senile dementia, and, as Chapter 8 explores, mental disorder continues to divide professional doctors, neurologists, psychiatrists, and psychoanalysts. Medicine may express confidence about the 'medical model'; within that model, however, enormous scope remains for disagreement and controversy. This is nowhere better seen in our own time than with the question of AIDS.

Some religious fundamentalists have contended that AIDS is a divine punishment for sin. Early in the epidemic speculation was rife that it might be the consequence of disastrously injurious lifestyles: drug abuse and rampant sexual promiscuity, notably amongst the male homosexual community ('the gay plague'). Once again, medical hypotheses and moral judgments had seemingly become confused. There was therefore great relief when a viral source (HIV) was identified in 1984. Not God, not lifestyles, but a neutral, scientific microorganism was responsible – one that could fell the supposedly 'innocent' (such as recipients of blood transfusions) no less than the 'guilty' (promiscuous gays).

Once AIDS was recast as a communicable disease, however, a Pandora's Box was opened, loosing all those destructive fears that fester when diseases are regarded as being caused by unseen agents spread by 'other people'. In particular, punitive, guilt-ridden fantasies have been rampant, associating AIDS with a sexual malaise in our midst (a 'social cancer') that needs to be controlled, policed, segregated, and eradicated.

Notions of contagion evoke spectres of pollution and defilement. In a study of the representation of disease, the American historian Sander Gilman has drawn attention to pervasive tendencies to construct schemes of Self and Other, Us and Them, in which self-definition is strengthened through stereotyping and scape-goating of those who are 'different' and (therefore) dangerous. It is easy to cast the sick as Other and label the Other as sick. This has happened throughout history, especially with disease conditions involving peculiar appearances, for visible abnormalities are held to bespeak moral defects – the marks of Cain, Ham, or the Devil. Regarded as singled out by God, lepers, for example, were forced to the fringes of medieval society, beyond contaminating contact, made to wander, ringing bells: they were 'unclean' or even socially 'dead'.

On leprosy's decline, the stigmata of uncleanness became transferred to syphilitics – moral lepers who wore their pocky skin like a convict's uniform, advertising their carnal sins. Lunatics, too, were similarly stigmatized. In art, medical texts, and the popular imagination, maniacs were standardly shown as savage, bemired, unkempt, locks dishevelled and straw-matted, near naked or raggledy-taggledy: William Blake depicted King Nebuchadnezzar, demented by God, reduced to shaggy brutishness, lower than the animals. By setting the sick apart – in our mental pictures, but also behind institutional walls – we uphold the fantasy that we are whole. Purity is maintained by driving away pollution. In other words, 'scientific' disease theories can frequently reinforce, yet hide, collective moral prejudice and personal stigma.

When cholera swept Europe and the Americas from the 1830s, physicians blamed the outbreaks on the low morals and drunkenness of the poor. Writing in the late eighteenth century, a leading American physician, Benjamin Rush, suggested that blackness (negritude) was a disease, akin to leprosy. Victorian doctors proposed that women with robust sexual appetites were suffering from 'nymphomania' and sometimes recommended surgical cures – removal of the ovaries, womb, very occasionally, the clitoris. Published case histories reveal all too clearly the sexual atrocities committed on female patients in the name of medicine. For a nineteenth-century German physician, Gustav Broun, physical 'anomalies' in the female genitalia were caused by an overactive sexual sensibility: 'Under the influence of a salacious imagination, which is stimulated by obscene conversations or by reading poorly selected novels, the uterus develops a hyperexcitability which leads to masturbation and its dire consequences', he wrote. With one 25-year-old patient, Broun's concern was to prevent her from touching her outer genitalia, as had been her custom:

on November 11, 1864, a good part of the labia minora and the foreskin of the clitoris were cauterized with a cauterizing instrument. To limit the copious discharge from the uterus, the uterine cavity was cauterized with Chiari's caustic solution. At the same time, the patient was given Lupulin, in dosages of three grains to combat her sexual excitement, and lactic iron.

When that and other treatments brought no benefit, 'the amputation of the clitoris and the major portions of the labia minora was proposed to the patient as the only possible cure'.[7]

Ever since the Greeks, medical writers have implied that the female gender is, in itself, an abnormality (Aristotle called women 'monsters'), and that, on account of their gynaecological disorders, women were inherently pathological. In short, physicians' accounts of the causes of diseases have, in reality, doubled as sagas of condemnation.

The aim here is not to ridicule or castigate doctors: blaming doctors for victim-blaming would be singularly futile. Rather, two points deserve consideration. First, we must remain sceptical about claims that medicine has ever been, or has finally become, 'value-free' in its accounts of diseases and their causation. For one thing, medicine has largely embraced the model of the physical sciences, a materialist reductionism – which is by no means self-evidently right for comprehending the true character of all kinds of human sickness. For another, as the graveyard of discarded 'diseases' shows, medicine has often stuffed into disease envelopes strange collections of clinical symptoms, social phenomena, and prejudices. Second, we must see that this apparent 'frailty' of medicine arises from the fact that sickness is not simply the work of pathogens; it is a function of social relations. For this reason, physic necessarily goes beyond the bounds of the paradigms of physics.

Stories of Disease

It is easy to come across evidence of the medical profession weaving moral fantasies around the sick and around diseases: if you masturbate you will go blind or mad (medicine has often been guilty of creating this kind of pseudoscientific folklore). It has enabled doctors to sound off their prejudices, and also to camouflage their ignorance behind plausible fabrications and just-so stories.

The need to cope with ignorance is all the greater with the sick themselves, especially those suffering from mysterious, incurable, and fatal conditions. It may appear doubly dreadful (reflected the American writer Susan Sontag in her book *Illness as Metaphor*) to succumb to a virus if it seems a bolt from the blue, without rhyme or reason, for life is thus reduced to an irrational chapter of accidents. And so the dire explanatory void ('Why me? What have I done to deserve it?') is filled by fabricating stories of the meanings of disease. The diseased organ may be deemed 'bad', or one's personality may be accused of precipitating the malady. Thus, Susan Sontag argued, it has commonly been said that such-and-such person got cancer due to a 'cancer personality', a supposed proclivity to bottle-up feelings and drive anger inside, the thwarted passions finally taking self-destructive vengeance on the flesh. It is no accident that the most feared disease of the twentieth century, the 'Big C' (significantly, the disease cannot speak its name) has been associated with 'dirty' parts – the colon, rectum, womb, scrotum, and breast – or that, in the popular imagination, AIDS has acquired an identity as a disease associated with anal intercourse. Another instance is offered by tuberculosis.

Nineteenth-century physicians regarded tuberculosis primarily as a female disease. Simply being a woman was itself 'a condition favourable to the development of tuberculization', said one doctor. The tubercular state was the female ideal taken to the limit. Romantic fashions expected ladies to be slim – their delicacy expressed a child-like air. Satirists insinuated that young belles or their mothers even courted tuberculosis by swanning around in flimsy attire or deliberately undereating, so as to grow slender enough to snare a husband. Around 1800, the English physician Thomas Beddoes bantered that tuberculosis had become *à la mode* amongst the fair sex. 'Writers of romance', he grumbled, 'exhibit the slow decline of the consumptive, as a state . . . in which not much more misery is felt, than is expressed by a blossom, nipped by untimely frosts.' The preposterous idea had thus got about, he protested, that 'consumption must be a flattering complaint', radiating mystery and allure.[8]

Yet chic tubercular cadaverousness was not wholly confined to women of a pre-Raphaelite look. Because leanness betokened high-minded refinement, the triumph of mind over matter, male poets and poseurs equally liked to display an aetherial presence. 'When I was young', recalled the French writer Théophile Gautier in the mid-nineteenth century, 'I could not have accepted as a lyrical poet anyone weighing more than ninety-nine pounds.'[9] Ideally, flesh simply melted into the imagination.

The consumptive look signalled the becoming petiteness of the feminine, but, paradoxically, it also conveyed a thrilling eroticism. Consumptive beauties like Mimi in Puccini's *La Bohème* and Marguerite Gauthier in Verdi's *La Traviata* were fragile, yet they were also feverish with passion. It was part of the mythology, confirmed by doctors, that tuberculosis was an aphrodisiac. The tubercular woman was bewitching in appearance, with her prominent eyes, pallid skin, and the hectic flush of the hollow cheeks. And the disease supposedly triggered inner erotic cravings too. For public-health experts, tuberculosis was, alongside syphilis, the principal disease of the prostitutes thronging Paris – the result of 'venereal excesses', according to René Laënnec, the leading hospital physician in Paris in the early nineteenth century.

It was thus poetic justice that tuberculosis was lethal, yet it was an affliction that destroyed in a distinctive way. There was something serenely rapturous about the consumptive's deathbed. The body, it was said, almost vanished away, the flesh dissolved, leaving just the parting smile, freeing the spirit. The sufferer died, but his or her agony was the relinquishing of mortal flesh that permitted the soul to breathe. So death was not just an end, it was atonement; suffering was morally redeeming.

Such moralizing with sickness (what I have said applies equally to many diseases, not just tuberculosis) has a *prima facie* appeal: it rationalizes menacing maladies and renders adversity less mysterious. Compensatory comfort was thus offered by the Romantic myth that bodies wasting away with tuberculosis were actually being refined into pure, angelic 'spirituality'. Better a tale with a barbed moral and a tragic ending than no story at all. Yet such labels may mainly serve to 'blame the victim': disease fantasies are usually punitive.

It is worth glancing at a different condition and a separate set of metaphors: gout, a condition chronic and painful, though rarely fatal. Gout was widely esteemed as a disease, because of the myth that the gout-ridden were thereby protected from worse disorders. Gout was thus a kind of immunization. A gouty foot might even be a sign of health, since the big toe typically affected was far distant from the vital organs. Secure in his 'gouty bootikins' (slippers), the mid-eighteenth-century English man of letters Horace Walpole thus recommended sitting it out stoically. 'It prevents other illnesses and prolongs life', he maintained: 'Could I cure the gout, should not I have a fever, a palsy, or an apoplexy?'[10]

Influential here was the old saw that diseases were jealous of each other and mutually exclusive. So long as gout was in possession, no deadlier enemy could gain invade. 'To the Gout my mind is reconciled', Samuel Johnson informed his friend, Mrs Thrale, for he had been assured by his physician 'that the gout will secure me from every thing paralytick.'[11]

Paradoxical as it may seem, gout was thus regarded as a disease that protected – a prophylactic. Charles II's Archbishop of Canterbury, Gilbert Sheldon, reportedly offered '£1,000 to any person who would "help him to the gout"', looking upon it as the only remedy for the distemper in his head, which he feared might in time prove an apoplexy; as in time it did and killed him'.[12] In short, being gout-ridden was preferable to being rid of gout. All that needed to be ensured, according to Jonathan Swift, was that it never got deep into the innards:

> As if the gout should seize the head,
> Doctors pronounce the patient dead,
> But if they can, by all their arts;
> Eject it to the extreamest parts,
> They give the sick man joy, and praise
> The gout that will prolong his days.[13]

Gout is thus an exemplary case of how disease is rationalized. In these sufferers' accounts, gout is neither the focus of a Romantic, punitive, or sadomasochistic fiction, in the manner of the 'cancer personality'; nor is it reduced to a laboratory specimen, alien and meaningless. Rather, gout is a malady that is humanized, accepted as the other face of life, and integral to the human condition.

A radical critic of modern medicine, Ivan Illich, argued in *Limits to Medicine* (1977) that the progress of scientific medicine, or at least the success of its propaganda, has been creating Promethean expectations of an almost infinite prolongation of healthy, fit, and fully functioning existence. Cosmetic and spare-part surgery feed these fantasies. Such dreams, Illich argued, are, finally, unrealistic: all must age and die, and longer life may mean greater pains. Hence these utopian myths of perfect, endless health are disabling, because they impair our ability to come to terms with fates that are inevitable. Moreover, they prove heartless, because they provoke the young, healthy, fit, sexy, and beautiful to distance themselves from the aged, decrepit, and dying.

Illich's analysis may suggest, in short, that we have moved – partly thanks to the philosophy of scientific medicine and partly because of genuine health improvements – from the morbid sickness culture of medieval Christianity to one in which disease is denied, becoming either meaningless or featuring only in punitive moral tales. By contrast to the traditional myths of gout, the triumph of scientific medicine, reinforced by the inflation of unrealistic health expectations (above all in the USA), has challenged the legitimacy of traditional stories of sickness and discounted our capacity to cope.

The Sick Role

Modern life thus creates various binds. It produces claims, or illusions, of freedom from sickness and positive health, thanks to the benign intervention of the medical profession. Yet that also fosters preoccupations with sickness. Indeed, the growth of medicine has encouraged what has been called 'medicine-mongering'.

Medicine enjoyed a golden century from around 1850. Before the Victorian era, medicine had but paltry power to cure disease and save the sick, and few entertained great expectations of it. Thereafter, surgery leapt ahead, thanks to anaesthetics and antiseptics; public health improved hygiene; bacteriology explicated aetiology; laboratory medicine flowered; and, at long last, sulphonamides and antibiotics wrought a pharmaceutical revolution. Lethal diseases were overcome, life expectations soared. Medicine and society enjoyed a honeymoon era.

Since around the 1960s, however, the marriage has soured. Cancer and many other major diseases remain embarrassments, even scandals; medicine itself is increasingly held responsible for pain and sickness, through 'iatrogenic' (doctor-created) complaints. Above all, modern critics accuse medicine of embarking upon what Ivan Illich has called the 'medicalization of life'. For various reasons – some would say genuine compassion, others would blame professional 'imperialism' – medicine is allegedly set on course to put all aspects of living into the hands of the doctors. Pregnancy and childbirth are nowadays seen, if not precisely as diseases, at least as conditions requiring professional medical attendance, by law in advanced Western societies. Many geriatricians argue that ageing is a pathological process; and, like birth, dying is becoming routinely hospitalized. During the past couple of centuries, all manner of personal habits, vices, and idiosyncrasies have been redefined by the medical profession as ailments or medicopsychiatric disorders; for instance, heavy drinking has been medicalized as alcoholism.

Such medicalization requires subtle interpretation. In some ways, it might be viewed as emancipatory, as it has been for suicide. Traditionally, the Church regarded self-murder (*felo de se*) as a mortal sin. From the late seventeenth century, doctors, with public approval, began to contend that suicide was typically, almost by definition, committed in an unbalanced state of mind. Thereby the censure of sin and crime was avoided, as also was forfeiture to the state of the suicide's property.

Often, however, medicalization has involved stigmatization, as feminists have noted, protesting against medical accounts of menstruation, menopause, and anorexia nervosa. And it may be particularly perilous as medicine increasingly serves as an arm of the state, through compulsory health insurance, the National Health Service, and the use of medical records to monitor employment, criminality, delinquency, and so forth. Political dissidence has been called 'sick' and subjected to medical and psychiatric correction as a matter of policy in the former Soviet Union and Communist China. In subtler ways, similar pressures exist elsewhere.

In part, medicalization spreads because the public colludes in it: medicine promises benefits. Moreover, in a secular society where the Church no longer explains fate and directs behaviour, the culture of sickness offers a surrogate. Being ill becomes a way of life accorded social sanction and medical encouragement. Two facets are worth examining: the sick role and the psychosomatic complaint – frequently, it is obvious, two sides of the same coin.

The idea of the sick role was formulated in the 1950s by the American sociologist Talcott Parsons, who regarded it as a tacit deal between sufferer and society by which John or Joan Citizen would be allowed occasionally to retire from social demands under the cover of being ill. Temporarily relieved of social responsibilities, he (or she) could stay off work, take to his bed, and luxuriate in tea and sympathy. In return, he must abstain from drink, sex, sport, and other pleasures, and would be honour-bound to recover as quickly as possible, so his 'well role' could be resumed. A legitimate 'time out' was thus offered, a sort of joyless extra holiday or Scottish Sunday, begirt by conventions of reciprocity.

Parsons's account of 'legitimate deviance' affords insight into society's perennially ambiguous attitudes towards the sick. It also expresses a 'victim-blaming' of its own, reducing the social actor who avails himself of the role to a sort of *malade imaginaire* or at least a manipulative game-player.

The existential side of playing sick is psychosomatic illness, whose intriguing history has been traced by Edward Shorter.[14] He focused on what he calls 'somatizers' – that is, people suffering from 'pain and fatigue that have no physical cause'. These are patients frustrating to no-nonsense physicians such as the early-twentieth-century Kentucky doctor who thought a 'good spanking, sometimes even a good "cussing"', was the surest way with such evident hypochondriacs'. Most of those suffering in the past two centuries from conditions variously called 'nervous spine', 'neurasthenia', 'fits', and nowadays myalgic encephalomyelitis or ME (also called 'yuppie flu' or chronic fatigue syndrome) and perhaps repetitive strain injury (RSI) have had nothing intrinsically organically wrong with them, argued Shorter, but have been consciously or unconsciously seeking solace, attention, or social excuses. Such somatizers have produced a fascinating succession of phantom diseases, Shorter suggested, the 'unconscious', selecting convenient suits of somatoform manifestations from a wider 'symptom pool'.

Early in the nineteenth century, motor disorders were prominent. Archetypal Victorian ladies collapsed on their beds, literally incapable of standing on their own two feet, from fits, convulsions, spasms, or paralysis. By 1900, such operatic displays softened into a symptomatological chamber music, and motor defects were superseded by more discreet sensory complaints: neuralgia, headache, and fatigue. Each made sense in context. In the claustrophobic milieu of the Victorian family, only a melodramatic acting out of abnormalities could command attention. Amidst the twentieth-century 'lonely crowd', by contrast, the introspective ego finds expression in private pain.

Somatizers act ill, and a melancholy collusion has entangled 'somatizers' and doctors – above all, those physicians grasping or cynical enough to spy rich pickings in pandering to insatiable, well-heeled valetudinarians. And in the succession of medical alibis tacitly negotiated between profession and patient in the Victorian era and subsequently, the constant was a gentleman's agreement that the complaint was truly physical. Sufferers were relieved to hear that their ailments were organic, requiring medical or surgical treatment. For the entrenched 'medical model' presupposed that a somatic malady was real; all others might be fictional and fraudulent. With an organic complaint, patients lost no face: there was no hint that they were shamming, and no risk that they be thought crackers. Medical men maintained the charade by cooking up innovations in minor surgery, spa regimes, coloured waters, and health-retreat regimes, relying on the desperate gullibility of patients prepared to believe that each and every organ could spawn dozens of defects.

The presence – indeed, growing incidence – of psychosomatic disorders, and hence of people enacting the sick role and reaping its secondary gains, speaks volumes about the profound ambiguities of disease concepts and sickness strategies. In our secular, atomized environment, illness is one of the relatively few ways of expressing social complaints and the ambiguities of self. Yet it is riven with ambiguity: publicly distrusted, freighted with stigma, and often mocked by the very professionals who massage it.

Alternative Medicine

One apparent escape from such impasses lies in positing radically different ideas of disease, sickness, and healing. Over the centuries, alternative medicine and holistic theories have tended to reject materialist, ordinary (allopathic), or mechanical theories of disease, and to espouse the belief that health and sickness involve the whole person – often the whole cosmos. Sickness is a malady not of the body but of the complete self; within that self the cure lies, through acts of will or lifestyle changes. Such ideas were extensively developed in nineteenth-century North America, through such movements as Christian Science. Health reform was championed not by regular physicians but by lay people, disaffected equally with official churches and with regular medicine, and seeking to replace both with a unified, holistic philosophy of spiritual and bodily health, carved out of personal experience.

Among the medical botanists (called Thomsonians after Samuel Thomson, an early Victorian health reformer in New Hampshire) and similar sects, certain convictions were widely shared. They promoted a medical version of original sin, arguing that civilized man had 'fallen', bringing disease on himself by greed, speed, excessive meat-eating, and alcohol abuse. By way of remedy, they advocated a return to 'natural' living – vegetarianism, sexual restraint, temperance, abandonment of such stimulants as tea and tobacco, and an end to artificial drugs, trusting to herbal remedies. Homeopaths for their part insisted on ultra-pure medicaments, taken in minute quantities.

Influenced by the teachings of the mystic Emmanuel Swedenborg, some groups went further, discarding medicines altogether, and trusting to the healing powers of Nature, aided by water, prayer, self-control, and spiritual illumination. With its 'a plague on both your houses' attitude, the Christian Science movement exemplifies all these features. Its founder, Mary Baker Eddy, spent much of her New Hampshire youth in the 1830s sick with obscure nervous disorders. She rejected her parents' strict Congregationalism. Regular physicians did her no good. Relieved by homeopathy and mesmerism, she then undertook self-healing, and her success led her to adumbrate her own system, in which 'there is but one creation, and it is wholly spiritual'. Matter therefore was an illusion; hence, there could be no such thing as somatic disease, the marrow of medical science. As explained in her best-selling *Science and Health* (1875), sickness and pain were illusions that true 'mind healing' would dispel.

In England, the Moses of alternative medicine at the dawn of the Victorian era was James Morison. A businessman first in Aberdeen and later in London, who had suffered gastric disorders and consulted numerous ordinary doctors, he despised regulars with evangelical fervour. Doctors, he contended, were not merely ignorant and mercenary, but also dangerous. Their polypharmacy and heavy dosing habits were little less than criminal. Morison proposed new institutes for medicine, encapsulated in Ten Commandments:

- The vital principle is contained in the blood.
- Blood makes blood.
- Everything in the body is derived from the blood.
- All constitutions are radically the same.

- All diseases arise from the impurity of the blood or, in other words, from acrimonious humours lodged in the body.
- This humour, which degenerates the blood, has three sources – the maternine, the contagious and the personal.
- Pain and disease have the same origin; and may therefore be considered synonymous terms.
- Purgation by vegetables is the only effectual mode of eradicating disease.
- The stomach and bowels cannot be purged too much.
- From the intimate connexion subsisting between the mind and the body, the health of the one must conduce to the serenity of the other.[15]

There was a single cause for all disease – bad blood – and a single therapeutics: heavy and frequent purgation, using vegetable laxatives. In 1825, Morison marketed the perfect purge, his 'Vegetable Universal Pills', that would cure all diseases.

The early Victorian age saw myriad medical movements, such as homeopathy, naturopathy, medical botany, and spiritualism. Phrenology – the belief that character is determined by the relative size of the different parts of the brain and hence can be known by feeling the bumps of the head – and mesmerism (and their hybrid form, phreno-mesmerism) were others. All made a break with regular medicine. Each argued in its own language that the whole system of allopathic medicine was radically wrong. Characteristically, they accused the orthodox of striving to blitz disease with poisonous drugs. Each offered a new plan of life based on Nature's way, and claimed to use more natural modes of healing – using herbs alone or pure water. Each professed to invest the individual with new control over his health as part of a culture of self-improvement and realization. Medical heretics typically doubled as heretics in politics and faith as well, while cultivating unorthodox lifestyles.

Holism is back in fashion. Promising not the 'pill for every ill' approach but rather positive health, alternative healing holds out glowing prospects: life-enhancing organic gentle remedies fresh from Mother Nature's bosom – therapies free of hi-tech impersonality. But, as is evident, in attacking the scientific simplicities of regular medicine, alternative medicine creates a simplistic, black-and-white philosophy of its own. *They* are threatening your well-being with chemicals and pesticides, processed food, and pollution. *You* can safeguard it by following Nature – eating natural fare and, in so doing, discovering your natural energies and vital forces.

What is this but junk rhetoric? Moreover, alternative cults often carry unsavoury, victim-blaming hidden agendas. Sickness proves you are not in touch with yourself. So the fault lies within. Luckily, you can put youself right by working on yourself. But this turns out to be another variant on sturdy Protestant self-help, masquerading as a radical alternative: working-out is the old Protestant work ethic in a new guise.

What Is Disease?

It might be thought that we live in an age in which the questions of illness and disease should be sewn up as never before. Medicine has enjoyed exceptional success: of special symbolic significance was the final global eradication of smallpox in 1979. Life expectations continue to rise. The realities are, however, more murky. Many diseases continue to thwart scientific medicine. Public dissatisfaction grows; dreams fade, promises are broken, people vote with their feet and try alternative medicines and psychotherapies. New conditions appear, such as ME, which do not merely resist ready cure but which challenge the categories of established medicine. Faced with 'yuppie flu', chronic fatigue, strange allergies, and today's sickness salad-bar, the medical profession has made hostile and dismissive noises: all was psychosomatic, whingeing. Then the doctors jumped on the bandwagon, medicalized ME as a real condition, and railroaded it. Yet they proved no nearer to resolving its nature or satisfying its sufferers.

Such developments offer windows onto history. The past presents a changing disease panorama, in several senses. For one thing, diseases, like empires, rise and fall: plague has declined – although occasional localized outbursts remain severe – but cancer has worsened. For another, there have been shifts in perceptions of diseases. One does not need to embrace a modish sociological scepticism to recognize that diseases, like beauty, are somewhat in the eye of the beholder: people see what they want or are programmed to see. Particular anxieties, academic training, new technologies, and so forth cause conditions to come into focus and create pressures to create labels. People doubtless died of heart complaints in earlier centuries, but it took the outlooks and diagnostic apparatus of modern medicine to create the modern categories of the heart attack and coronary thrombosis, or to perceive how the condition long seen as 'dropsy' (oedema) was actually due to heart disease; weaknesses depicted in earlier medicine became crystallized into diabetes. Diseases become 'framed' at particular times and for particular reasons.[16]

'Disease', and its complex interplay with sickness, has its history, too. Different circumstances lead to different facets of life – pains, fevers, bad habits, impairments – being called disease. The fit between what someone experiences as sickness and what doctors deem disease may be close or it may be loose. Wider issues are often at stake: quests for research funds, insurance company regulations, medical exoneration before the law or at the workplace, social excuses. This volume examines the rise of medicine. But it must be remembered that medicine has always been embedded both in human cultural milieux and in the diverse needs of intelligent warm-blooded bodies.

4. Primary Care

Edward Shorter

The first doctor that one sees when one is ill offers 'primary care'. The doctor might be in a hospital emergency room or in a local clinic, but, historically, general practitioners have been the first point of call. This is a story of how patients and general practitioners have collided and colluded over the past two centuries. The story could, of course, be extended much further back in time than the late eighteenth century. Yet that is when the practice of medicine, which had been fairly constant in its humoral theories and drastic treatments over the centuries, began to change. Although medical theories had been in flux over the seventeen centuries from Galen of Pergamum to Herman Boerhaave of Leiden, the actual practice of medicine, or primary care, had changed little. With the infusion of science into medicine late in the eighteenth century, however, the story begins to change. Many of the subsequent travails of primary care may be understood as the confused efforts of doctors and patients to come to grips with the ever-changing realities of medicine imposed on them by science, on the one hand, and by subjective views of 'medical correctness' on the other.

What the Traditional Patient Wanted

In the past (and even today in countries lacking a National Health Service), doctors competed against one another for the custom of patients, for they practised medicine to make a profit. To attract patients, they often felt obliged to offer whatever it was the patients wanted. As George Bernard Shaw wrote in his preface to *The Doctor's Dilemma* (1911),

The doctor who has to live by pleasing his patients in competition with everybody who has walked the hospitals, scraped through the examinations, and bought a brass plate, soon finds himself prescribing water to teetotallers and brandy or champagne jelly to drunkards; beefsteaks and stout in one house, and 'uric acid free' vegetarian diet over the way; shut windows, big fires, and heavy overcoats to old Colonels, and open air and as much nakedness as is compatible with decency to young faddists, never once daring to say either 'I don't know', or 'I don't agree'.[1]

This desire to placate patients' ideas of what constitutes good medicine is one of the basic motors of change in primary care.

'Traditional' means the prescientific phase of medical practice, before doctors became 'men of science' and before patients acquired respect for that science. Traditional patients often had (to us) bizarre notions of what was wrong with them and how it might be fixed. One popular idea in the eighteenth century stressed ridding the body of the poisons that cause disease by drawing them out through the skin. This entailed sweating cures, and patients cherished the idea – as did physicians to a lesser extent – of sweating a patient with a fever. Edinburgh physician William Buchan wrote in his best-selling medical guide *Domestic Medicine* in 1769, 'It is a common notion that sweating is always necessary in the beginning of a fever... The common practice is to heap clothes upon the patient, and to give him things of a hot nature, as spirits, spiceries, &c. which fire his blood, increase the spasms, and render the disease more dangerous.'[2]

How else might one get those poisons, or bad humours, out of there? Bleeding was much beloved by the common people, extending past the time when it lost popularity with physicians. There were many other popular strategies for eliminating toxins. One was vomiting, relinquished relatively early by academic medicine but cherished until the twentieth century by patients.

Taking emetics was intended to produce therapeutic puking, ridding the stomach of toxicity that was supposedly making the whole body sick. The German physician Adolf Kussmaul himself took emetics therapeutically until around the age of forty in 1864. He recalled many patients whose faith in their efficacy was deeply held. One day a peasant in the practice of Kussmaul's father sent word that he was ailing, weak, losing weight, and unable to arise from bed. The father, busy at that moment, sent on by messenger some remedy containing a sweet syrup that could at least do no harm.

Arriving at the peasant's cottage, the doctor found the man restored, at that very moment delecting a roasted dove and drinking a glass of wine. 'Herr Doktor, you prescribed that very well. It was really tough medicine but it cleaned me out and drove out the illness. But I don't think I could get the ants down a second time.' The ants? Apparently, the messenger had fallen asleep *en route*, and as he snoozed under a tree the cork had popped out of the bottle, giving a local ant colony a chance to check out the syrupy prescription by climbing into the bottle. The peasant, so implicitly convinced of the restorative powers of emetic therapy, had vomited heartily after downing the ants – and was well again.[3]

The point is that sweating, bleeding, and vomiting, in addition to salivating, urinating, purging, and many other ways of getting the bad humours out, had a hold on the popular mind that reached back for centuries, existing alongside medical doctrines of belief in such procedures. Thus the patients arrived in primary care with their own definite views of what was needed.

What Traditional Physicians Offered

Before the threshold of the twentieth century, physicians in primary care were surrounded by fever. Fever, a symptom of the body's response to invasion by bacteria and viruses, occupies a minor role in Western medicine today, mainly in the form of initial childhood encounters with common microorganisms and of colds and coughs (upper respiratory infections). Being a doctor before 1900 meant spending the bulk of one's time on fever. Fever was the axis about which the traditional consultation turned – the hot bedridden patient, his pulse quickened and respiring rapidly, the doctor making a house call.

The diary of Richard Kay, a doctor who lived near Bury in Lancashire in the mid-eighteenth century, shows how immersed in fever was the typical practitioner.

July 10. Kay visited Mrs. Chippingdale at Ewood, 'she being very bad', ill apparently with typhus, a tick-born bacterial infection characterized by malaise, severe headache, and sustained high fever.

July 11. 'In the evening as I returned home I visited Miss Betty Rothwell at Ramsbottom who is dangerously bad of a miliary fever [one causing skin eruptions, again, probably typhus].'

July 13. Mrs. Chippingdale was now dying.

July 14. Miss Rothwell was now dead. 'I visited a young man in Rossendale who is dangerously bad of a fever.' Another patient, John Mills, was also ill with fever.

July 15. He visited John Mills again.

July 16. 'This last night about midnight a messenger came with a letter... I was to come to Manchester to visit Mr William Blythe.' 'I found Mr Blythe very dangerously bad of a miliary fever.' Dr Kay also received word that Mrs. Chippingdale and John Mills were dead.

July 17. William Blythe had now died of the fever.[4]

By the time another year would pass, the author's father, his sister Rachel, and his sister Elizabeth were also dead of fever. Dr Kay himself died of fever in October 1751.

Infection means pus. Late in the nineteenth century Arthur Hertzler, a small-town doctor on the Kansas frontier, was called to a case of empyema, or pus in the lungs. 'To answer the call eight miles from town I battled mud for three hours. As I entered the sick-room I saw a boy fourteen years of age half sitting up in bed in deep cyanosis [caused by lack of oxygen], with grayish-blue skin and heaving chest, his mouth open and his eyes bulging. It seemed that each gasp would be his last.'

Dr Hertzler threw down his medical bag and sat flat on the floor with his legs under the bed.

Grabbing a scalpel I made an incision in his chest wall with one stab – he was too near death to require an anesthetic. As the knife penetrated his chest, a stream of pus the size of a finger spurted out, striking me under the chin and drenching me. After placing a drain in the opening, I wrapped a blanket about my pus-soaked body and spent another three hours reaching home.[5]

In medical practice well into the twentieth century, fever was omnipresent. Pneumonia, for example, counted as 'the old person's friend', because it was so common in the elderly and often fatal after a short illness. And few physicians would not face the sadness of death in the young from the epidemic diseases of childhood. James Herrick, a doctor in Chicago, recalled what it was like to treat diphtheria before the introduction of the antitoxin to the USA in the early 1890s. In diphtheria, the growth of bacteria in the throat interferes with breathing.

In the case of an attractive seven-year-old child in whom the disease had invaded the larynx, I had inserted an O'Dwyer intubation tube [Herrick had practised the technique in the morgue of the Cook County Hospital]. This gave relief for several hours; then it was evident that the tube was becoming clogged. The parents begged me not to let the child strangle. I explained the desperate nature of the trouble, the extreme weakness of the circulation due to the toxaemia, and the danger of even mild manipulative treatment. They understood. The mother left the room, the father took the child in his arms, and with little difficulty the tube was removed. As the father uttered a 'Thank God', the child gave a feeble gasp and was gone. In memory I can still see the room, the exact location of the bed, the chair, the limp child in the father's lap, the adjustment of the light.[6]

Herrick himself was so upset at the loss that he nearly broke into tears.

Before the twentieth century, therefore, infectious diseases dominated over all others. Tuberculosis, syphilis, diphtheria, plague, meningitis, malaria, and post-partum sepsis were the diseases against which medical graduates and physicians everywhere had to struggle. That is what primary care was all about.

For this task, the doctrines of traditional physicians had singularly ill-equipped them. In the middle of the nineteenth century, medical theories about the causes of disease would be turned inside out. But before that time notions of disease causation were constructed along 'humoral' lines, attributing illness to imbalances of the fluids, or humours, which the Ancients believed to be the constituents of the body: black bile, yellow bile, phlegm, and blood. By the eighteenth century, these Galenic humoral doctrines had undergone considerable modification.

The Dutch physician Herman Boerhaave, for example, added to the ancient theories baroque elaborations that distinguished between disorders of 'the solids' and those of 'the blood and humours'. Tuberculosis was an example of weakness of the solid parts, thrombosis and blood clots examples of overly rigid fibres. Give milk and iron for weak fibres; do bloodletting for rigid ones, Boerhaave counselled in the early eighteenth century. Yet virtually all theorizing about the mechanisms of disease before 1800 was like a castle built in the air: it had little empirical foundation and was completely false in modern scientific terms.

Therapies derived from these humoral theories were almost without exception injurious to the patient. Little was cured and much damage caused by depleting the body of its natural physiological constitutents and dosing it with toxic metals. Bloodletting was a mainstay of medical therapy in treating fever. A variety of mechanical contrivances, from the little folding knife called the 'lancet' to the elaborate 'scarificators' of the early nineteenth century – fiendish devices whose multiple blades would cut simultaneously into the skin – testify to its commonness. To be a surgeon or 'medical man' before the 1870s meant bloodletting.

A proper physician (as opposed to a surgeon or an apothecary) might disdain such procedures as bloodletting and setons in favour of giving 'physic', or medicine. The aim of traditional therapeutics was getting the bowels open. To the extent that the traditional pharmacopoeia used drugs that were active in the body at all, the medicines were mainly laxatives, or purgatives – a more powerful laxative. One treated fever with laxatives, getting those bad humours out of the bowels by procuring an 'opening'.

Towards 1800, Edward Sutleffe, a medical man of long experience in London's Queen Street, called on Mrs. W. of Finsbury. Her fingers were painful and swollen, 'thickly studded with eruptions, from which issued a semi-transparent excoriating ichor. I suspected the latent cause, and told her she had neglected her bowels in particular'. She confessed to having done so. Sutleffe prescribed for her 'a tepid bath and mild aperients [laxatives]'.[7] Quite dramatic substances were used to get those bowels open, those bladders peeing. Philadelphia's Benjamin Rush popularized the use of mercury, calling it in 1791 'a safe and nearly a universal medicine'.[8] Calomel, or mercurous chloride, appeared in every physician's bag throughout the nineteenth century, and was an active ingredient in the 'blue pills' that distinguished nineteenth-century English therapeutics.

Traditional medical therapeutics therefore amounted to making patients anaemic through bloodletting, depleting them of fluids and valuable electrolytes via the stool, and poisoning them with compounds of such heavy metals as mercury and lead. Even some contemporary physicians had the wit to notice what damage traditional therapeutics inflicted. Boston's William Douglass observed in 1755: 'In general, the physical practice [giving medications] in our colonies is so perniciously bad, that excepting in surgery and some very acute cases, it is better to let nature under a proper regimen take her course (*naturae morborum curatrices*) than to trust the honesty and sagacity of the practitioner... Frequently there is more danger from the physician than from the distemper.' When Douglass had first arrived in New England he had asked a colleague, 'what was their general method of practice; he told me their practice was very uniform, bleeding, vomiting, blistering, purging, anodyne [relieving pain], etc. If the illness continued, there was repetendi, and finally murderandi'.[9] These murderous methods were characterized in general as 'heroic medicine'.

Patients, generally speaking, adored some bloodletting and some purging. But heroic medicine went beyond the bounds of what patients found acceptable. It was the excesses of traditional therapeutics, not its basic principles, that caused unease among sufferers, making primary care seem more a last resort than a route to wellbeing. 'If we look into the profession of physic', said Joseph Addison in *The Spectator* in 1711, 'we shall find a most formidable body of men. The sight of them is enough to make a man serious, for we may lay it down as a maxim, that when a nation abounds in physicians it grows thin of people.'[10]

Two centuries later Baltimore physician Daniel Cathell, in an 1882 work aimed at fellow physicians called *The Physician Himself and What He Should Add to the Strictly Scientific*, captured less laconically this loathing of the excesses of traditional medicine: 'So great, indeed, is the popular dread of what doctors *might do*, that in choosing an attendant from among regular physicians, the nervous and the timid, who constitute nine-tenths of all the sick, are greatly inclined to shun all who treat heroically, and seek those who use moderate, even though less efficient, means.' Hence the popular fondness for 'irregulars', such as homeopaths, who, Cathell mocked, 'cure by Mild Powers or Harmless Methods'.[11]

At the outset of the story of primary care, therefore, we find the doctors in the grips of (to us) ludicrous and dangerous theories, the patients terrified and in search of alternatives. Science, however, brought the two opposing parties together.

The Making of the Modern Doctor

The modern general practitioner, the guarantor of primary care in the USA until the 1920s and in the UK until the present day, evolved more from surgery and pharmacy than from academic medicine, and was called into being as much for social as scientific reasons. Before the Napoleonic years most medical care in Britain was furnished by men who were not qualified physicians but had trained as apprentices and passed the examinations of the Society of Apothecaries or the Company of Surgeons. With an act in 1815 these surgeon-apothecaries began to be recognized as general practitioners, a term legitimized in 1826 when the Association of Apothecaries and Surgeon-Apothecaries renamed itself 'The Associated General Medical and Surgical Practitioners'.

Among middle-class families, the demand was rising for a single practitioner who would be able to fulfil all of the family's medical and surgical needs, from bleeding and lancing boils to dispensing physic. These families, according to one observer in 1815, 'had long wished for a class of the faculty to whom they could apply with confidence in any description of case in which medical or surgical aid was necessary'.[12] Thus, 'medical man' came to mean apothecary-surgeon or general practitioner, and 'doctor' meant a qualified member of the Royal College of Physicians in London, a tiny elite of physicians who supplied health care to the rich and consulted in difficult cases.

A Medical Reform Act of 1858 created a single overseeing council for the entire UK, and stipulated that only the universities and the established corporations (Surgeons, Apothecaries, Physicians) of England and Wales, Scotland, and Ireland could grant medical licences (and no longer the Archbishop of Canterbury, for example). Henceforth only those registered by a General Medical Council, which the Act set up, would be considered 'qualified medical practitioners'. This Act gave general practitioners the same legal though not social status as the elite consultant physicians of London, and established the framework within which primary care would grow for the next century.

In the USA, the regulation of physicians remained chaotic until far later in time. Until the beginning of state licensing in the 1880s anybody could call him- or herself a 'doctor' (for there were numerous women doctors as well). Typically, these doctors would apprentice for 3 years to a 'preceptor', who would supply books, equipment, and a certificate at the end. In the first half of the apprenticeship the aspirant would read basic medical textbooks and help compound drugs; in the second, he would go riding with the doctor on house calls. Medical schools had existed in the USA since the middle of the eighteenth century, but they tended to be 2-year affairs, the students repeating in the second year the lectures they had heard in the first. There was little opportunity to do dissections or to see patients. Once medical licensing systems were established, many of these earlier medical men, who had qualified without undergoing examinations, came to be known under the embarrassing title of 'Y-of-P' men, standing for years of practice – their sole qualification for the practice of medicine.

There were scientific reasons, too, for the emergence of the modern family doctor. Awareness was dawning that medicine was something more than an art, that it possessed a scientific basis with a corpus of knowledge from such disciplines as physiology that must be mastered before one could diagnose or treat patients effectively. And this *prise de conscience*, in addition to the social needs of the middle classes, also drove forward medical reform on both sides of the Atlantic. Once medicine had something to teach other than anatomy and get-those-poisons-out-of-there-style therapeutics, medical competence would be acquired in a stepped programme of study and verified with qualifying examinations. The point about the onrush of science is important, because the physician's new scientific attainments transformed the nature of the relationship between doctor and patient and thus the nature of primary care.

Consider how the style of practice changed under science. The traditional physician was casual about history-taking; he limited himself in the physical examination to looking at the tongue, feeling the pulse, and inspecting the countenance to establish the patient's constitution. The typical consultation concluded with the drawing up of elaborate prescriptions for laxatives. The physician who practised scientifically, by contrast, would take a systematic history of the present illness, perform a physical examination by pounding, listening and poking, consider all the possible diseases the patient might have on the basis of the signs and symptoms hitherto gathered (this is called the 'differential diagnosis'), then finally select the one disease most likely afflicting the patient by doing further examinations and laboratory tests (making the 'clinical' diagnosis). In this scientific practice, the clinical investigation as well as the differential diagnosis were historically quite new. It was a style that swept the traditional approach to primary care out the window.

The modern style of practice assumed that similar signs and symptoms of illness could be caused by a wide range of different disease mechanisms. Mechanism is a key word in modern medicine. It refers to the pathological processes leading to tissue changes in the body. We are, for example, dealing with a blue-ish, coughing patient who reports a history of blood-flecked sputum. The traditional doctor might conclude it was an excess of the humour phlegm. The scientifically oriented modern doctor approached the problem quite differently. He would have learned in medical school that vastly different mechanisms can cause this bedside ('clinical') picture. In pathology class, he would have studied slides of tuberculosis, pneumonia, and lung cancer, each with a different mechanism and producing its own unique changes in lung tissue, which were visible under the microscope.

The scientifically practising physician would proceed from this differential diagnosis to listen carefully to the chest, then take an X-ray (after 1896) or perform other tests that would pin down which of the three diseases was causing this patient's problems. At the end of the consultation the physician would be able to give the patient his or her prognosis, and determine a rational plan of treatment.

Traditional physicians had, of course, an instinct for prognosis, knowing generally what happened to patients who coughed up a lot of blood. But their therapeutics were based on humoral doctrines that totally lacked any kind of scientific basis. Thus, even if modern doctors could not cure their patients, at least an understanding of disease mechanisms and drug action *kept them from doing harm.* This ability to refrain from doing harm stands as one of the major acquisitions of primary care for the period from around 1840, when bloodletting began to go out of use, to 1935, when the first of the wonder drugs was introduced.

For modern doctors to draw up their differential diagnoses, a score of scientific advances had to occur. The science of microscopy and of different stains for making tissues visible under the microscope had to develop. The whole anatomical-clinical technique of identifying specific diseases had to be elaborated, in which researchers reason back and forth from autopsy findings to the patient's signs and symptoms before death. A germ theory of disease was required to put the understanding of fever on a scientific basis, the knowledge that specific kinds of infectious illnesses are caused by specific kinds of microbes. In other words, advances in many areas of background knowledge were required to transform medicine from being just an art to an art and a science.

How was all this science imported into primary care? The link between the doctor's scientific knowledge and the patient's subjective symptoms was the physical examination. To establish which disease mechanism was at work inside the body, the doctor would, in the first line, have to look at the patient's body, and touch and press him. The physical examination consisted of three innovations: palpating the patient's abdomen, percussing his chest, and listening – at first with one's ear against the major body cavities, later using a stethoscope – to the movement of blood, gas, and air within the limbs and major body cavities. All three innovations were first put into practice by the elite physicians of the Parisian teaching hospitals during the Napoleonic years, then spread outwards to other centres of medicine in the years before 1850, finally diffusing into general practice in the second half of the nineteenth century.

Whereas traditional medical students memorized lists of herbal infusions and the kind of fevers for which each was appropriate, the modern medical student learned to observe the patient. Here is young Karl Stern, a resident physician in Frankfurt in the early 1930s, at the lectures of Professor Franz Volhard. Volhard, who himself had trained in the pathology department of a Berlin teaching hospital in the 1890s, was very much the image of the modern scientifically practising physician. Frequently, Stern said, Volhard would bring the patient in 'without any preliminary introduction'. 'The professor raised his hand in an imploring manner, glanced all over the audience, and then looked long and pensively at the patient. Presently there was a hush over the big room, and one could have heard a pin drop. The only thing one heard was the patient's breath. This silence went on for several minutes which seemed like half an hour.'

Suddenly, Stern continued, Volhard would call out, 'What do you see?' Again silence, because at first none of the medical students saw anything. Yet soon someone would call out, 'There is dyspnoea [shortness of breath]. The respiration is thirty-five per minute.' Volhard would remain silent, as if he had not heard. Someone else would say, 'Pallor around the area of the mouth' (a sign of lack of oxygen). Another would call, 'Club-shaped fingers', also an index that the lungs are poorly oxygenating the blood.

The students would be permitted to feel and touch only after having described what they had seen. 'It was quite extraordinary', Stern continued, 'to experience the varieties of tactile sensation.'

There was, quite aside from the world of sight, an entire world of touch which we had never perceived before. In feeling differences of radial pulse [at the wrist] you could train yourself to feel dozens of different waves with their characteristic peaks, blunt and sharp, steep and slanting, and the corresponding valleys. There were so many ways in which the margin of the liver [just below the right ribs] came up towards your palpating finger. There were extraordinary varieties of smell. There was not just pallor but there seemed to be hundreds of hues of yellow and gray.[13]

When these young physicians later entered primary care, everything they noted about the patient would be filtered through this riot of hues and sounds and touches.

The contrast between old and new could not be more striking. Young Arthur Hertzler in Kansas described traditionally oriented colleagues making a house call in the 1890s: 'The usual procedure for a doctor when he reached the patient's house was to greet the grandmother and aunts effusively and pat all the kids on the head before approaching the bedside. He greeted the patient with a grave look and a pleasant joke. He felt the pulse and inspected the tongue, and asked where it hurt. This done, he was ready to deliver an opinion and prescribe his pet remedy.'

Hertzler by contrast did as he had learned in medical school.

I examined my patients as well as I knew how. My puerile attempts at physical examination impressed my patients and annoyed my competitors...Word went out that the young doctor 'ain't very civil but he is thorough'. Only yesterday one of my old patients recalled that when I came to see her young son I 'stripped him all off and examined him all over'. Members of that family have been my patients for the intervening forty years, so impressed were they. Incidentally, it may be mentioned that in this case I discovered a pleurisy with effusion [an inflammation of the lining of the lungs producing serum] which had not been apparent to my tongue-inspecting colleague.[14]

Being a country doctor at the turn of the nineteenth century did not necessarily mean being traditional: Hertzler was practising medicine based on science.

Something more than a lust for science lay behind these new clinical reflexes. As a result of the lax entry standards previously in effect, the medical profession had become quite overcrowded before the First World War. Being known as somebody who practised scientifically represented for young physicians a drawing card. So there was perhaps a public-relations tactic as well as a scientific motive in all this apparent meticulousness – the need to offer what the public demanded rather than what the practitioner deemed just. But, now, the public was demanding science.

Writing in 1924 with more than 50 years of medical practice under his belt, Daniel Cathell reflected how important this aura of science was in medical success. 'Working with the microscope and making analyses of the urine, sputum, blood, and other fluids as an aid to diagnosis, will not only bring fees and lead to valuable information regarding your patient's condition, but will also give you reputation and professional respect, by investing you, in the eyes of the public, with the benefits of being a very scientific man'.[15]

The ascendancy of science thus added a hands-on dimension to the doctor–patient relationship. The doctor now touched the patient, percussed, palpated, and listened. In addition to gathering important information for making a diagnosis, this physical contact also conveyed psychologically the impression of giving care, and fortified the psychological bond between physician and patient.

New Medications

In the traditional doctor's medical bag, very little of the 'physic' had the power to do good. Of the hundreds of drugs listed in 1824 in the *Pharmacopoeia* of the Royal College of Physicians of London, only opium, dispensed as a deep-brownish 'tincture', or solution in alcohol, conferred much therapeutic benefit. Yet it lost much of its punch when taken orally (dissolved by stomach enzymes), and even though opium had been known in Europe since the sixteenth century to be effective against pain, a tincture of opium supplied little relief of severe pain. The college also proposed various forms of iron to its members, calling them useful, among other things, as a 'tonic'. Physicians did give iron for conditions that later would be diagnosed as iron-deficiency anaemia, but they did not do so systematically and 'chlorosis' – the term of the day for iron-deficiency anaemia – was not mentioned.

What other genuine good could the Fellows of the Royal College of Physicians achieve in 1824 with drugs? It was very little. To say that they were able to relieve constipation is equivalent to saying that a shotgun may be used as a fly swatter: they purged ruthlessly with the many plant-based purgatives, such as aloes and senna, for every condition imaginable. In 1785, the Birmingham physician William Withering had disseminated within medicine the knowledge – already long known in folk culture – that the foxglove plant was useful against certain forms of 'dropsy', or oedema caused by congestive heart failure (foxgloves contain digitalis). The college's *Pharmacopoeia* does mention a foxglove tea, or infusion, as a helpful diuretic, meaning a drug to stimulate the kidneys. This shows at least that they were in the right ballpark, since a strengthened heart causes the kidneys to start making urine. Yet medicine as a whole in the nineteenth century lost sight of digitalis as a cardiac drug, using it against tuberculosis and everything else, until London physicians James Mackenzie and Thomas Lewis reintroduced it before the First World War.

Therewith the list of genuinely useful drugs was at end. The physician practising before the middle of the nineteenth century had nothing against infectious disease, cancer, arthritis, diabetes, asthma, heart attacks, or vaginitis (inflammation of the vagina). The list of conditions he could not relieve (although he believed that he could) is much longer than those which he could. Arthur Hertzler, the Kansas frontier doctor, said in 1938 of his earlier colleagues, 'I can scarcely think of a single disease that the doctors actually cured during those early years...The possible exceptions were malaria and the itch [scabies]. Doctors knew how to relieve suffering, set bones, sew up cuts and open boils on small boys.'[16]

During the nineteenth century, some important new drugs became available, principally as a result of the growth of the organic chemical industry in Germany, which synthesized new molecules from coal tar (benzene). By 1935, the list of useful drugs in the GP's bag would be much longer. In the area of pain relief, the nineteenth century saw the introduction of the alkaloids of opium, which are much more concentrated than raw opium. After Alexander Wood made it known in 1855 that morphine could be administered with the hypodermic needle he had perfected, they could be injected directly into the blood stream, bypassing the stomach. The hypodermic syringe and the injectible opioids in the nineteenth-century medical bag became the subject of much mischief, for while they offered undoubted pain relief, they also were highly addictive. The old family doctors gave morphine at the drop of a hat, and tales are legion of patients whom these physicians casually addicted.

The aspirin family represented another innovation in pain relief. Members of this family, all synthesized in the laboratory, cut pain effectively as well as reducing fever and inflammation. This is part of the larger story of the search for antifever drugs, or antipyretics. In the absence of a germ theory, earlier physicians had directed their attention to bringing down fever rather than to overcoming the underlying infection. Such efforts went back to experiments with quinine as a general febrifuge, not just an antimalarial drug. But quinine was ineffective against other fevers, and unbeloved among patients because of its bitter taste and side-effects.

Since its introduction in 1899, aspirin (acetylsalicylic acid) has been the most popular drug of all time. In the USA alone, some

10,000 to 20,000 tons of aspirin are used annually. If the members of the aspirin family had been consumed mainly over-the-counter, bought at the pharmacy without a prescription, they might not figure so prominently in the history of primary care. Yet many doctors themselves dispensed aspirin and its relatives, and wrote out prescriptions for them. By 1909, aspirin and the antipyretic phenacetin (another member of the acetanilid family) ranked among the ten items most prescribed by American physicians. The aspirin family had come to symbolize medicine's new therapeutic accomplishments.

An enduring problem in primary care is patients who cannot sleep, or are nervous, irritable, depressed, or agitated. The nineteenth-century German chemical industry had presents to offer them as well. In 1869, a foul-tasting hypnotic called chloral hydrate (made by adding water to chloral) came into medical use. Known popularly as a 'Mickey Finn', chloral hydrate was in reality a mild sleeping potion, one that starts to lose its efficacy after about the third night. (It has the potential for addiction, however, and 'chloral' addicts were a familiar sight in late-nineteenth-century private nervous clinics.)

In 1888, a more powerful hypnotic called sulphonal came into medical use. Sulphonal was the first really popular drug of the Bayer Company's laboratories in Germany, and helped finance research on a further cascade of hypnotics. Bayer's final stroke in this area was to take barbituric acid, first synthesized in 1864, and add on several small hydrocarbon sidechains. The result, generically called barbital (barbitone in the UK), was marketed in 1903 under the trade name Veronal. The barbiturates virtually put an end to all the earlier hypnotics except for chloral hydrate. A relative of barbital named phenobarbital was introduced in 1912 as Luminal, and has attained epic status in novels about psychoneurosis among the middle classes. Amytal, Seconal, Nembutal, and fifty or so other barbiturates followed later.

A detailed history of these sedatives and hypnotics would be more appropriate in a history of psychiatry were it not for the fact that general practitioners prescribed them so often. One Canadian family doctor, William Victor Johnston, wrote of the interwar years that Luminal, alongside aspirin, morphine, and digitalis, had been 'indispensable'. 'I bought Luminal tablets in five-thousand lots every few months', Johnston wrote, looking back on decades of practice.[17]

There were other advances, too – drugs such as amyl nitrite (Thomas Brunton discovered its usefulness in 1867) and nitroglycerine (William Murrell in 1879) to dilate the arteries of the heart in patients enduring anginal pain. These drugs tended to be administered more by specialists than by family doctors. What caused a sensation in primary care, a virtual revolution in the image of the physician, occurred in the realm of infectious diseases such as diphtheria.

Of all the new drugs before 1935, that most to astonish the world was the antitoxin against diphtheria, developed in 1891 in Robert Koch's laboratory in Berlin. Emil Adolf von Behring and Shibasaburo Kitasato showed that the serum of a horse immunized against diphtheria (using techniques developed at the Pasteur Institute in Paris) could be used to immunize other horses. In 1892, the first commercial vaccines against diphtheria began to be produced. The introduction of the diphtheria antitoxin sharply upgraded the doctor's image in the eyes of the public. For the first time, medicine was truly capable of curing an infectious disease that threatened the children of every home in the nation.

Apart from the diphtheria antitoxin, however, it would be unwise to exaggerate the therapeutic accomplishments of the modern doctor before 1935. Syphilis was treatable with Salvarsan from 1910 but the reality of clinical practice reduced itself more to tonics and laxatives than to finely calibrated doses of Bayer's pharmaceutical products. In 1869, one observer described the scene at the casualty department of St Bartholomew's Hospital in London: '120 patients were seen by the physician and dismissed in an hour and ten minutes, or at the rate of 35 seconds each... [The patients] were dismissed with a doubtful dose of physic, ordered almost at random, and poured out of a huge brown jug'.[18] Ten years later the medications dispensed at Bart's had scarcely become more sophisticated. 'They consist essentially,' said an anonymous contributor to *The Lancet*, 'of purgatives; a mixture of iron, sulphate of magnesia, and quassia [both laxatives], and cod-liver oil, fulfilling the two great indications of all therapeutics – elimination, and the supply of some elements to the blood.' The anonymous writer criticized Bart's for supplying medicine 'out of jugs, and patients seen at the rate of one a minute, for sixpence or a shilling'.[19]

What did the old-time US doctor around 1900 have in the saddlebags that he threw atop his horse as he made housecalls? 'In his case there are but few drugs', said Joseph Mathews, past-president of the American Medical Association in 1905, 'but he knows the quality of each one of them.' 'Calomel, opium, quinine, buchu [a diuretic to stimulate the kidneys], ipecac [an emetic], and Dover's powder [a laxative] constitute his armamentarium. He has never heard of many of the "new-fangled" remedies that are in the case of his young competitor, but he has managed to "get along" these many years without them'. Mathews felt that in time young physicians, too, would discover that all they really needed in their bags were drugs to make the patients defaecate and vomit.[20] Over a 12-month period in 1891–2 Americans consumed, among other drugs, 255,000 pounds (115,700 kg) of aloes (a laxative), 113,000 pounds (51,250 kg) of jalap (another laxative), 1,400,000 pounds (635,040 kg) of nux vomica (an emetic), and 13,000 pounds (5,900 kg) of 'calomel and other mercurial medicinal preparations'.[21] Thus medical therapeutics had clearly not experienced the same kind of scientific revolution as medical diagnostics.

Technology and Primary Care

When 'Dr Stark Munro', one of Arthur Conan Doyle's fictional characters, set up medical practice in the 1890s, he had little with him by way of equipment. 'In my box were a stethoscope, several medical books, a second pair of boots, two suits of clothes, my linen and my toilet things.'[22] Was that really all that one needed for the practice of medicine in those days? One must distinguish between innovations that remain the monopoly of a small group of specialists, and those that diffuse widely among general practitioners.

The panoply of new technology in primary care that emerged in the late nineteenth century was reassuring to the patients, and extended the range of medical diagnosis far beyond what the simple techniques of physical examination permitted. One US study between the two world wars found, for example, that of 100 cases of heart disease seen in general practice sixty-five were chronic cases requiring no new visits for a diagnosis and, in thirty-five, the general practitioner should require no more than a single visit of 30 minutes to make the diagnosis. 'For 30 cases, this is sufficient; 2 need an additional visit of 20 minutes; the remainder are referred to a specialist after the first visit to the general practitioner.'[23]

The study was focused on medical economics, but it assumed that a general practitioner would be able competently to determine what the heart was doing in a single surgery visit of half an hour. By contrast the great English heart specialist James Mackenzie had complained just a decade previously about the 'utmost confusion prevailing as to the significance of the signs detected in the heart'.[24]

Scepticism and the Patient-as-a-Person Movement

The combination of scientifically trained physicians thinking systematically about the mechanisms of disease, together with the persistence of tides of laxatives dispensed from big brown jugs, made it inevitable that doctors would become sceptical about the possibilities of drug treatment in general. This scepticism was called therapeutic nihilism. In the second half of the nineteenth century the nihilists ruled the roost in academic medicine, teaching generations of medical students, quite correctly, that the decoctions and infusions then available in the formulary were either useless or harmful, that physicians could do relatively little to cure disease (although they could relieve suffering with opium), and, by implication, that the real function of medicine was to accumulate scientific information about the human body rather than to heal.

Therapeutic nihilism had begun in the big European medical centres in the 1840s. The term itself is associated with the Viennese academic Joseph Dietl, a pupil of the famous physician Josef Škoda. Dietl wrote in 1841: 'Medicine as a natural science cannot have the task of inventing panaceas and discovering miracle cures that banish death, but instead of discovering the conditions under which people become ill, recover, and perish, in a word, of deepening a doctrine of the human condition that is based scientifically upon the study of nature, physics and chemistry.'[25] Thus the task of medicine was to be not healing at all, but research into scientific mechanisms. Bernhard Naunyn, who later became a professor of internal medicine in Germany, remembered of his professors in Berlin in the 1860s: 'They knew that the healing part of medicine rested upon the discipline's scientific basis, and that the physician's compulsion to cure [*Drang zum Heilen*] had to be reigned in.'[26]

In the USA, therapeutic nihilism surfaced as praise of 'nature's healing ways', or the *vis medicatrix naturae*, and a rejection of the classic heroic therapies of bleeding and purging. In 1844, Harvard's Jacob Bigelow cautioned medical students against 'always thinking that you must make your patients worse before they can be better. I believe that much of the medical imposition of the present day is sustained in places where practice has previously been overheroic, and because mankind are gratified to find that they and their families can get well without the lancet, the vomit, and the blister, indiscriminately applied'.[27]

Another Harvard professor in the mid-nineteenth century, Oliver Wendell Holmes, would rescue only opium, wine, and anaesthesia from the formulary. The rest of it could be sunk to the bottom of the sea. 'The best proof of it is, that no families take so little medicine as those of doctors.'[28] By the 1890s this kind of dubiety about heroic therapy had gathered enough steam to plough up not just bleeding and purging but virtually the entire traditional pharmacopoeia. William Osler, Canadian-born professor of medicine at Johns Hopkins University and one of the most influential physicians in the English-speaking world, limited himself in his 1892 textbook to a handful of drugs and said that for many diseases there was no treatment at all. For example, for malignant scarlet fever, 'The disease cannot be cut short. In the presence of the severer forms we are still too often helpless'.[29]

But family doctors do not want to be helpless. In primary care, the doctrine of therapeutic nihilism was anathema because physicians enjoy the feeling of helping and because patients crave a prescription at the end of the consultation. It was entirely unacceptable that patients should be sent away with the news that medicine was powerless in their case. Kansas doctor Arthur Hertzler summed up the position of the general practitioner around the turn of the century,

> In some cases I knew, even in the beginning, that my efforts would be futile in the matter of rendering service to anyone ... Often I knew before I touched harness that the trips would be useless ... Of course, one left some medicine in case of a recurrence of the trouble; this was largely the bunk, but someone had to pay for the axle grease and just plain advice never was productive of revenue unless fortified by a few pills. It was about as important as the deacon's 'Amen' during the preacher's sermons – it did no harm and it was an evidence of good faith.[30]

So what was the family doctor to do? His medicines were mainly 'the bunk' and he realized that in scientific terms either the patient would recover spontaneously from the infectious illness or he would not. Organically based medicine could do little save yield a diagnosis and prognosis. But the patients craved help.

In this logical dilemma was born the patient-as-a-person movement, a doctrine that would run through primary care from the 1880s until the Second World War. The patient could not be helped with medicines, although these would be given anyway, but with the psychological support of the doctor. In seeing the patient as 'a person' and not just as 'a case of disease' the physician was able to approach him in an understanding and sympathetic manner that was *in and of itself therapeutic*. Here was born the reputation of the 'old-time GP' as being someone willing to sit and listen to his patients, to give them time to tell their stories, and advise them patiently about how to cope with their problems. It was not that the old-time doc was necessarily a more sensitive and humane individual than his predecessors or his successors, merely that he was therapeutically desperate and realized that he had nothing to give them except such psychological benefits as inherently resided in the consultation.

The patient-as-a-person movement originated within the commanding heights of medical science in Europe, but among physicians, whose particular bent was healing, rather than anatomical pathology. In Vienna, Hermann Nothnagel, professor of medicine after 1882, embodied the new philosophy. As he said in his 1882 inaugural lecture, 'I repeat once again, medicine is about treating sick people and not diseases'.[31] Nothnagel was well known for his views about 'being a friend to the patient', and fought for their best interests, even at the cost of harsh words with the family doctor. He emphasized to the house staff at the Vienna General Hospital the importance of history-taking in the consultation – a key theme in the movement as a whole because in taking a long and careful history the doctor has the chance to establish an emotional rapport with the patient.

Nothnagel was fond of quoting a saying from an earlier prince of German medicine, Christoph Wilhelm Hufeland, to the effect that, 'Only a truly moral person can become a physician in the truest sense of the term'. (Interestingly, it was the nihilist Josef Škoda who had turned the whole world of romantic medicine that Hufeland embodied upside down.) Nothnagel's good nature did indeed shine through: he was unfavourably known among the generally anti-Semitic Viennese medical faculty as being philo-Semitic. Nothnagel, who had a huge consulting practice in the Vienna hotels, prescribed great quantities of the useless medications of the time, but established close rapport with his patients and was much loved by them.

Among the significant professors of medicine in Germany was Adolf Kussmaul. Towards 1880 at Strasbourg, Kussmaul admonished the medical students. A young American physician, who was sitting in, recalled his words: 'the physician examines and treats the "patient" and not the "case". It was this insistence on the human and the humane side of medicine that made the deepest impression on me', wrote New York neurologist Barney Sachs many years later.[32]

Noted American physicians also kept up a drumfire of support for seeing the patient as a person, which was not incompatible with a scientific disbelief in drugs. Most notably, William Osler embodied these humanistic values, teaching the medical students on rounds at Johns Hopkins University that, 'The good physician treats the disease but the great physician treats the patient who has the disease'.[33] One of his young students, Clarence B. Farrar who later became a psychiatrist, noted: 'Osler was instinctively practising psychotherapy without ever having studied it'.[34]

Another Osler student who went on to become a Hopkins clinician, developing all the while a successful private practice, was Lewellys Barker. Why has your practice been so successful, Dr Barker? 'I am of the opinion that to make patients like him, a doctor must himself have a real liking for people; he must be interested in *them* as well as in their *diseases*'.[35] In 1939, George Canby Robinson, another Osler student, wrote a book entitled *The Patient as a Person*, deploring that 'scientific satisfaction' was replacing 'human satisfaction' in medicine and urging the 'treatment of the patient as a whole'.[36]

Physicians in primary care found one aspect of the patient-as-a-person movement of particular interest: the utility of this approach in treating patients whose symptoms were 'functional' or 'psychosomatic' – in other words, symptoms that had arisen in the absence of any organic lesion but were defined by the patient as organic in nature. Such symptoms constituted – and constitute today – a huge amount of what was seen in primary care: a third or more of all patients. Here the patient-as-a-person movement had stellar advice to offer. As Francis Weld Peabody, the professor of internal medicine at Harvard University, volunteered in 1927, 'The successful diagnosis and treatment of these patients... depends almost wholly on the establishment of that intimate personal contact between physician and patient which forms the basis of private practice. Without this, it is quite impossible for the physician to get an idea of the problems and troubles that lie behind so many functional disorders'.[37]

Harvard even started a course in 1941 on the 'Treatment of patients as persons'. Writing in 1936, William Houston, a professor of medicine in Georgia, commented that this kind of psychological sensitivity was what distinguished the doctor from the veterinarian: 'All that part of a doctor's work that rises above the veterinary level, that part in which the personality of the doctor is the therapeutic agent and the personality of the patient is the object acted upon, may properly be called "psychological treatment".' But the psychology consisted in spending lots of time with patients and talking to them, and having some 'awareness of what [one] is about'.[38]

There is no doubt that this message was picked up by physicians in primary care. Daniel Cathell, in the 1924 edition of his famous doctors' guide, said 'It is often very satisfying to the sick to be allowed to tell, in their own way, whatever they deem important for you to know. Give a fair, courteous hearing, and, even though Mrs Chatterbox, Mr Borum, and Mrs Lengthy's statements are tedious, do not abruptly cut them short, but endure and listen with respectful attention, even though you are ready to drop exhausted'.[39] In Guy de Maupassant's novel *Mont-Oriol* (1887) about spa life, the newly arrived 'Docteur Black' draws the custom of all the wealthy elderly ladies at the spa. Why was this successful? Among other things, 'He heard their stories out without interruption, taking notes of all their observations, of all their questions, of all their wishes. Every day he would increase or decrease the dosage of water drunk by his patients, which gave them complete confidence in the care he was taking of them'.[40]

Hermann Nothnagel was probably wrong that to be successful in medicine a physician had to be a good person. Dr Black and countless other physicians doubtlessly used the show of concern as a marketing tactic in primary care. But why not? It was a tactic of great therapeutic effectiveness that responded to the patient's desire to be cared for, in the face of diseases that could not be cured.

Shifting the Site of Primary Care

In 1950, after finishing a study of Britain's National Health Service, Joseph Collings announced that the day of the horse-and-buggy doctor was gone: 'It is absurd to try to recapture the 19th-century concept of the benign old doctor in his frock coat and silk hat sitting through the night, awaiting the pneumonia crisis or the delayed arrival of the first-born'.[41] Two things were killing off this old-style family doctor – a shift in the locus of medical practice from general practitioner to specialist, and a shift in the physical site of primary care from the patient's home to the doctor's surgery and the hospital outpatient department.

The rise of specialism at the end of the nineteenth century was in part pushed by public demand, in part pulled by medical supply. To specialists even more than to general practitioners clung the mantle of science, a powerful attraction for a public with implicit confidence in the wonders of progress. 'The inexorable public', mocked Walter Rivington in 1879, a surgeon at the London Hospital, 'will not believe in a man who is good all round. With the public a physician who can treat the liver is not good for the stomach, certainly not for the kidneys. The heart has no connexion with the lungs, and all the organs of the body are totally independent of one another.' Rivington spoke of patients who would 'come up from the country, and consult four or five separate practitioners – one for his general state, one for his ear, another for his chest, and another for his throat... The force of subdivision of the human body can no further go'.[42] Rivington mirrored the traditional distaste of British doctors for specialism.

But physicians followed the internal logic of their own interests to specialism, not just the fancy of the public. Subjects such as ophthalmic surgery did indeed possess demanding cores of knowledge that could not be mastered while staying abreast of the information needed for general practice. 'The line of skirmishers advancing into the No Man's Land of fresh knowledge is always radiating outwards, and breaking up into smaller groups', said Wilmot Herringham, himself a London physician, in 1920. 'First there is a continual invention of fresh instruments of precise observation or treatment' that called for specialized skill. He cited the laryngoscope and the urethral catheter. Then came inventions that called for specialized knowledge, such as the electrocardiograph.[43] All these specialists had something to offer the general practitioner in their function as consultants (giving opinions or doing procedures) but not – at this point – taking the family doctor's patients away.

The 1870s saw the flourishing of societies devoted to specialized knowledge on the East coast of the USA. New York City had, for example, a dermatological society, an obstetrical society, and a forensic-medicine society by the 1870s. London saw in the 1880s the formation of six specialty societies, including dental surgery, opthalmology, dermatology, gynaecology, neurology, and ear-nose-and-throat surgery. London's Harley Street, which had three doctors in 1840, had acquired ninety-seven by 1890, becoming the centre of gravity of London's consultant and specialty practice.

Now at this point an interesting divergence between the UK and the USA occurred. In Britain, family doctors retained an important share of primary care whereas, in the USA, they became a vanishing breed. In Britain, a fairly strict line had already been drawn by the turn of the century between primary care in the hands of general practitioners and specialist care in hospitals, for GPs lost the right to attend patients in hospital. As one writer commented, 'the demarcation of responsibilities between the urban GP and consultant was to take place at the gates of the city hospital'.[44] This cut GPs off from hospital science and hospital care, but preserved them as a group because a letter from a family doctor was essential for referral to a hospital outpatient department or to a consultant. The National Health Insurance Act of 1911 then safeguarded the GP's survival by creating a system of 'panel doctors' in which GPs were paid to take on state-insured workers. By 1939 there were some 2,800 full-time consultants and specialists and 18,000 general practitioners in Britain. Among the 43,000 physicians in the UK in 1980, 65 per cent were still GPs.

In the USA, by contrast, general practitioners began disappearing around 1900, the result of the pressure of the specialists from above and the hospital outpatient departments from below. By the mid-1920s perhaps a quarter of the population of the largest cities was receiving its medical care in clinics and outpatient departments. In 1928, of some 152,000 physicians in the USA, 27 per cent had either limited themselves entirely to a specialty or were interested in one. By 1942 only 49 per cent of all doctors were GPs. The American public flocked to the specialists, shunning the 'old-time family doctor'. Daniel Cathell commented in 1924: 'Today a specialist wisely located in any large city must be but an ordinary man, not to get considerable business. While a general practitioner in a large city must be an extraordinary man to get much or any good, desirable business at all.'[45]

This drift away from general practice continued inexorably in the following decades in the USA. By 1989, of 469,000 physicians in active patient care, only 12 per cent were in general and family practice. Within the speciality practices, the great bulk of care was primary care. Several medical specialities were surveyed in 1977: only 3.5 per cent of all patient visits in internal medicine were referrals, the others were walk-ins; in obstetrics and gynaecology, only 4.4 per cent were referrals, in opthalmology 7.7 per cent, and so on. In no medical specialty were more than 13 per cent of the patients referred (urology), meaning that these doctors were giving primary care to most of their patients.

In a second change in locus, medical practice shifted from the patient's home to the doctor's surgery. Although the figure of the kindly old doc making housecalls retains its nostalgic appeal, one forgets easily how tough this work was on the physicians themselves, especially the arduousness of night calls, when a note that simply said 'come at once' could mean anything from a headache to a ruptured appendix.

Bernhard Naunyn recalled from the time of his general practice in the late 1860s in Berlin being hauled from bed in the wee hours three nights in a row. On the first night he had to climb up the stairs of some tenement in Kreuzberg to the bedside of a 'healthy looking young lad who was sleeping'. Naunyn woke him up. The boy looked about a bit dazed. 'So you see', said the father, 'that's the way he looked before too.' Naunyn assured the father that nothing was wrong with the boy and went home.

On the second night at 3 a.m., there was another, similar occurrence, 'completely unfounded anxiety on the part of a worried mother'. 'When on the third night 1 was supposed to go out again between three and four, because the child was said to have "internal fits" I didn't go at once. I said I'd come as soon as I was up. Of course I couldn't then go back to sleep. I thought about the sick child, and soon I did get up, and went over there, and I found the child dead.'[46]

The maddening thing about housecalls, therefore, was that one could not tell which were emergencies: all summonses had to be answered. Then there was the sheer exhaustion of being on the road in a horse and buggy or on horseback, and spending the night on top of tables in the waiting rooms of railway stations.

Wasn't there a better way? The telephone made it possible for the physician to establish whether an emergency existed before going out. Motor transport, of course, let the doctor get about more easily on housecalls but, more important, it permitted the patient to come to the doctor, or to the hospital emergency department. The first rudimentary telephone exchange on record, built in 1877, connected the Capital Avenue Drugstore in Hartford, Connecticut, with twenty-one local doctors.

Motorcars first became available in the 1890s, and physicians were among the earliest customers for them. Ecstatic doctors talked of making housecalls in 'half the time', and increased their business as well by broadening their range. By 1928, one small-town doctor in New Hampshire, USA, was covering 30,000–35,000 miles a year. 'With a single exception, it is five years since I have driven a horse', Ralph Tuttle wrote. 'This increased facility of transportation not only helps the doctor get to his patients but makes it possible to take the patients to a hospital'.[47] It had even become possible for a physician 'to keep office hours'. There was one more consequence. Because it was now possible for patients to get about easily, doctors stopped settling in rural areas in the USA. In 1926, physicians polled in 283 counties reported that in 100 of those counties no new medical graduate had settled within the previous 10 years. Cars had stimulated the urbanization of medical practice and the denuding of the countryside.

Urban medical practice itself became increasingly office- and hospital-based. Although in the USA as a whole in the late 1920s 50 per cent of all medical calls took place at home, big cities saw somewhat less home visiting. In 1929, in Philadelphia, only 39 per cent of the average GP's 64 hours a week was spent on housecalls. (Of the 50 hours that full-specialists put in a week, only 12 per cent were spent doing housecalls.) In the early 1950s, in 'Regionville' – an anonymous community selected for research – of 1,318 illnesses treated by doctors, only 22 per cent were seen at the patient's home, 71 per cent in the doctor's surgery (and the others in a variety of settings). By 1990, only 2 per cent of all physician contacts in the USA took place in the patient's home, 60 per cent in the surgery, and 14 per cent in a hospital outpatient department.

In Britain, home visiting remained more intact, doubtlessly because the National Health Service, enacted in England and Wales in 1946 and coming into being on 5 July 1948, had fortified the position of the general practitioner. According to one survey, as late as 1977, 19 per cent of all patient contact still took place in the form of home visits.

The Changing Nature of the Consultation

In primary care during the twentieth century, serious infectious disease has become much less common, at least in the Western world; the subjective sensations of illness on the other hand have become more frequent, but they are cared for less intensively. These are the major changes over the past hundred years in patterns of help-seeking and care-giving.

The dominance of fever in general practice lasted right up to the years between the world wars. Describing in 1927 his own practice in Leeds, England, over a period of several years, Stanley Sykes put influenza as the commonest complaint with 335 cases: six of his patients had died of it. Then came acute bronchitis, tonsilitis, measles, whooping cough, and impetigo (a bacterial skin infection). Each of these, all major infectious illnesses, had occurred fifty or more times. Of Dr Sykes's thirty-two tuberculosis patients, ten had died. Pneumonia on his list (twenty-four patients with twelve deaths) beat cancer (twenty-three patients with twelve deaths). Only thirty-nine of his patients had heart disease, twenty of whom died. Dr Sykes was still seeing patients with typhoid fever, rheumatic fever, and erysipelas (a streptococcal infection causing redness and swelling under the skin).[48]

This picture of disease in general practice in the developed world would soon change radically. The major infections would fall away – a result of improvements in public health (such as more effective quarantining), of apparently spontaneous changes in the virulence of some infectious agents (such as the organisms causing scarlet fever and tuberculosis), and, finally, of improved therapy (such as the introduction of the sulpha drugs in 1935). A practice like Stanley Sykes's soon became a thing of the past. One British family doctor, Keith Hodgkin, wrote in 1963: 'Tuberculosis, meningitis, polio ... rheumatic fever, chilblains [reddening of fingers and toes from mild frostbite] and lobar pneumonia continue to decline and are disappearing from practice in Western countries.'[49]

In a report published in 1963 it was noted that the average general practitioner in the developed world 'might wait eight years to see a case of rheumatic fever in a child under the age of fifteen; sixty years to see a case of typhoid or paratyphoid fever; and as long as 400 years to see a case of diphtheria'.[50] Replacing the former major infectious illnesses in Western countries have been diseases related to modern lifestyles – lung cancer and coronary artery disease. Because upper respiratory infections – coughs and colds – also count as infectious illnesses, it is difficult to make the claim that infectious illness as a whole has declined. Yet the conclusion is justified that among serious medical problems in the Western world, the major infectious diseases of the past have given way to chronic degenerative diseases today, such as cancer, heart disease, and arthritis.

In spite of the decline of acute infectious illness, the population seems to be feeling worse than better. Systematic door-to-door surveys of the USA in 1928–31 and again in 1981 make it possible to compare rates of illness, or the sense of well-being, of the population over this 50-year period. The annual number of self-reported illnesses per hundred population rose from 82 in 1928–31 to 212 in 1981, a 158 per cent increase. This increase was not the result of a rise in chronic illness, for among children aged 5–14 (an age group generally not subjected to chronic disease) the rate of reported illness rose by 233 per cent. The explanation of this striking rise in the subjective sensation of illness, at a time when major infectious disease in the developed world has declined, may be that individuals as a whole have become more sensitive to bodily symptoms and more inclined to seek help for physical sensations that earlier generations would have dismissed as trivial.

With this increase in the perception of illness, there has been an increase in medical help-seeking. In the USA, in 1928–31, the average person visited the doctor only 2.9 times a year; by 1964, this had risen to 4.6 times a year, and to 5.5 times in 1990. In Britain, in 1975, the average person had three NHS consultations a year; by 1990, this had risen to five.

But these rising global rates of consultation do not necessarily mean that each individual illness is intensively seen. In the years before 1940, doctors would see an ill patient quite often. How many home calls were necessary for a typical illness? An American survey done in 1928–31 found that for a cold, the doctor would consult 2.4 times (either at home or the surgery), for a reportable communicable disease, 3.6 times, and for a digestive disease 6.2 times. On the whole, 3.6 home calls would be necessary for a typical illness.

In England, patients expected the doctor to visit often. It was, explained Stanley Sykes, so easy for the family doctor to get backlogged. Of a hundred patients on your visiting list, 'You see perhaps fifteen on the first day. The arrears accumulate with alarming rapidity, and the inevitable result is that indignant messages or relatives are arriving every day demanding to know why the doctor hasn't been. It is futile to explain that you are busy. To a sick man there is only one patient in the universe, and that is himself.'[51] This adds up to an extraordinary intensity of care in illness.

Although we do not have comparable statistics on the intensity of treatment today, people sometimes lack the feeling that their woes are being looked after. The much higher annual rates of consultation today, combined with the decline in acute infectious illness, suggests that patients of today consult more regularly over the course of the year, in a kind of ongoing anxiety about wellness, rather than demanding the doctor's presence at the bedside on the odd occasion when they are genuinely ill.

But even if today's patient did lie febrile, he or she would probably see the doctor only in the surgery or in the hospital emergency department, and not at home. Physicians have many techniques for keeping the patient at bay, including unlisted phone numbers, answering services, and nurse-receptionists who have their own notions of the hierarchy of urgency in medical diagnosis. Hence, as one observer said, 'There is a longing on the part of patients for that old doctor – one always available, ever kindly, modest in fees, and inspiring in manner'.[52]

Primary Care and Medicine Today

In February 1935, a German biochemist, Gerhard Domagk wrote an article in a German medical journal on the subject of a brick-red sulphonamide dye called 'Prontosil Rubrum' that combated staphylococcal and streptococcal infections. At last, a medication had been found that was effective against many different bacterial killers. Prontosil and its relatives became known as the 'sulpha' drugs, and their appearance marked the beginning of the postmodern period of medicine. The discovery of prontosil represented a turning of the page. For the first time in history medicine could really heal diseases that were common and affected large numbers of the population – the many fevers and bacterial infections of the past. They became known as the 'wonder drugs': the long list of sulpha drugs introduced after 1935 and then penicillin and the many antibiotics used for the first time on the civilian population after the Second World War. They gave to medicine enormous new therapeutic power.

The antibiotics were just the beginning. In the explosion of bio-chemical and pharmacological research that followed the Second World War, drugs were discovered that relieved arthritis, that fought cancer, that reduced high blood pressure, and that dissolved clots in blocked coronary arteries. These drugs caused a transformation not just of clinical medicine, but of doctors' attitudes towards patients, and towards the consultation. The introduction of these drugs and the investigation of the biochemical mechanisms that lie behind their success represented the beginning of medicine's post-modern period. If the modern period had been characterized by the doctor's ability to diagnose disease scientifically while being therapeutically powerless against it, the post-modern period was characterized by the ability to triumph over the classic killers of humankind and to relieve suffering on a scale hitherto undreamt of.

A basic theme in the history of primary care has been the necessity of giving the patients what they want. The irony of post-modern medicine is that, although doctors have become therapeutically far more awesome than ever before, they have ceased giving the patients what they want. Effective against disease at an organic level, doctors have often found it no longer necessary to enlist the psychological benefits of the doctor–patient relationship in bolstering the patient through an illness. The whole patient-as-a-person movement fell into desuetude after 1950, replaced by a new generation of physi-cians filled with an overweening therapeutic self-confidence. The aspects of the doctor–patient relationship to which patients had once thrilled, such as the physician's show of interest in the history-taking or the laying on of hands in the physical exam, became down-played in favour of using the resources of diagnostic imaging and of laboratory tests in the diagnosis of disease. It was not that physicians became somehow more inhumane, merely that the previous display of apparent humanity had now become therapeutically unnecessary.

Thus post-modern medicine has become haunted by a grow-ing dissatisfaction among patients with primary care. The sympa-thetic old doc, always willing to turn an apparently attentive ear, has become a totemic figure in tirades against the impersonality of the health-care system. Grateful as patients have been for the new drugs, they have become increasingly resentful of those who prescribe them, hurling showers of malpractice suits against physicians perceived as remote and arrogant. Alternative medicine, with its confidence in the therapeutic benefits of stroking the soles of the feet or getting those poisons out of there with colonic irrigation, has undergone a rebirth.

This failure to supply what is psychologically required to gratify the patient has thus produced a supreme irony. At the very moment that science has conferred success over much of the vast range of disease that plagues humanity, the crown of victory has been snatched from the physician's head. An adversarial note has entered the doctor–patient relationship, and it has become, rightly or wrongly, increasingly anachronistic to claim of a post-modern doctor what the patients of an old family doctor in Chicago once said to him, with a hug about the neck: 'Oh, you dear, good man, how we all love you!'[53]

5. Medical Science

Roy Porter

In medieval times, the educated physicians of the Islamic East and the Christian West practised medicine on the basis of the teachings of the Ancient Greeks. By the late Middle Ages, however, there was growing dissatisfaction with certain deeply entrenched doctrines, and the new intellectual ferment we call the Renaissance – the quest to purify old doctrines and discover new truths – encouraged fresh biomedical inquiry. During the Renaissance, medicine was put on a surer footing, particularly once the Scientific Revolution brought glowing success to the mechanical sciences, physics, and chemistry.

Laying the Anatomical Foundations

Of fundamental importance in enhancing the standing of medicine was the pursuit of systematic human anatomy. Doctors in ancient Athens had treated the human body as sacred, and honoured it by refraining from cutting up dead bodies. In spite of their many contributions, therefore, Hippocratic and the later Galenic medicine were anatomically weak. Analogous views about the sanctity of the body (the belief that it belonged to God not man) later led the Roman Catholic Church to voice some opposition to dissecting the dead. Common people also felt deep misgivings. Grassroots hostility to dissection made itself felt in Britain even as late as the passing of the Anatomy Act in 1832. This was not surprising, given the notorious activities of William Burke and William Hare and other 'resurrection men'. In Edinburgh, Burke and Hare murdered the subjects they then sold for research to the medical school.

A sound anatomical and physiological basis is to us essential to scientific medicine, but it could develop only out of systematic dissection. Ecclesiastical opposition to dissection slowly melted away in medieval times. During the Black Death in the mid-fourteenth century, the Papacy sanctioned postmortems to search for the cause of the pestilence, but it was not until 1537 that Pope Clement VII finally accepted the teaching of anatomy by dissection. From the fourteenth century, however, dissections grew more common, especially in Italy, which was then the centre of scientific inquiry. Early anatomical demonstrations were public occasions, almost spectacles, for the purpose not of research but instruction – they allowed the professor to parade his proficiency. Dressed in long robes he would sit in a high chair reading out relevant passages from the works of Galen, while his assistant pointed to the organs alluded to and a dissector did the knifework. Early in the sixteenth century Leonardo da Vinci produced some 750 anatomical drawings. These were done in a purely private capacity, perhaps in secret, and made no impact at all on medical progress.

The real breakthrough came with the work of Andreas Vesalius. Born in 1514 the son of a Brussels pharmacist, Vesalius studied in Paris, Louvain, and Padua, where he took his medical degree in 1537, becoming at once a professor there; later, he became court physician to the Holy Roman Emperor Charles V and to Philip II of Spain. In 1543, he published his masterwork, *De Humani Corporis Fabrica* (On the Structure of the Human Body). In the exquisitely illustrated text, printed in Basel, Vesalius praised observation and challenged Galenic teachings on various points, recognizing that Galen's beliefs rested on knowledge of animals rather than humans. He criticized other doctors for describing the *plexus reticularis* because they had seen it in Galen's writings but never actually in a human body. He chided himself for once believing in Galen and the writings of other anatomists.

Vesalius's great contribution lay in creating a new atmosphere of inquiry and in setting anatomical study on solid foundations of observed fact. Although his work contained no startling discoveries, it induced a shift in intellectual strategy. After Vesalius, appeals to ancient authority lost their unquestioned validity, and his successors were compelled to stress precision and personal, first-hand observation. Vesalius's work was quickly honoured: Ambroise Paré, the leading surgeon of the day, used it for the anatomical section of his classic work on surgery, published in 1564.

Vesalius presented exact descriptions and illustrations of the skeleton and muscles, the nervous system, the viscera, and the blood vessels. His followers developed his techniques in greater depth and detail. In 1561, his student and successor as professor of anatomy at Padua, Gabrielle Falloppio (Fallopius), published a volume of anatomical observations that elucidated and corrected aspects of Vesalius's work. Falloppio's findings included structures in the human skull and ear, and research into the female genitalia. He coined the term vagina, described the clitoris, and was the first to delineate the tubes leading from the ovary to the uterus. Ironically, however, he failed to grasp the function of what became known as the Fallopian tubes; only two centuries later was it recognized that eggs were formed in the ovaries, passing down those tubes to the uterus. Early anatomy thus outran physiology.

By the close of the sixteenth century, Vesalian anatomy had become the golden method for anatomical investigations. Another Italian pioneer, Bartolommeo Eustachio, discovered the Eustachian tube (from the throat to the middle ear) and the Eustachian valve of the heart; he also examined the kidneys and explored the anatomy of the teeth. In 1603, Falloppio's successor at Padua, Girolamo Fabrizio (Fabricius ab Acquapendente), published a study of the veins that contained the first descriptions of their valves; this was to prove an inspiration to the English physician William Harvey. Slightly later, Gasparo Aselli of Padua drew attention to the lacteal vessels of the mesentery and identified their function as carrying chyle from food. This led to further studies of the stomach; Franz de le Boë (Franciscus Sylvius) of Leiden was later able to outline a chemical theory of digestion. Work also proceeded on the structure of the kidney, while Regnier de Graaf, a Dutch physician, was able to provide by 1670 a high-quality description of the reproductive system, discovering the Graafian vesicles of the female ovary.

Thus the work of Vesalius lent impetus to explorations of the organs of the body, although it must be said that Renaissance researchers generally had a better grasp of structure than function. A climate of opinion had, however, been created in which anatomy became the foundation of medical science.

William Harvey and the New Science

The growing prestige of anatomical knowledge began to change the orientation of study of the body and its disorders. The humoral theories of Hippocrates and his followers had viewed health and disease in terms of overall fluid balance. This was challenged in the Renaissance by a new concern with precise bodily mechanisms.

From earliest times, blood had been viewed as a life-giving fluid, perhaps the most significant of the four humours: it was recognized to nourish the body, although when disordered it was the cause of inflammation and fever. Galen's theory of the production and motion of blood long held sway. He believed that the veins that carried blood originated in the liver (the arteries stemmed from the heart). Blood was concocted (literally 'cooked') in the liver; it then migrated outwards on a kind of tidal motion through the veins into organs, where it carried nourishment and was consumed. The part of the blood proceeding from the liver to the right ventricle of the heart divided into two streams. The former passed along the pulmonary artery to the lungs, the latter traversed the heart through 'interseptal pores' into the left ventricle, where it mingled with air (*pneuma*), became heated, and proceeded from the left ventricle to the aorta, to the lungs and the periphery. The linkage of arteries with veins permitted some *pneuma* to enter the veins, while the arteries received some blood.

Galen's characterization of the blood system carried authority for fifteen hundred years. By 1500, however, his teachings were beginning to be questioned. Michael Servetus, a Spanish theologian and physician, offered a hypothesis about a 'smaller circulation' through the lungs, and implied that blood could not (Galen notwithstanding) flow through the septum of the heart but must find its way across the lungs from the right to the left side of the heart. In 1559, Servetus's hints about the pulmonary circulation of the blood were reiterated by the Italian anatomist, Realdo Colombo. In his *De Re Anatomia* Colombo showed, against Galen, that there were no openings in the heart's dividing wall between its auricles and ventricles. Colombo's theory became widely known, but in the short term it did not produce any serious threat to Galen's doctrines. In his 1603 treatise, Girolamo Fabrizio described venous valves but drew no inferences regarding the operations of the blood system. That was left to William Harvey.

Harvey's revolutionary work was not universally accepted. Parisian physicians, notoriously conservative, remained loyal for some time to Galenic teachings, and Harvey supposedly complained that his medical practice 'fell off mightily' after he published *De Motu Cordis* in 1628 because patients, too, were suspicious of new-fangled teachings. Nevertheless, Harvey's inspiration spurred and guided further physiological inquiry. A clutch of younger English researchers continued his work on the heart, lungs, and respiration.

One was Thomas Willis, who became a founder member of London's Royal Society (1662) and Sedleian Professor of Natural Philosophy at Oxford, and was also a fashionable London physician. Willis pioneered study of the anatomy of the brain, and of diseases of the nervous system and muscles, discovering the 'circle of Willis' in the brain. The most brilliant of the English Harveians, however, was Richard Lower. Born into an old Cornish family, he studied at Oxford and followed Willis to London. He collaborated with the mechanical philosopher Robert Hooke in a series of experiments, exploring how the lungs changed dark-red venous blood into bright-red arterial blood, and publishing his findings in *Tractatus de Corde* (Treatise on the Heart) in 1669. Lower earned a certain immortality by conducting at the Royal Society the first blood-transfusion experiments, transferring blood from dog to dog, and from person to person.

Physicians met scientists (or 'natural philosophers' as they were then called) at such venues as the Royal Society and exchanged ideas and techniques. Physicians felt there was all to gain from making their doctrines more 'scientific'. A new aid was the microscope, developed by Antoni van Leeuwenhoek in the Netherlands and taken up by Robert Hooke. Another lay in the startling contemporary advances in natural philosophy in general, above all in the physical sciences. The mechanical philosophy promoted by René Descartes, Robert Boyle, Hooke, and others presented the idea of the machine (with its levers, cogs, pulleys, and so forth) as the model for the body. Building on Harvey, many suggested a hydraulic understanding of its pipes, vessels, and tubes. Fashionable philosophers now rejected the old humoral theories as nothing but verbal flimflam, lacking any basis in material reality.

The mechanical philosophy stimulated new research programmes. In Italy, Marcello Malpighi conducted a remarkable series of microscopic studies of the structure of the liver, skin, lungs, spleen, glands, and brain, many of which were published in early numbers of the *Philosophical Transactions* of the Royal Society. Giovanni Borelli of Pisa and other 'iatrophysicists' (doctors convinced that the laws of physics offered the key to the body's operations) studied muscle behaviour, gland secretions, respiration, heart action, and neural responses. Working in Rome under the sponsorship of Sweden's Queen Christina, Borelli's main contribution was a treatise, *De Motu Animalium* (On Animal Motion), published in 1680–1. He made remarkable observations on birds in flight, fish swimming, muscular contraction, the mechanics of breathing, and a host of similar subjects, and attempted, more boldly than any before him, to comprehend body functions primarily in terms of the laws of physics.

Exploring what made the body machine work, Borelli postulated the presence of a 'contractile element' in the muscles; their operation was triggered by processes similar to chemical fermentation. He viewed respiration as a purely mechanical process that drove air through the lungs into the bloodstream. Familiar with the air-pump experiments conducted by Otto von Guericke and Robert Boyle, in which small animals expired in 'rarefied' air (that is, a vacuum), he maintained that 'aerated blood' included elements vital to life. Air possessed, he said, a life-sustaining function because it served as a vehicle for 'elastic particles' that entered the blood to impart internal motion to it. In Borelli's highly innovative work, physics and chemistry together promised to unravel the secrets of life.

Another innovative attempt to analyse the body in scientific terms lay in iatrochemistry. Whereas iatrophysics read the human frame through the laws of physics, iatrochemists applied chemical analysis.

Repudiating the humours as archaic and fanciful, certain investigators looked back to the chemical theories of the sixteenth-century Swiss iconoclast, Paracelsus, dismissed by some as a quack but respected by many as a major medical reformer. Paracelsus harked back to the simplicity of Hippocrates, learned from folk medicine, and believed in the power of nature to cure the body and heal the mind.

Devotees of Paracelsus also drew on the opinions of his Netherlandish follower, Johannes (Jean) Baptiste van Helmont. Van Helmont rejected Paracelsus's notion of a single *archeus* (or indwelling spirit), developing instead the idea that each organ has its own specific *blas* (spirit) regulating it. His concept of 'spirit' was not mystical but material and chemical. He held all vital processes to be chemical, each being due to the action of a particular ferment or gas. These ferments were imperceptible spirits capable of converting food into living flesh. Transformative processes occurred throughout the body, but particularly in the stomach, liver, and heart. Van Helmont deemed body heat a by-product of chemical fermentations, arguing that the whole system was governed by a soul situated in the pit of the stomach. Chemistry, broadly understood, was thus the key to life. Views like these were radical. Gui Patin, leader of the ultra-orthodox medical faculty in Paris, denounced van Helmont as a 'mad Flemish scoundrel'.

One of van Helmont's chief followers was Franciscus Sylvius. A supporter of William Harvey who taught at Leiden, Sylvius emphasized the salience of blood circulation for general physiology. He disparaged van Helmont's ideas as too esoteric, seeking to substitute for his gases and ferments notions of bodily processes that combined chemical analysis with circulation theory. Even more than van Helmont, Sylvius concentrated on digestion, arguing that this fermentive process occurred in the mouth, in the heart – where the digestive fire was kept burning by chemical reactions – and in the blood, moving outwards to the bones, tendons, and the flesh.

By 1700, in other words, advances in gross anatomy – and, after William Harvey, in physiology also – had created the dream of a scientific understanding of the body's structures and functions, drawing on and matching those of the new and highly prestigious mechanics and mathematics. Scientific medicine during the following century fulfilled certain of these goals, but also saw them frustrated.

Theories of Life in the Age of Enlightenment

During the eighteenth century, the Age of Enlightenment, research into general anatomy – bones, joints, muscles, fibres, and so on – continued along lines developed by Andreas Vesalius and his followers. Demonstrating supreme artistic skill and capitalizing on improvements in printing, many splendid anatomical atlases were published, including folios such as the *Osteographia* (1733) of the London surgeon-anatomist William Cheselden.

Careful investigation into individual organs continued, spurred by the fascination shown by Marcello Malpighi and other exponents of the 'new science' in bellows, syringes, pipes, valves, and similar contrivances. Anatomists struggled to lay bare the form/function relationship of minute (sometimes microscopical) structures, in the light of images of the organism as a system of vessels, tubes, and fluids. The laws of mechanics thus underwrote anatomical inquiry.

The Dutch anatomist Herman Boerhaave, the greatest medical teacher of his times, proposed that physical systems operating throughout the body comprised an integrated, balanced whole in which pressures and liquid flows were equalized and everything found its own level. Spurning the earlier 'clockwork' models of René Descartes as too crude, Boerhaave treated the body as a plumbing network of pipes and vessels, containing, channelling, and controlling body fluids. Health was explained by the movement of fluids in the vascular system; sickness was largely explained in terms of its obstruction or stagnation. The old humoral emphasis on balance had thus been preserved but translated into mechanical and hydrostatic terms.

Yet the fascination felt by Boerhaave and others in the mechanics of the body does not mean that medicine had become dogmatically reductionist or materialist. The presence of a soul in human beings could be taken for granted, but (Boerhaave judiciously maintained) inquiry into the essence of life or the immaterial soul was irrelevant to the nitty-gritty of medicine, whose business lay in the investigation of tangible physiological and pathological structures and processes. Considerations of the soul, in Boerhaave's opinion, were best left to priests and metaphysicians: medicine should study secondary causes not primary causes, the 'how', not the 'why' and 'wherefore'.

Certain aspects of Newton's natural philosophy, however, encouraged investigators to dismiss narrowly mechanistic views of the body and to pose wider questions about the properties of life. That meant reopening old debates over historic subjects, such as the doctrine of the soul. Highly significant was the work of the German chemist and physician Georg Ernst Stahl.

The founder of the distinguished Prussian medical school at the University of Halle in 1693, Stahl advanced classic anti-mechanistic arguments. Purposive human actions could not, he maintained, be wholly explained in terms of mechanical chain-reactions – like a stack of dominoes toppling over or balls cannoning round a billiard table. Wholes were greater than the sum of their parts, he claimed. Purposive human activity presupposed the presence of a soul, understood as a constantly intervening, presiding power, the very quintessence of the organism. More than a Cartesian 'ghost in the machine' (present but essentially separate), Stahl's *anima* (soul) was the ever-active agent of consciousness and physiological regulation, and a bodyguard against sickness. For disease, in his view, was a disturbance of vital functions provoked by maladies of the soul. The body, strictly speaking, was guided by an immortal spirit. Because the soul acted directly at bottom – that is, without need for the mediation of the *archæi* (ferments) of van Helmont or any other physical intermediaries – neither gross anatomy nor chemistry had much explanatory power: to fathom the operations of the body required understanding the soul and life itself.

Friedrich Hoffmann, Stahl's younger colleague at Halle, looked rather more favourably upon the new mechanical theories of the body. 'Medicine', he pronounced, 'is the art of properly utilizing physico-mechanical principles, in order to conserve the health of man or to restore it if lost.'[1]

Experimental researches into living bodies in the eighteenth century continually raised the question: is the living organism essentially a machine, or something different? Certain discoveries revealed the phenomenal powers possessed by living beings, not least a wonderful capacity to regenerate themselves in a manner unlike clocks or pumps. In 1712, the French naturalist René Réaumur demonstrated the ability of the claws and scales of lobsters to grow again after being severed. In the 1740s, the Swiss investigator Abraham Trembley divided polyps or hydras, and found that complete new individuals grew; he got a third generation by cutting up the latter. There was obviously more to life than the mechanists suspected.

Experimentation led to new opinions regarding the character of vitality – and, by implication, the relations between body and mind, body, and soul. The premier figure in these debates was a Swiss polymath, Albrecht von Haller, who produced a pathbreaking text, the *Elementa Physiologiae Corporis Humani* (Elements of the Physiology of the Human Body) in 1757–66. Building on Boerhaave's concern with the fibres, Haller's finest contribution was his laboratory demonstration of the hypothesis proposed by Francis Glisson in the mid-seventeenth century that irritability (also known as contractility) was a property inherent in muscular fibres, whereas sensibility (feeling) was the exclusive attribute of nervous fibres. Haller thus established the fundamental division of fibres according to their reactive properties. The sensibility of nervous fibres lay in their responsiveness to painful stimuli; the irritability of muscle fibres was their property of contracting in reaction to stimuli. Haller thereby advanced a physical explanation – something William Harvey had lacked – of why the heart pulsated: it was the most 'irritable' organ in the body. Composed of layers of muscular fibres, it was stimulated by the inflowing of blood, responding with systolic contractions.

On the basis of experimental procedures used on animals and humans, Haller's theories thus differentiated organ structures according to their fibre composition, ascribing to them intrinsic sensitivities independent of any transcendental, religious soul. Like Newton when faced with the phenomenon of gravity, Haller believed that the causes of such vital forces were beyond knowing – if not completely unknowable, at least unknown. It was sufficient, in true Newtonian fashion, to study effects and the laws of those effects. Haller's concepts of irritability and sensibility achieved widespread acclaim and formed the basis for further neurophysiological investigation.

A Scottish school of 'animal economy' (the contemporary phrase for physiology) also arose, centred on the impressive new Edinburgh University medical school, founded in 1726. Like Haller, Robert Whytt, a pupil of Alexander Monro *primus*, explored nervous activity, but Whytt contested Haller's doctrine of the inherent irritability of the fibres. In *On the Vital and Other Involuntary Motions of Animals* (1751), he argued that the reflex involved 'an unconscious sentient principle . . . residing in the brain and spinal cord', although he denied that his teaching entailed any undercover reintroduction of the *anima* of Stahl or the Christian soul. Whytt's view that body processes involved insensible purposive activities may be seen as an early attempt to grapple with the problem of what Sigmund Freud would later call the unconscious.

One who built on Haller's concept of irritability as a property of fibres was William Cullen, professor of medicine at the University of Edinburgh and, at the time, the most influential medical teacher in the English-speaking world. Born in 1710, Cullen taught chemistry in Glasgow before moving to Edinburgh to teach chemistry, materia medica, and medicine. He was the leading light of the Edinburgh Medical School during its golden age, publishing the best-selling nosologically arranged *First Lines of the Practice of Physic* (1778–9).

Cullen interpreted life itself as a function of nervous power and emphasized the importance of the nervous system in disease causation, coining the word 'neurosis' to describe nervous diseases. His one-time follower but later foe, John Brown, a larger-than-life figure who radicalized Scottish medicine (his followers were called Brunonians) but died an alcoholic, was to go further than Haller by reducing all questions of health and disease to variations around the mean of irritability. In place of Haller's concept of irritability, however, Brown substituted the idea that fibres were 'excitable'. Animation was hence to be understood as the product of external stimuli acting on an organized body: life was a 'forced condition'. Sickness, he ruled, was disturbance of the proper functioning of excitement, and diseases were to be treated as 'sthenic' or 'asthenic', depending on whether the body was over- or underexcited.

In France, graduates of the distinguished University of Montpellier – more go-ahead than Paris – led the vitality debate. Francois Boissier de Sauvages denied that mechanism on the Boerhaave model could explain the origin and continuation of motion in the body. Rather like Haller, he maintained that anatomy made little sense on its own; what was needed was physiological study of the structure of a living (not a dissected) body, endowed with a soul. Later Montpellier teachers such as Théophile de Bordeu adopted a more materialist stance, stressing the inherent vitality of living bodies rather than the operation of an implanted soul.

Comparable researches were pursued in London. John Hunter, who was Scottish-born but had trained in the dissecting-rooms of his brother William, proposed a 'life-principle' to account for properties distinguishing living organisms from inanimate matter: the life-force was in the blood. Thus philosophies of the 'machine of life' characteristic of the age of Descartes gave way to the more dynamic idea of 'vital properties' or vitalism. It is no accident that the very term 'biology' was coined around 1800, by, amongst others, Gottfried Reinhold Treviranus, a professor at Bremen, and the French naturalist and trailblazing evolutionist Jean-Baptiste Lamarck.

Debates about the nature of life were not conducted simply by armchair philosophers. They were advanced by particular researches into human and animal bodies: conjectures were put to the test. The processes of digestion, for example, earlier raised by Johannes van Helmont and Franciscus Sylvius, were subjected to sophisticated experimentation. Was digestion performed by some internal vital force, by the chemical action of gastric acids, or by the mechanical activities of churning, mincing, and pulverizing by the stomach muscles? The digestion debate had rumbled on since the Greeks, but eighteenth-century inquiries were characterized by striking experimental ingenuity, pioneered by René Réaumur. Having trained a pet kite to swallow and regurgitate porous food-filled tubes, Réaumur demonstrated the powers of gastric juices, and showed that meat is more fully digested in the stomach than are starchy foods.

As studies of digestion suggest, medicine fruitfully interacted with chemistry. A Scottish chemist, Joseph Black, formulated the idea of latent heat and identified 'fixed air' or what came to be known, in the new chemical nomenclature, as carbon dioxide. Major advances followed in understanding respiration. Black had noted that the 'fixed air' given off by quicklime and alkalis was also present in expired air; while non-toxic, it was physiologically incapable of being breathed. It was the French chemist Antoine-Laurent Lavoisier who best explained the passage of gases in the lungs. He showed that the air inhaled was converted into Black's 'fixed air', whereas the nitrogen ('azote') remained unchanged. Respiration was, Lavoisier believed, the analogue within the living body to combustion in the external world; both needed oxygen, both produced carbon dioxide and water. Lavoisier thus established that oxygen was indispensable for the human body, showing that, when engaged in physical activities, the body consumed greater quantities of oxygen than when at rest. Alongside chemistry, advances in other physical sciences, such as electricity, also promised medical payoffs.

The Origins of Clinical Science

Anatomy and physiology thus forged ahead in the eighteenth century, and the new-found faith in science probed the laws of life. But the relations between basic biological knowledge and medical practice remained opaque, and few scientific breakthroughs had direct payoffs for the mastery of disease. Many eminent physicians recorded their opinions on disease. William Heberden, who trained in Cambridge and practised in London, developed an impressive grasp, in the Hippocratic manner, of the characteristic disease syndromes. Heeding the advice of the great seventeenth-century clinician Thomas Sydenham, that clinical symptoms should be described with the same minuteness and accuracy observed by a painter in painting a portrait, Heberden emphasized the importance of distinguishing symptoms that were 'particular and constant' from those due to extraneous causes such as ageing. The fruit of 60 years' conscientious bedside notetaking, his *Commentaries* (1802) debunked hoary errors (for instance, the supposed prophylactic qualities of gout) and offered shrewd diagnostic and prognostic counsel.

Certain new clinical skills emerged. In his *Inventum Novum* (New Discovery) of 1761, Leopold Auenbrugger, physician-in-chief to the Hospital of the Holy Trinity at Vienna, advocated the technique of percussion of the chest. An innkeeper's son, Auenbrugger had been familiar since childhood with the trick of striking casks to test how full they were. Switching from barrels to patients, he noted that when tapped with a finger's end, a healthy subject's chest sounded like a cloth-covered drum; by contrast, a muffled sound, or one of unusually high pitch, indicated pulmonary disease, especially tuberculosis.

In general, eighteenth-century physicians rested content with the traditional diagnostic uses of the 'five senses'; they would feel the pulse, sniff for gangrene, taste urine, listen for breathing irregularities, and attend to skin and eye colour – looking out for the *facies Hippocratica*, the cast on the face of a dying person. These time-honoured methods were almost exclusively qualitative. Thus, what standardly counted in 'pulse lore' was not the number of beats per minute (as later), but their strength, firmness, rhythm, and 'feel'. Some attention was given to urine samples, but the historic art of urine-gazing (uroscopy) was now repudiated as the trick of the quackish 'pisse prophet': serious chemical analysis of urine had barely begun. Qualitative judgments dominated, and the good diagnostician was he who could size up a patient by acuity and experience.

Concepts of Disease

The good clinician thus knew his patients, but he also knew his diseases. Eighteenth-century practitioners trod in the footsteps of Thomas Sydenham and ultimately of Hippocrates, amassing comprehensive empirical case records, especially of epidemic disorders. Sydenham was much admired in England. 'The English Hippocrates' had served as captain of horse for the Parliamentarian army in the Civil War. In 1647, he went to Oxford and from 1655 practised in London. A friend of Robert Boyle and John Locke, he stressed observation rather than theory in clinical medicine, and instructed physicians to distinguish specific diseases and find specific remedies. He was a keen student of epidemic diseases, which he believed were caused by atmospheric properties (he called it the 'epidemic constitution') that determined which kind of acute disease would be prevalent at any season.

Following Sydenham's teachings, a Plymouth doctor, John Huxham, published extensive findings about disease profiles in his *On Fevers* (1750); and a Chester practitioner, John Haygarth, undertook analysis of smallpox and typhus epidemics. John Fothergill, a Yorkshireman and a Quaker who built up a lucrative London practice, was another avid follower of Sydenham. In *Observations of the Weather and Diseases of London* (1751–4), Fothergill gave a valuable description of diphtheria ('epidemic' sore throat), which was then growing more common especially among the urban poor. His friend and fellow Quaker, John Coakley Lettsom, was the driving-force behind the clinical investigations pioneered by the Medical Society of London, founded in 1778. Such medical gatherings, developing also in the provinces, collected clinical data and exchanged news. The birth of medical journalism also helped pool experience and spread information.

Systematic epidemiological and pathological research programmes did not develop until the nineteenth century; yet many valuable observations on diseases were made before 1800. In 1776, Matthew Dobson demonstrated that the sweetness of the urine in diabetes was due to sugar; in 1786, Lettsom published a fine account of alcoholism; Thomas Beddoes and others conducted investigations into tuberculosis, which was already becoming the great 'white plague' of urban Europe. But no decisive breakthroughs followed in disease theory. Questions as to true causation (*vera causa*) remained highly controversial. Many kinds of sickness were still attributed to personal factors – poor stock or physical endowment, neglect of hygiene, overindulgence, and bad lifestyle. This 'constitutional' or physiological concept of disease, buttressed by traditional humoralism, made excellent sense of the uneven and unpredictable scatter of sickness: with infections and fevers, some individuals were afflicted, some were not, even within a single household. It also drew attention to personal moral responsibility and pointed to strategies of disease containment through self-help. This personalization of illness had attractions and pitfalls that are still debated today.

Theories that disease spread essentially by contagion were also in circulation. These had much common experience in their favour. Certain disorders, such as syphilis, were manifestly transmitted person-to-person. Smallpox inoculation, introduced in the eighteenth century, offered proof of contagiousness. But contagion hypotheses had their difficulties as well: if diseases were contagious, why didn't everyone catch them?

Such misgivings explain the popularity of long-entrenched miasmatic thinking – the conviction that sickness typically spread not by personal contact but through emanations given off by the environment. After all, everyone knew that some locations were healthier, or more dangerous, than others. With intermitting fevers like 'ague' (malaria), it was common knowledge that those living close to marshes and creeks were especially susceptible. Low and spotted fevers (typhus) were recognized as infecting populations in the overcrowded slum quarters of great towns, just as they also struck occupants of gaols, barracks, ships, and workhouses. It was thus plausible to suggest that disease lay in poisonous atmospheric exhalations, given off by putrefying carcases, food and faeces, waterlogged soil, rotting vegetable remains, and other filth in the surroundings. Bad environments, the argument ran, generated bad air (signalled by stenches), which, in turn, triggered disease. Late in the century, reformers directed attention to the 'septic' diseases – gangrene, septicaemia, diphtheria, erysipelas, and puerperal fever – especially rampant in slum quarters and in ramshackle gaols and hospitals. The Hôtel Dieu in Paris had an atrocious reputation as a hotbed of fevers.

Disease theory greatly benefited from the rise of pathological anatomy. The trail was blazed by the illustrious Italian, Giovanni Battista Morgagni, professor of anatomy at Padua, who built on earlier postmortem studies by Johann Wepfer and Théophile Bonet. In 1761, when close to the age of eighty, Morgagni published his great work *De Sedibus et Causis Morborum* (On the Sites and Causes of Disease), which surveyed the findings of some 700 autopsies he had carried out. It quickly became famous, being translated into English in 1769 and German in 1774.

It was Morgagni's aim to show that diseases were located in specific organs, that disease symptoms tallied with anatomical lesions, and that pathological organ changes were responsible for disease manifestations. He gave lucid accounts of many disease conditions, being the first to delineate syphilitic tumours of the brain and tuberculosis of the kidney. He grasped that where only one side of the body is stricken with paralysis, the lesion lies on the opposite side of the brain. His explorations of the female genitals, of the glands of the trachea, and of the male urethra also broke new ground.

Others continued his work. In 1793, Matthew Baillie, a Scot and a nephew of William Hunter practising in London, published his *Morbid Anatomy*. Illustrated with superb copperplates by William Clift (they depicted, among other things, the emphysema of Samuel Johnson's lungs) Baillie's work was more of a textbook than Morgagni's, describing in succession the morbid appearances of each organ. He was the first to give a clear idea of cirrhosis of the liver, and in his second edition he developed the idea of 'rheumatism of the heart' (rheumatic fever).

Pathology was to yield an abundant harvest in early nineteenth-century medicine, thanks to the publication in 1800 of the *Traité des Membranes* by François Xavier Bichat, who focused particularly on the histological changes produced by disease. Morgagni's pathology had concentrated on organs; Bichat shifted the focus. The more one will observe diseases and open cadavers, he declared, the more one will be convinced of the necessity of considering local diseases not from the aspect of the complex organs but from that of the individual tissues.

Born in Thoirette in the French Jura, Bichat studied at Lyon and Paris, where he settled in 1793 at the height of the Terror. From 1797 he taught medicine, working at the Hôtel Dieu. His greatest contribution was his perception that the diverse organs of the body contain particular tissues or what he called 'membranes'; he described twenty-one, including connective, muscle, and nerve tissue. Performing his researches with great fervour – he undertook more than 600 postmortems – Bichat formed a bridge between the morbid anatomy of Morgagni and the later cell pathology of Rudolf Virchow.

Medicine Becomes Scientific

The seventeenth century had launched the New Science; the Enlightenment propagandized on its behalf. But it was the nineteenth century that was the true age of science, with the state and universities promoting and funding it systematically. For the first time, it became essential for any ambitious doctor to acquire a scientific training. Shortly after 1800, medical science was revolutionized by a clutch of French professors, whose work was shaped by the opportunities created by the French Revolution for physicians to use big public hospitals for research. Among physicians, they acquired a heroic status, not unlike Napoleon himself. Perhaps the most distinguished was René-Théophile-Hyacinthe Laënnec, a pupil of François Bichat. In 1814, he became physician to the Salpêtrière Hospital and two years later chief physician to the Hôpital Necker. In 1816, Laënnec invented the stethoscope. Here is how he described his discovery:

> In 1816 I was consulted by a young woman presenting general symptoms of disease of the heart. Owing to her stoutness little information could be gathered by application of the hand and percussion. The patient's age and sex did not permit me to resort to the kind of examination I have just described (direct application of the ear to the chest). I recalled a well-known acoustic phenomenon: namely, if you place your ear against one end of a wooden beam the scratch of a pin at the other extremity is distinctly audible. It occurred to me that this physical property might serve a useful purpose in the case with which I was then dealing. Taking a sheet of paper I rolled it into a very tight roll, one end of which I placed on the precordial region, whilst I put my ear to the other. I was both surprised and gratified at being able to hear the beating of the heart with much greater clearness and distinctness than I had ever before by direct application of my ear.
>
> I saw at once that this means might become a useful method for studying, not only the beating of the heart, but likewise all movements capable of producing sound in the thoracic vacity, and that consequently it might serve for the investigation of respiration, the voice, rales and possibly even the movements of liquid effused into the pleural cavity or pericardium.[2]

By experiment, his instrument became a simple wooden cylinder about 23 centimetres (9 inches) long that could be unscrewed for carrying in the pocket. It was monaural (only later, in 1852, were two earpieces added – by the American George P. Cammann – for binaural sound). The stethoscope was the most important diagnostic innovation before the discovery of X-rays in the 1890s.

On the basis of his knowledge of the different normal and abnormal breath sounds, Laënnec diagnosed a multiplicity of pulmonary ailments: bronchitis, pneumonia, and, above all, pulmonary tuberculosis (phthisis or consumption). His oustanding publication, *Traité de l'Auscultation médiate* (1819), included clinical and pathological descriptions of many chest diseases. Ironically, Laënnec himself died of tuberculosis.

Laënnec's investigations paralleled those of his colleague, Gaspard Laurent Bayle, who in 1810 published a classic monograph on phthisis, on the basis of more than 900 dissections. Bayle's outlook was different from Laënnec's. He was more interested in taxonomy, and distinguished six distinct types of pulmonary phthisis. Laënnec had no interest in classification; rather, his ability to hear and interpret breath sounds made him primarily interested in the course of the diseases he examined. Like other contemporary French hospital physicians, he was accused of showing greater concern for diagnosis than for therapy – but this stemmed not from indifference to the sick but from a deep awareness of therapeutic limitations. Translations of Laënnec's book spread the technique of stethoscopy, as did the foreign students drawn to Paris. A man with a stethoscope draped round his neck became the prime nineteenth-century image of medicine: the instrument had the word science written on it.

Laënnec remains the one famous name amongst the generation of post-1800 French physicians who insisted that medicine must become a science and who believed that scientific diagnosis formed its pith and marrow. At the time, however, the most illustrious was Pierre Louis, whose writings set out the key agenda of the new 'hospital medicine'. Graduating in Paris in 1813, Louis spent 7 years practising in Russia. On returning home, he plunged into the wards of the *Pitié* hospital and published the results of his experiences in a massive book on tuberculosis (1825), followed 4 years later by another on fever.

Louis' *Essay on Clinical Instruction* (1834) set the standards for French hospital medicine. He highlighted not only bedside diagnosis but also systematic investigation into the patient's circumstances, history, and general health. He deemed the value of the patient's *symptoms* (that is, what the patient felt and reported) secondary, stressing the far more significant *signs* (that is, what the doctor's examination ascertained). On the basis of such signs, the lesions of the pertinent organs could be determined, and they were the most definite guides to identifying diseases, devising therapies and making prognoses. For Louis, clinical medicine was an observational rather than an experimental science. It was learned at the bedside and in the morgue by recording and interpreting facts. Medical training lay in instructing students in the techniques of interpreting the sights, sounds, feel, and smell of disease: it was an education of the senses. Clinical judgment lay in astute explication of what the senses perceived.

Louis was, furthermore, a passionate advocate of numerical methods – the culmination of an outlook that had begun in the Enlightenment. Louis' mathematics were little more than simple arithmetic – quantitative categorizations of symptoms, lesions, and diseases, and (most significantly) application of numerical methods to test his therapies. To some degree, Louis sought to use medical arithmetic to discredit existing therapeutic practices: he was thus a pioneer of clinical trials. Only through the collection of myriad instances, he stressed, could doctors hope to formulate general laws.

Overall, the leading lights among French hospital doctors were more confident about diagnosis than cure, although Laënnec highlighted the Hippocratic concept of the healing power of nature – the power of the body to restore itself to health. But in the French school, therapeutics remained subordinate to pathological anatomy and diagnosis. The meticulousness with which Laënnec, Louis, Bayle, and others delineated disease reinforced the nosological concept that diseases were discrete entities, real things. The move from reliance upon symptoms (which were variable and subjective) to constant and objective lesions (the sign) supported their idea that diseased states were fundamentally different from normal ones.

The 'Paris school' was not a single cohesive philosophy of medical investigation. Nevertheless, there was something distinguished about Paris medicine; and during the first half of the nineteenth century students from Europe and North America flocked to France. Young men who studied in Paris returned home to fly the flag for French medicine. Disciples in London, Geneva, Vienna, Philadelphia, Dublin, and Edinburgh followed the French in emphasizing physical diagnosis and pathological correlation. They often also took back with them knowledge and skills in basic sciences such as chemistry and microscopy. Several leading English stethoscopists, including Thomas Hodgkin (of Hodgkin's disease), learned the technique directly from Laënnec himself.

Imitating the French example, medical education everywhere grew more systematic, more scientific. Stimulated by teachers who had studied in Paris, medical teaching in London expanded: by 1841, St George's Hospital had 200 pupils, St Bartholomew's 300. There were hundreds of students in other London hospital schools as well, and from the 1830s London also boasted a teaching university, with two colleges, University and King's, each with medical faculties and purpose-built hospitals.

London become a major centre of scientific medicine. Amongst the most eminent investigators was Thomas Addison, who became the leading medical teacher and diagnostician at Guy's Hospital where he collaborated with Richard Bright and identified Addison's disease (insufficiency of the suprarenal capsules) and Addison's anaemia (pernicious anaemia). Bright for his part was a member of the staff at Guy's Hospital from 1820. His *Reports of Medical Cases* (1827–31) contain his description of kidney disease (Bright's disease), with its associated dropsy and protein in the urine.

Vienna also grew in eminence. The University of Vienna had well-established traditions: the old medical school had bedside teaching on the model espoused by Herman Boerhaave in the early eighteenth century, but decay had set in towards 1800. However, new teaching was introduced by the Paris-inspired Carl von Rokitanski, who made pathological anatomy compulsory. The age's most obsessive dissector (supposedly performing some 60,000 autopsies in all), Rokitanski had a superb mastery of anatomy and pathological science, and left notable studies of congenital malformations and reports of numerous conditions, including pneumonia, peptic ulcer, and valvular heart disease.

In the USA, by contrast, high-quality medical schools and clinical investigations developed more slowly. In its *laissez-faire*, business-dominated atmosphere, many schools were blatantly commercial, inadequately staffed, and offered cut-price degrees.

Medicine in the Laboratory

Influenced by the Paris school, hospitals became the key sites for medical science. Remarkable advances also started taking place in the laboratory. By 1850, laboratories were transforming physiology and pathology and beginning to make their mark on medical education. Laboratories were not new – they had grown up with seventeenth-century science – nor was experimental medicine; the Revd Stephen Hales, for instance, conducted experiments on blood circulation in the early eighteenth century. Nevertheless, nineteenth-century practitioners of organic chemistry, microscopy, and physiology rightly believed they were giving birth to a new enterprise, based on the laboratory and its stress on vivisection. The hospital was a place to observe, the laboratory to experiment.

Science went from strength to strength in the nineteenth century, winning greater public funds and a place in the sun. German universities, in particular, became associated with the research ethos. Justus von Liebig's Institute of Chemistry at the University of Giessen established the mould for German laboratory science. Liebig studied chemistry at Bonn and Erlangen before spending 2 years in Paris, gaining laboratory experience. In 1824, at the tender age of twenty-one, he was appointed professor of chemistry at Giessen, where his institute became a magnet, attracting students seeking practical instruction in qualitative analysis. It proved a huge success, being enlarged to house more students and research facilities before the University of Munich lured him away in 1852 with an offer he could not refuse.

Liebig's goal was to subject living beings to strictly quantified chemical analysis. By measuring what went in (food, oxygen, and water) and what came out (urea, various acids and salts, water, and carbon dioxide in the excretions and exhalations), vital information would be discovered about the chemical processes occurring within. Liebig thought of the body in terms of chemical systems. Respiration brought oxygen into the body, where it mixed with starches to liberate energy, carbon dioxide, and water. Nitrogenous matter was absorbed into muscle and comparable tissues; when it was broken down, urine was the final product, together with phosphates and assorted chemical by-products.

Becoming the age's great breeder of chemists, Liebig encouraged his students to undertake chemical analyses on such animal tissues as muscle and liver, or on blood, sweat, tears, urine, and other fluids. They attempted measurement of the relationship in living organisms between food and oxygen consumption and energy production.

In short, Liebig's school launched energetic investigation of nutrition and metabolism, developing what was later to be called biochemistry.

Liebig's career proved crucial. He trained scores of students in research methods and organized systematized laboratory research. He emphasized the cardinal importance of physicochemical thinking in understanding biological processes, developing the reductionist ambition of applying the physical sciences to living organisms. As early as 1828 his lifelong friend, Friedrich Wöhler (from 1836 professor of chemistry at Göttingen), synthesized the organic substance urea from inorganic substrates: this served as a persuasive proof that no categorical barrier separated 'vital' compounds found in living beings from ordinary chemicals. Such findings gave impetus to the programme known as scientific materialism, whose adherents were engaged in a militant repudiation of the speculative, idealistic philosophy (*Naturphilosophie*) that, in the musings of Goethe and others, had achieved much prestige in-German culture in the Romantic era. Liebig and his followers were sober experimentalists scornful of mystical and poetic aspirations to understand the Meaning of Life.

The enshrinement of physiology as a high-status experimental discipline was a key feature of nineteenth-century medical science. Johannes Müller was its trailblazer. Born in Coblenz, Müller became professor of physiology and anatomy at Bonn and from 1833 at Berlin. Gifted at neurophysiological research, Müller's enormous two-volume *Handbuch der Physiologie des Menschen* (1833–40) was fundamental to the progress of the discipline. He was above all an inspiring teacher, and his students – Theodor Schwann, Hermann von Helmholtz, Emil du Bois-Reymond, Ernst Brücke, Jacob Henle, Rudolf Virchow, and many others – became trendsetters in scientific and medical research.

Four promising young physiologists associated with Müller – Helmholtz, du Bois-Reymond, Karl Ludwig, and Brücke – published a manifesto in 1847 proclaiming that physiology's goal was to explain all vital phenomena in terms of physicochemical laws. Before he turned to physics in the 1870s, Helmholtz devoted himself to central physiological problems, including measurement of animal heat and the velocity of nerve conduction, and investigation of sight and hearing. He invented the ophthalmoscope, aiding work on vision. Ludwig for his part did pioneer research on glandular secretions, notably the manufacture of urine by kidneys. Du Bois-Reymond, professor of physiology in Berlin, was mainly immersed in electrophysiology, studying muscles and nerves. Brücke went to Vienna, where his concerns spanned physiological chemistry, histology, and neuromuscular physiology. Tough-mindedly committed to scientific naturalism, Brücke became one of Sigmund Freud's teachers and heroes.

The thrust of the experimental physiology carried out by such field-leaders was, in Ludwig's words, to understand functions 'from the elementary conditions inherent in the organism itself'.[3] It required the use of experimental animals and drew on new instruments to record data. In 1847, Ludwig introduced the technological device that epitomized physiological research: the kymograph – the machine designed to trace body alterations onto a line on a graph. Growing technological sophistication was central to modern medical science. There were other developments in instrumentation. The design of the microscope was greatly improved, correcting distortion and so enabling histology to create a bridge between anatomy and physiology. Learn to see microscopically, Rudolf Virchow insisted, summing up the message that Müller taught all his pupils.

Microscopy was intimately linked with the new study of cells, in 1838 begun by another of Müller's pupils, Theodor Schwann. Schwann discovered the enzyme pepsin in the stomach, investigated muscle contraction, and demonstrated the role of microorganisms in putrefaction. But he is chiefly remembered for extending the cell theory, previously applied to plants, to animal tissues. His model was reductionist: cells, he believed, were the fundamental units of zoological and botanical activity. Incorporating a nucleus and an outer membrane, they could be formed (in a manner he compared to crystals growing within solutions) out of a formless organic matrix that he called the blastema.

Schwann's views were modified by Rudolf Virchow, professor of pathological anatomy at Würzburg (1849) and later Berlin (1856). His microscopical work carried profound biological significance. In his *Cellularpathologie* (1858), he disputed Schwann's notion of the blastema, and developed the maxim: *omnis cellula e cellula* (all cells from cells). If François Bichat's *Traité des Membranes* (1800) put tissues on the map, Virchow's treatise did the same for cells: it established a new, productive unit for making inferences about function and disease. Virchow's hypothesis had special pertinence for such biological events as fertilization and for pathophysiological ones, such as the source of the pus cell in inflammation. Diseases arise (he argued) from abnormal changes within cells; such abnormal cells multiply through division. Virchow thus regarded the study of cells as basic to the understanding of cancer, on which he lavished great attention, describing leukaemia for the first time. His view of disease was essentially an internal one, and he proved distrustful of the bacteriology of Louis Pasteur, which he regarded as rather shallow. German laboratories attracted students from all over Europe and North America. In the 1830s, the migration was a trickle: chemists went to Justus von Liebig in Giessen and microscopists to Johannes Müller in Berlin. Half a century later, it had become a deluge, with medical students flocking to complete their education in the German-speaking universities.

French hospital medicine in its heyday had not relied on laboratory-based inquiries, although foreign medical students sometimes gained instruction in microscopy as well as experience in hospital wards and morgues. France gradually slipped behind Germany because it failed to create the new laboratories necessary for physiological research. Nevertheless, France continued to produce eminent researchers. For example, François Magendie, professor of anatomy at the Collège de France (1831), made important studies of nerve physiology, the veins, and the physiology of food. His real distinction lay in helping to launch the career of Claude Bernard.

Born near Villefranche, Bernard failed as a dramatist and so studied medicine at Paris, in 1841 becoming Magendie's assistant at the Collège de France. Thereafter, all was success, including chairs at the Sorbonne and the Museum of Natural History, a seat in the Senate, and the presidency of the French Academy. Bernard's brilliance lay in his superb operative techniques and the simplicity of his experiments. His earliest researches were on the action of the secretions of the alimentary canal, pancreatic juice, and the connection between the liver and nervous system. Later researches were, for example, on changes of temperature of the blood, levels of oxygen in arterial and in venous blood, and the opium alkaloids. He reached major physiological findings: the role of the liver in synthesizing glycogen and in keeping blood-glucose levels within a healthy range; the digestive functions of the secretions of the pancreas; the vasodilator nerves and their role in regulating the flow of blood in blood vessels; and the effects on muscles of carbon monoxide and curare (the South American arrow poison).

Bernard's most famous book, *Introduction à la Médecine expérimentale* (1865), was a systematic exposition of the experimental method for biomedical sciences. Traditional hospital medicine, Bernard maintained, had two key limitations. As an observational science, it was purely passive, akin to natural history. The progress of physiology required the active observation of the experimentalist under controlled conditions. At the sickbed, there were too many imponderables to allow precise understanding. Moreover, he argued (contradicting Pierre Louis, René Laënnec, and their school), the pathological lesion itself was not the origin but the end point of disease. Pathophysiological knowledge could be fulfilled only in the laboratory, and only through use of laboratory animals in controlled environments. No pathology without physiology, he insisted. The interplay of physiology, pathology, and pharmacology constituted for him the foundations of experimental medicine, and each had to be a laboratory science.

Yet Bernard was no crass materialist or physical reductionist. Animals and human beings, he maintained, were not automata at the mercy of the external environment. And the reason for this was because higher organisms did not live solely in the exterior environment; they actively created their own internal environment, the *internal milieu*, the home of live communities of cells. Numerous physiological mechanisms, mediated through fluids such as blood and lymph, were devoted to balancing concentrations of sugar, salt, and oxygen in the blood and tissue fluids; it was their job to preserve a uniform body temperature in relation to the fluctuations of variable external ones. It was through these mechanisms – later to be called 'homeostasis' by the Harvard physiologist Walter Bradford Cannon – that higher organisms achieved a degree of autonomy within the more fundamental determinism of the natural order.

Scientific medicine developed later in Britain and the USA, owing profound debts to developments in France and Germany. By the 1880s, droves of Americans were studying biology and medicine in German-speaking universities: there were perhaps 15,000 between 1850 and the First World War, mostly in Vienna, Göttingen, Berlin, and Heidelberg. They primarily went for clinical instruction, but some, like the pathologist William Henry Welch, homed in on the laboratories. It was Welch who introduced the Germanic spirit into American experimental medicine, building his career at the most Germanic of American universities, Johns Hopkins in Baltimore, Maryland. The Johns Hopkins Hospital opened its doors to patients in 1889, although the medical school – unusual in admitting women – was delayed for a further four years because of a short-age of funds. The emphasis was on advanced teaching and research. British medical students also went in droves to Germany, but institutions in Britain supporting medical research remained small all through the Victorian age – British medicine was mainly practical and geared to private practice. Research achieved little status in the universities, and there was hardly any state support. Moreover, the British situation was not helped by public hostility to vivisection to a degree not experienced elsewhere.

The antivivisection campaign grew vocal at the 1874 Norwich meeting of the British Medical Association after a demonstration by a French physiologist – he injected alcohol into two dogs – made headline news. A summons for wanton cruelty was issued. Although unsuccessful, the prosecution put animal experimentation on the political agenda, leading to the setting up of a Royal Commission to examine experimental medicine. The resultant 1876 Cruelty to Animals Act was a compromise that satisfied neither antivivisection-ists nor the science lobby. It permitted medically trained investiga-tors to conduct vivisection experiments under licence and strictly stipulated conditions. No other nation passed legislation regulating animal experimentation before the twentieth century.

Neither the 1876 Act nor the activities of the antivivisectionists prevented British physiology from increasing its international sta-tus in the decades before the First World War. Working first in

London and then in Edinburgh, Edward Schafer (later Sharpey-Schafer) achieved fame for his researches on muscular contraction. Around the same time, Michael Foster and his pupils John Newport Langley and Walter Holbrook Gaskell created a research school in Cambridge that produced a number of future Nobel Laureates and boosted Cambridge's reputation as Britain's most enterprising medical school. Foster set himself the problem of determining whether the heartbeat was muscular or neurological in nature; and his Cambridge protégés in due course broadened out this question to explore the anatomy and physiology of the autonomic nervous system, the chemical transmission of nerve impulses, and the control of reflexes and movement.

Tropical Medicine in the Era of Imperialism

During the nineteenth century medicine grew international, indeed global: the Red Cross was established by the Geneva Convention of 1864, and international medical congresses were inaugurated in 1867 in Paris. The specialism of tropical medicine emerging from the 1870s reflects the spirit of the era of imperialism, when the great powers battled to settle the less 'civilized' parts of the globe. Scientists became embroiled in an uneasy mix of competition and cooperation.

Imperial expansion had long been thwarted by diseases such as malaria (from the Italian *mala aria*, bad air) that remained troublesome around the Mediterranean and continued to thwart colonial endeavours in Asia, Africa, and Latin America; and generations of experience had taught that the tropics were the white man's grave. Yet the relations between climate, disease, and victims had long been a puzzle. Some 'tropical' diseases, such as sleeping sickness and schistosomiasis, primarily affected natives. Others, like malaria, afflicted Europeans too. And from the 1830s, cholera had moved beyond its traditional home in the Indian subcontinent, circling the globe in great pandemics. Malaria remained. Plague had never disappeared from Asia and the Near East; as late as the 1890s an outbreak in China inaugurated a pandemic that spread catastrophically to India and beyond; in 1900, the USA itself was hit by an epidemic in San Francisco.

Each of the diseases just mentioned was 'tropical' in the sense that it was more frequent in hot climates; and certain diseases – for example, schistosomiasis in the Nile Valley – seemed to be restricted almost exclusively to hot climates and the native inhabitants. Not surprisingly, traditional explanations of diseases of hot climates had drawn on the general framework of miasmatic environmentalism: heat produced severe fevers and tendencies to putrescence. But new explanations emerged in the last quarter of the nineteenth century; their pioneer was Patrick Manson.

A Scot, Manson had gone to the Far East in 1866 as a Customs Medical Officer. During a dozen years in Amoy (now Xiamen) off the south-east China coast, he studied elephantiasis, the chronic disfiguring disease that through blockage of lymph flow leads to massive swelling of the genitalia and limbs. He was also able to demonstrate that it was caused by a parasite – a nematode worm called *Filaria* or *Wuchereria* – spread through mosquito bites. This was the first disease shown to be transmitted by an insect vector. Returning to London in 1890, he became the leading consultant on tropical diseases, in 1899 helping to found the London School of Tropical Medicine. His *Tropical Diseases* (1898) delineated the new specialism, emphasizing that entomology, helminthology, and parasitology were the keys to understanding diseases exclusive to tropical climates.

Building a reputation as a scientific parasitologist, Manson stamped his vision on the emergent specialism, not just in Britain but also throughout Europe and the Americas. Assimilating but going beyond bacteriology, his work led to the spotlighting of a new class of parasitic organisms as the precipitants of tropical diseases: schistosomiasis was found to be produced by the trematode worms *Bilharzia*; tropical dysentery was caused by an amoeba; sleeping sickness by a trypanosome protozoan; and malaria by another sort of protozoan, *Plasmodium*.

Other diseases were mastered, in theory if not in practice, by extending the new parasitological model. The Spanish-American War in Central America led to shocking mortality from yellow fever and hence to the foundation in 1900 of a US Army Yellow Fever Commission. A local Havana doctor, Carlos Finlay, was already championing a mosquito-borne theory of yellow fever, based on experiments in which healthy volunteers were bitten by mosquitoes that had fed on yellow-fever victims: they then typically fell sick. The Yellow Fever Commission enlisted the help of Finlay and the Chief Sanitary Officer in Havana, the American military doctor, Colonel William Gorgas, and, building on the work of the British parasitologist Ronald Ross and Giovanni Grassi, it followed up Finlay's mosquito hypothesis, subjecting healthy volunteers under supervised conditions to mosquitoes that had previously bitten yellow-fever patients. This time a different species of mosquito, *Aedes aegypti*, proved to be responsible. Laboratory and field studies led Gorgas to inaugurate a successful mosquito-eradication programme in Havana.

A similar scheme followed in the Panama Canal Zone. The French had begun to construct the Panama Canal, but they had abandoned the enterprise because losses from yellow fever had been exorbitant. Through draining marshes, oiling ponds over, and reducing stagnant water in townships, the number of mosquitoes was reduced, with significant decline in the incidence of mosquito-borne diseases. The construction of the canal then went ahead between 1904 and 1914 – a dramatic vindication of the potential of medical science in the tropics.

Twentieth-Century Breakthroughs

Building on the developments of the nineteenth century, the past hundred years have brought unparalleled developments in biology, chemistry, and physiology and the opening up of new specialities within medical science. It would be quite impossible even to list here all the main twentieth-century breakthroughs in medical science, but a few fields and salient advances may be outlined.

The microbiological research promoted by Louis Pasteur and Robert Koch led to the creation around 1900 of immunology. The word 'immunity' – exemption from a particular disease – was popularized as researchers grew more familiar with the enigmatic relations of infection and resistance. Fascinated by the nutritional requirements of microorganisms, Pasteur had suggested a nutritional dimension to the resistance of a host and the attenuation of a parasite: the microorganism lost its power to infect because it could no longer flourish and reproduce.

Pasteur was more concerned with vaccine production than with the theoretical reasons why vaccines protected (or immunized). In 1884, however, a Russian zoologist, Elie Metchnikoff, observed in the water flea (*Daphnia*) a phenomenon he termed phagocytosis (cell-eating), subsequently developing his observations into a comprehensive cellular view of resistance. Metchnikoff saw amoeba-like cells in these lower organisms apparently ingesting foreign substances like vegetable matter. He deduced that these amoeba-like cells in *Daphnia* might be comparable to the pus cells visible in higher creatures. Microscopic examination of animals infected with various pathogens, including the anthrax bacillus, showed white blood cells assaulting and appearing to digest the disease germs. Metchnikoff likened white blood cells to an army that was 'fighting infection'. Extrapolating from these hypotheses, Metchnikoff subsequently turned into a scientific guru, expounding striking beliefs on diet, constipation, ageing, and humanity's biological future. He became noted for his advocacy of eating yoghurt, arguing that the bacilli used in producing it inhibited the bacteria in the gut that caused harmful putrefactive by-products.

Metchnikoff's cellular theory of immunity gained prominence within the French scientific community; in an era of tense scientific rivalry, German researchers proposed chemical theories. Robert Koch's scepticism about the immunological significance of phagocytosis carried great weight in Germany, and two of his younger colleagues, Emil Adolf von Behring and Paul Ehrlich, argued that immunological warfare was waged less by the white blood cells than in the blood serum. Their chemical hypothesis had important factors in its favour. It was known that the cell-free serum of immunized creatures could destroy lethal bacteria, and that protection could be transmitted via serum from animal to animal: this implied there was more to immunity than the operation of white blood cells alone. Moreover, two of Pasteur's own pupils, Emile Roux and Alexandre Yersin, showed in 1888 that cultures of diphtheria bacilli were toxic even when the cells themselves had been filtered out. This seemed to suggest that it was not necessarily the bacterial cell itself that bred disease but rather some chemical toxin the cell manufactured.

On the strength of these observations serum therapy was developed. Working with a Japanese associate, Shibasaburo Kitasato, Behring claimed in 1890 that the whole blood or serum of an animal, rendered immune to tetanus or diphtheria by injecting the relevant toxin, could treat another creature exposed to an otherwise fatal dose of the bacilli. Serum therapy had some genuine triumphs, but it never proved a wonder cure – not least because epidemic diseases such as diphtheria were notoriously variable in their virulence. Nevertheless, serum therapies grew in popularity after 1890, and antitoxins were prepared for diseases other than tetanus and diphtheria, including pneumonia, plague, and cholera. Many, however, remained convinced of the superior protective possibilities of vaccines. Vaccines developed from the treated organisms of plague and cholera were introduced around 1900 by the Russian-born bacteriologist, Waldemar Haffkine.

From the 1880s Ehrlich had been exploring the physiological and pharmacological properties of various dyes, demonstrating, for example, the affinity of the newly discovered malaria parasite for methylene blue. Applying the stereochemical ideas of Emil Fischer and other organic chemists, Ehrlich devised a 'side-chain' notion to explain how antigens and antibodies interacted. His formulation was essentially a chemical interpretation of immunity, part of a molecular vision of reality that included the possibility of pharmacological 'magic bullets', the ultimate aim of chemotherapy. Ideas of immunity linked in various ways with the study of the relations between nutrition and health. Nutrition studies had various traditions on which to draw. Back in the eighteenth century, the problem of scurvy aboard ship had led to conjectures connecting diet and disease and to the first clinical trials by the Scottish doctor James Lind.

The researches of Justus von Liebig in Germany helped put the organic chemistry of digestion and nourishment on a sound footing. Liebig's pupils explored the creation of energy out of food and launched the idea of dietary balance. Notable work was done by German physiologist Wilhelm Kühne, a professor at Heidelberg from 1871, who introduced the term 'enzyme' to describe organic substances that activate chemical changes. There was a long tradition of explaining sickness in terms of absolute lack of food. Around

1900, however, a new concept was emerging: the idea of deficiency disease – the notion that a healthy diet required certain very specific chemical components. Crucial were the investigations of Christiaan Eijkman into beriberi in the Dutch East Indies. The first to produce a dietary deficiency disease experimentally (in chickens and pigeons), Eijkman proposed the concept of 'essential food factors', or roughly what would later be called vitamins. He demonstrated that the substance (now known as vitamin B_1) that gives protection against beriberi was contained in the husks of grains of rice – precisely the element removed when rice is polished. Through clinical studies on prisoners in Java, he determined that unpolished rice would cure the disorder.

Eijkman's researches were paralleled by the Cambridge biochemist Frederick Gowland Hopkins, who similarly discovered that very small amounts of certain substances found in food (his name for them was 'accessory food factors') were requisite for the body to utilize protein and energy for growth. An American physiologist, Elmer Verner McCollum, showed that certain fats contained an essential ingredient for normal growth: this provided the basic research for the understanding of what became known as vitamins A and D. In 1928, Albert von Szent-Györgyi isolated vitamin C from the adrenal glands, and it became recognized that that was the element in lemon juice that acted as an antiscorbutic. The idea of deficiency disease proved highly fruitful. In 1914, Joseph Goldberger of the US Public Health Service concluded that pellagra, with its classic pot-bellied symptoms, was not an infectious disorder but was rather caused by poor nutrition. Goldberger was able to relieve pellagra sufferers in the southern states by feeding them protein-rich foods. By the 1930s the pellagra-preventing factor was proved to be nicotinic acid (niacin), part of the B vitamin complex.

Study of nutrition could broadly be seen as part of the programme of research into the 'internal environment' launched by Claude Bernard. So, too, was another new specialty – endocrinology or the investigation of internal secretions. Its key concept was that of the hormone, which arose out of the energetic research programme in proteins and enzymes pursued at University College London, by William Bayliss and Ernest Starling. In 1902, an intestinal substance called secretin that activates the pancreas to liberate digestive fluids was the first specifically to be named a hormone (from the Greek: I excite or arouse). It opened up a new field: the study of the chemical messengers travelling from particular organs (ductless or endocrine glands) to other parts of the body in the bloodstream.

The relations between the thyroid gland, goitre (an enlargement of the gland), and cretinism (defective functioning of the gland) were early established, and surgical procedures followed (their mixed success is examined in Chapter Six). The pancreas, ovaries, testes, and the adrenals were all recognized to be endocrine glands, like the thyroid. Researchers sought to ascertain precisely what metabolic processes they controlled, and which diseases followed from their imbalances. Once it was discovered that the pancreas releases into the circulation a material contributing to the control of the blood sugar it became clear that diabetes was a hormone-deficiency disease. With a view to treating diabetes, a race followed to extract the active substance (called 'insuline' by Edward Sharpey-Schafer) produced by the 'islets of Langerhans' in the pancreas.

Attention was also given to the pituitary gland, which was recognized to secrete growth hormone. In his *The Pituitary Body and Its Disorders* (1912), an American surgeon, Harvey Cushing, showed that its abnormal functioning produced obesity (he described the sufferer as a tomato head on a potato body with four matches as limbs). As with thyroidism, surgery was used to remove the adrenal gland or the pituitary tumour. Further endocrinological researches led to the isolation of the female sex hormone, oestrone. By the 1930s the family of the oestrogens had been elucidated, as had the male sex hormone, testosterone. Twenty years later, on the basis of these discoveries, an oral contraceptive for women was developed.

Some of the most fundamental advances in the biomedical sciences have arisen with the progress of neurology. Their potential significance for medical practice is still imperfectly understood. From René Descartes onwards, the importance of the nervous system for the regulation of behaviour was acutely recognized, but speculation long outran experimentation.

Experimental neurophysiology made great strides during the nineteenth century. The series of major studies stretching from Charles Bell (after whom Bell's palsy is named) to Charles

Sherrington cannot be described here. Sherrington's book, *The Integrative Action of the Nervous System* (1906), which is often called the 'Bible of neurology', clearly established that the operation of the brain cells involved two neurones with a barrier between one cell and the next, enabling the impulse to pass with differing degrees of ease (the synapse). What remained a subject of passionate debate was how the nerve currents, identified in the work of David Ferrier, Sherrington, and others, were transmitted from nerve to nerve, across synapses, to their targets. Evidence began to accumulate that chemical as well as electrical processes were at work. The English physiologist and pharmacologist, Henry Hallett Dale, found a substance in 1914 in ergot (a fungus), which he called acetylcholine. This affected muscle response at certain nerve junctions. In 1929, Dale isolated acetylcholine from the spleens of freshly killed horses, and showed it was secreted at nerve endings after electric stimulation of motor nerve fibres. Acetylcholine was thus the chemical agent through which the nerves worked on the muscles. This was the first neurotransmitter to be identified.

Meanwhile in 1921, the German physiologist, Otto Loewi, was investigating the chemical basis of the muscular actions of the heart. He was to record that

In the night of Easter Saturday, 1921, I awoke, and jotted down a few notes on a tiny slip of paper. Then fell asleep again. It occurred to me at six o'clock in the morning, that during the night I had written down something most important, but I was unable to decipher the scrawl. That Sunday was the most desperate day in my whole scientific life. During the night, however, I woke again, and I remembered what it was. This time I did not take any risk; I got up immediately, went to the laboratory, made the experiment on the frog's heart . . . and at five o'clock the chemical transmission of nerve impulses was conclusively proved.[4]

Loewi's experiments showed that the heart, when stimulated, secreted a substance directly responsible for certain muscular actions: this was the enzyme cholinesterase, a chemical inhibitor that interrupted the acetylcholine stimulator and produced the nerve impulse pattern.

Further work brought to light numerous other chemical agents that were found at work in the nervous system. At Harvard University, Walter Cannon identified the stimulative role of adrenaline, and this led to a classification of nerves according to their transmitter substances. More research provided evidence of monamines in the central nervous system, including noradrenaline, dopamine, and serotonin.

The transmitter–inhibitor pattern thus became known, stimulating fresh work on controlling or correcting basic problems in brain function. For instance, the action of tetanus and botulism on the nervous system could for the first time be explained. Parkinson's disease, a degenerative nervous condition identified in the nineteenth century, was considered largely untreatable until it was associated with chemical transmission in the nervous system. In the late 1960s, however, it was discovered that the adrenergic side could be stimulated with L-dopa, a drug that enhances dopamine in the central nervous system and acts on the precursor of noradrenaline, presumed to be the transmitter substance. Every further development in the understanding of neurotransmission and the chemicals involved therein opens new prospects for the control and cure of neurological disorders.

One other dimension of modern science and its medical applications that must be mentioned here is genetics. The establishment of Darwin's theory of evolution by natural selection inevitably gave prominence to the component of inheritance in human development. But Darwin himself lacked a satisfactory theory of inheritance, and specious concepts of degenerationism and eugenics achieved great and sometimes lethal consequence before modern genetics became soundly established from the 1930s.

Valuable advances were achieved, early in the twentieth century, in demonstrating the hereditary component of metabolic disorders. Archibald Edward Garrod, a physician at St Bartholomew's Hospital in London, investigated what he first called *Inborn Errors of Metabolism* (1909), using as a model for this concept alkaptonuria, an inherited metabolic disorder in which an acid is excreted in quantities in the urine. The real breakthrough came when the infant subdiscipline of molecular biology paved the way for the elucidation of the double-helical structure of DNA in 1953 by Francis Crick and James Watson, working at the Medical Research Council's laboratory in Cambridge. The cracking of the genetic code has in turn led to the Human Genome Project, set up in 1986 with the goal of mapping all human genetic material. Opinion remains divided as to whether this project will reveal that more diseases than conventionally thought have a genetic basis. Many believe that the next enormous medical breakthroughs will lie in the field of genetic engineering. In the meantime, a combination of clinical studies and laboratory research has firmly established the genetic component in disorders such as cystic fibrosis and Huntington's chorea. The latter was shown to run in families as long ago as 1872 by the American physician, George Huntington.

Clinical Science in the Twentieth Century

It is clear that the scientific pursuit of medical knowledge has undergone structural shifts during the past hundred years. Early nineteenth-century French medical science developed in the hospital, and German medical science pioneered the laboratory. New sites have emerged in more recent times to create and sustain clinical science. In some cases, this has meant special units set up by philanthropic trusts or by government. A key initiative in encouraging clinical research in the USA was the foundation in 1904 of the Rockefeller Institute for Medical Research in New York. Although the institute was at first entirely devoted to basic scientific studies, from the start the intention was to set up a small hospital alongside it, to be devoted to research in the clinic. The hospital was opened in 1910.

A vital influence on clinical research in the USA was Abraham Flexner's report on medical education, published in 1910. Flexner, educationalist brother of Simon Flexner, the first director of the Rockefeller Institute, drew attention to the parlous situation of many medical schools. An enthusiastic supporter of the German model then developing at Johns Hopkins in Baltimore, Flexner considered that there were only five US institutions that could be regarded as true centres of medical research – Harvard and Johns Hopkins, and the universities of Pennsylvania, Chicago, and Michigan. Soon after the publication of the Flexner report, the Rockefeller Foundation made funds available to Johns Hopkins for the establishment of full-time chairs in clinical subjects. This innovation spread throughout the USA, so that by the mid-1920s there were twenty institutions that could match the best in Europe. The system received a further boost with the foundation in 1948 of the National Institutes of Health. Research grants were awarded to clinical departments, which grew enormously.

Since the First World War, American clinical research has been notable both for quantity and for quality. The award of Nobel Prizes may be taken as some index. No British clinical research worker has won a Nobel Prize since Sir Ronald Ross, who won it in 1902 for the discovery of the role of the mosquito in the transmission of malaria. Nevertheless, numerous British individuals have made internationally recognized contributions to clinical research in the twentieth century, among them James Mackenzie, who pioneered the use of the polygraph for recording the pulse and its relationship to cardiovascular disease. His work was particularly important in distinguishing atrial fibrillation and in treating this common condition with digitalis. His *Diseases of the Heart* (1908) summarized his vast experience, although he never properly appreciated the possibilities of the electrocardiograph, then being taken up by the more technologically minded Thomas Lewis.

Thomas Lewis has been dubbed the architect of British clinical research. Born in Cardiff, Lewis went in 1902 to University College Hospital (London), where he remained as student, teacher, and consultant until his death. He was the first completely to master the use of the electrocardiogram. Through animal experiments he was able to correlate the various electrical waves recorded by an electrocardiograph with the sequence of events during a contraction of the heart, which enabled him to use the instrument as a diagnostic tool when the heart had disturbances of its rhythm, damage to its valves, or changes due to high blood pressure, arteriosclerosis, and other conditions. In later life, Lewis turned his attention to the physiology of cutaneous blood vessels and the mechanisms of pain, conducting experiments on himself in an attempt to work out the distribution of pain fibres in the nervous system and to understand patterns of referred pain.

Lewis fought for full-time clinical research posts to investigate what he called 'clinical science', a broadening of his interests signalled when in 1933 he changed the name of the journal he had founded in 1909 from *Heart* to *Clinical Science*. By the early

1930s, Lewis had become the most influential figure in British clinical research, and his department at University College Hospital was the Mecca for aspiring clinical research workers. He claimed that 'Clinical science has as good a claim to the name and rights of self-subsistence of a science as any other department of biology'.[5]

Britain lagged behind the USA in the funding and organization of medical research. Before the First World War, the medical schools, especially in London, were private and rather disorganized institutions, and there was little encouragement of clinical research. A Royal Commission on University Education in London initiated changes that led to the establishment of modern academic departments in clinical subjects with an emphasis on research. By 1925 five chairs of medicine were established among the twelve medical schools in London.

In the UK, financing of clinical research has come from two main sources – a government-funded agency, the Medical Research Council, and from medical charities, such as the Imperial Cancer Research Fund, the British Heart Foundation, and the Wellcome Trust. From its foundation in 1913, the Medical Research Committee – to become the Medical Research Council (MRC) in 1920 – sought to encourage 'pure' science and also clinical research and experimental medicine. The MRC also made other major contributions to clinical research, supporting, for example, Thomas Lewis in London.

In the immediate post-war era, the MRC was involved in two vital innovations in clinical research. The first was the introduction of the randomized controlled clinical trial. Advised by Austin Bradford Hill, professor of medical statistics and epidemiology at the London School of Tropical Medicine and Hygiene, in 1946 the council set up a trial of the efficacy of streptomycin in the treatment of pulmonary tuberculosis. The drug was in short supply and it was considered ethically justifiable to carry out a trial in which one group received streptomycin whereas a control group was treated with traditional methods. The MRC trial emphasized the importance of randomization in selecting subjects for study. This, the first randomized controlled trial to be reported in human subjects, served as a model for other such studies.

The second major development was the application of epidemiology to the analysis of clinical problems. The MRC set up a conference to discuss rising mortality from lung cancer. The MRC enlisted the aid of Bradford Hill and in 1948 he recruited the young Richard Doll, later Regius Professor of Medicine at Oxford University, to join him in analysing possible causes of lung cancer. Their painstaking survey of patients from twenty London hospitals showed that smoking is a factor, and an important factor, in the production of cancer of the lung. They went on to establish that the same conclusion applied nationally and, in an important study of members of the medical profession, they demonstrated that mortality from the disease fell if individuals stopped smoking.

These observations were not only important in showing the cause of a commonly occurring cancer in Britain, and subsequently in other countries such as the USA, but also in establishing the position of epidemiology in clinical research. As this last example shows, medical science now knows no bounds; its methods and scope sweep from the laboratory to the social survey, in helping to forge an understanding of the wider parameters of disease.

6. Hospitals and Surgery

Roy Porter

Today, surgery and hospitals go hand in glove. Without hospitals, no advanced surgery is possible; without surgery, or at least without a battery of invasive treatments, the hospital would lose its unique place in the medical system. These reciprocal ties reflect modern medical realities, but they provide a wholly misleading picture of the past.

Before 1700, the connections between hospitals and the surgeon's art were slight. The genesis of the hospital had little to do with the meeting of surgical needs; and the rise of surgery owed nothing to any special facilities that hospitals could provide. For centuries, surgery was performed on the kitchen table, on the field of battle, or below deck on the warship. In the eighteenth century and, above all, from around 1850, however, hospitals and surgery grew inseparable: they were destined to become utterly interdependent.

Traditional Surgery

Although the surgical art did not undergo revolution until the nineteenth century, surgery is almost as old as humanity. In antiquity and during the Middle Ages, surgeons performed a multitude of minor palliative services, such as lancing boils or bandaging wounds. Before 1850, however, serious surgical operations had to be short and sharp, although they were rarely sweet. Typically, they dealt with the exterior and the extremities while avoiding (except in the direst emergency, as with caesarian section) the abdomen and other body cavities and the central nervous system.

Archaeology reveals early surgical interventions. Evidence from skulls proves that trepanning was practised at least as early as 10,000 BC. Operators – they may have been shamans – used stone cutting tools to extract portions of the cranium to ease pressure created by depressed skull fracture, or to deliver sufferers from some tormenting 'devil' that had taken possession of the soul. Bonesetting and amputations were performed from early times, although these involved severe risks of haemorrhage, infection, and shock. Egyptian medical papyri dating from the second millennium BC refer to surgical procedures for abscesses and minor tumours as well as disorders of the ear, eye, and teeth.

The Hippocratic writings produced in Greece in the fifth and fourth centuries BC contain much that relates to surgery, including a treatise on wounds (*De Ulceribus*) and another on head injuries (*De Capitis Vulneribus*). In the latter, five different types of injury are recognized and trepanning is described: fractures are to be treated by reduction and immobilization with splints and bandages; the knife is to be used for excising nasal polyps and ulcerated tonsils; and cautery is recommended for haemorrhoids. In general, however, the picture that emerges is conservative: amputation of gangrenous tissue is accepted as a last resort. Catheterization is advocated for bladder stone; the removal of stones (lithotomy) is to be left to 'such as are craftsmen therein'. Vascular ligature was apparently unknown to the Greeks.

Hippocratic recommendations for the treatment of wounds proved influential for centuries. The theory was that suppuration was indispensable for healing to take place, because it was believed that pus derived from vitiated blood. This formed the basis for the later influential doctrine of 'laudable pus'.

The Hippocratic Oath stated that physicians should leave surgical interventions to others: this separation formed part of a medical division of labour, but surgery was also clearly viewed as an inferior trade, it being the work of the hand rather than the head. This is reflected in its name: the word 'surgery' derives from the Latin *chirurgia*, which comes from the Greek *cheiros* (hand) and *ergon* (work). Certain Greek physicians paid attention to surgery.

Soranus of Ephesus wrote extensively on obstetrics, discussing the use of the birthing-chair and giving instructions for difficult birth positions. Where the fetus was in a transverse position, for instance, he performed the procedure that was later called 'turning the foot' (podalic version), easing a hand into the womb and pulling down a leg, so that the baby would be born feet first. New operations gradually appeared in the literature. In the first century AD, Celsus gave the first full account of lithotomy.

Paul of Aegina in the seventh century, and al-Zahrawi (Albucasis) and lbn Sina (Avicenna), the illustrious Islamic physicians of the late tenth and early eleventh centuries, discussed cauterizing with a red-hot iron to stop bleeding. The Hippocratic *Corpus* and Celsus had earlier recommended cautery as a means of hindering putrefaction. In his great book, *Altasrif* (Collections), Albucasis discussed a multitude of surgical operations, but placed the greatest faith in cautery.

In the medieval West, the Salernitan school of medicine, which flourished in Salerno in southern Italy from the eleventh century, paid great attention to surgical handicraft, notably the treatment of skull wounds. It introduced the idea of dry wound management, a notion expanded in the distinguished treatises on surgery by the Frenchmen Henri de Mondeville and Guy de Chauliac, whose *Grande Chirurgie* (1363) – for two centuries the most influential textbook – contained discussion of the management of infected wounds. The importance of wound cleansing and closure was stressed, and the old doctrine of 'laudable pus' questioned: dissenting from orthodoxy, Guy de Chauliac suggested that wounds healed faster without pus formation.

Traditional surgery was performed by regular barber surgeons, for whom hair-cutting and shaving provided a solid day-to-day income. It was also undertaken by itinerants, often called quacks, specializing in one particular (and often intricate or hazardous) operation. Up to the nineteenth century there were itinerant tooth-drawers, precursors of modern dentists; travelling oculists would couch for the cataract; and lithotomists removed bladder stones. Surgical treatment of hernia was likewise long in the hands of such 'empirics' (regular licensed surgeons might be loath to handle hernia, in view of the almost inevitable castration that accompanied it). Itinerant 'hernia masters' were active until the eighteenth century.

From the sixteenth century, however, surgery was showing signs of becoming more methodical. Ambroise Paré, a towering figure, had sections of Vesalius's *De Humani Corporis Fabrica* (1543) translated into French as part of his *Anatomie universelle du Corps humain* (1561), to make the superior anatomical teachings of the Paduan professor available to barber-surgeons who had no Latin. Born in 1510 in northern France, Paré was apprenticed to a barber-surgeon and then saw extensive military service. Many of the treatments described in his *Oeuvres*, published in 1585 when he was seventy-five, were developed as a result of experience with battle-field wounds. The most important of these were the Paré ligature and his development of a substitute for hot-oil cauterizing of open wounds. As related in his *La Méthode de Traicter les Playes Faictes par Hacquebutes* (Method of Treating Wounds) of 1545, Paré concocted an ointment (or 'digestive') from egg yolk, rose oil, and turpentine, which he applied to the wound. The mixture proved successful. Wounds treated with Paré's digestive were less painful, did not swell up, and generally remained uninflamed. Concluding that gunshot wounds did not automatically require cautery – this should be reserved for gangrenous wounds or used as a means of stopping bleeding in infected wounds – Paré abandoned the hot-oil treatment.

Tudor and Stuart England also had competent surgeons. John Woodall's *The Surgeon's Mate* (1617) long served as a manual of naval surgery, and Richard Wiseman became known as the 'father of English surgery'. His *Several Chirurgical Treatises* (1676) dwelt particularly on military and naval surgery, while his *Treatise of Wounds* (1672) advertised itself as being specially intended for ships' doctors 'who seldom burden their cabin with many books'. Nevertheless, wound treatment retained a weird-and-wonderful penumbra. There was much ado, for instance, in the seventeenth century about the 'wound salve' developed by Sir Kenelm Digby and others. Designed to heal rapier wounds, this was an odd mixture of earthworms, iron oxide, pig brain, powdered mummy, and so forth. The salve was applied not to the wound but to the weapon that caused it. The idea clearly traded on magic.

Before the introduction of anaesthesia in the 1840s, all invasive surgery depended on the swift hand, sharp knife, and cool nerve of the operator, so as to minimize pain. Operations that were slow or demanded great precision were beyond the range of early surgeons. A few highly dangerous operations were performed, however, in dire emergency. One of the most controversial was caesarean section, which many authorities, Ambrose Paré included, believed was inevitably fatal. The first properly documented caesarian section was performed in 1610 by Jeremiah Trautman in the German town of Wittenberg. In 1689, in the French town of Saintes, Jean Ruleau performed a successful caesarian on a woman who could not give birth normally because of rickets. There is no record till the 1790s of a successful caesarian being performed in Britain with the mother surviving.

In such circumstances, the bulk of the traditional surgeon's work remained routine, small scale, and fairly safe (if often awesomely painful). It involved everyday therapeutics such as dressing wounds, drawing teeth, dealing with the chancres and sores of venereal disease (common from the sixteenth century), treating skin blemishes, and so forth. The most common surgical procedure – one that served as a symbol of the profession – was bloodletting, often performed at the patient's request. The normal method for bleeding (professionally known as 'venesection' or 'phlebotomy') was to tie a bandage around the arm to make the veins in the forearm swell up, and then open the exposed vein with a lancet: this was popularly called 'breathing a vein'. Cupping was another much-used procedure for drawing blood – it was also used to draw boils and similar eruptions; leeches have often been popular for the same purpose. Bleeding agreed with humoral doctrines, especially the theory of plethora – the idea that such illnesses as fevers, apoplexy, or headache followed from an excessive build-up of blood. As so often in the history of therapeutics, the 'cure' long outlived its original theoretical rationale, remaining ubiquitous, alongside purging and vomiting, until the mid-nineteenth century.

The Traditional Hospital

Although medically advanced, classical Greece had no hospitals. In Hippocratic times, a patient might occasionally be treated in the home of a physician or at shrines of Asclepius, the Greek healing god. In the Roman Empire, there were also facilities, termed valetudinaria, for the relief of slaves and soldiers and the provision of hospitality for wayfarers. There is no evidence, however, of buildings devoted to treatment of the sick among the population in general until well into the Christian era.

It is no accident that the triumph of the Christian faith brought the rise of nursing and the invention of the hospital as an institution of health care. Christ had performed healing miracles, giving sight to the blind and driving out devils from the insane. Charity was the supreme Christian virtue. In the name of love, service, and salvation, believers were enjoined to care for those in need – the destitute, handicapped, poor, and hungry, those without shelter, and the sick. Once the conversion of Constantine (died AD 337) made Christianity an official imperial religion, 'hospitals' sprang up as pious foundations, and with them religious orders dedicated to serving fellow humans.

Thus a hospital was founded in 390 by Fabiola, a convert to Christianity who dedicated the rest of her life to charity. A wealthy woman, she mixed among the sick and poor of Rome. Her teacher, Jerome, wrote that she

sold all that she could lay her hands on of her property (it was large and suitable to her rank), and turning it into money she laid out this for the benefit of the poor. She was the first person to found a hospital, into which she might gather sufferers out of the streets, and where she might nurse the unfortunate victims of sickness and want. Need I now recount the various ailments of human beings? Need I speak of noses slit, eyes put out, feet half burnt, hands covered with sores? Or of limbs dropsical and atrophied? Or of diseased flesh alive with worms? Often did she carry on her own shoulders persons infected with jaundice or with filth. Often too did she wash away the matter discharged from wounds which others, even though men, could not bear to look at. She gave food to her patients with her own hand, and moistened the scarce breathing lips of the dying with sips of liquid.[1]

This ideal of nursing and healing as an act of Christian charity remained influential throughout the Middle Ages, giving impetus to the foundation of hospitals.

Some hospitals were outgrowths of religious houses: after all, monasteries themselves needed medical facilities to tend sick brethren. Throughout the medieval centuries, thousands of such institutions were established by pious bequest under the rule of regular religious orders. These 'hospitals' (the term 'hospice' may sound more appropriate to our ears) were often ephemeral, and they were generally modest, with perhaps a dozen beds and a couple of brethren in charge.

Things were different in major cities, where hospitals put down more permanent roots. By the seventh century, there were some hospitals in Constantinople (then the capital of the Roman Empire) that were sufficiently well established to offer separate wards for men and women, and special rooms for surgical patients and for eye cases. The foundation charter (1136) of the Pantokrator hospital in Constantinople assumed that medical teaching would be offered within the hospital. From the tenth century, there were multifunctioned hospitals ('bimaristans') in Cairo, Baghdad, Damascus, and other Islamic cities. Some supported medical teaching. In the early medieval centuries, Byzantium and the Levant were far more medically developed than Latin Europe.

In the Christian West, provision of hospitals expanded from the twelfth century with the growth of population, trade, and towns. Medieval hospitals remained frequently associated with a church or monastery, and life within them was organized around the religious offices. It was more important to ensure that patients died in a state of grace, having received the sacraments, than to attempt heroic medical treatments to prolong temporal life. In medieval England and throughout the rural parts of continental Europe, hospices routinely provided care and hospitality for the indigent, elderly, infirm, and for pilgrims, without predominately being devoted to the sick.

In the twelfth and thirteenth centuries, hundreds of leper asylums were built. By 1225 there were around 19,000 such leprosaria in Europe. A high wall would separate the leprosary from the community, while small huts within provided shelter for the sick. As leprosy declined, the leprosaria were used for persons suspected of carrying infectious diseases, the insane, and even the indigent. Some became hospitals. Thus the Hôpital des Petits Maisons near the monastery of St Germain des Près outside Paris, which began as a leprosarium, was later used for indigent syphilitics and disordered pilgrims. St Giles in the Fields, west of the walls of London, was originally a leprosarium.

When bubonic plague struck Europe in the fourteenth century, the leprosaria were requisitioned as the first plague hospitals. Lazarettos (named after the protective patron, St Lazarus) began to be built in the later years of the century, to safeguard trade and to protect city populations. The first documented pesthouse was built at Dubrovnik (Ragusa) on the Adriatic coast of Croatia in 1377, followed by an infirmary in Marseilles in 1383. Venice built two lazarettos on islands of its lagoon in 1423 and 1468, respectively. Milan completed a pesthouse 20 years later, and the hospital of St Sebastian, built in Nuremberg in 1498, became the model for later German plague hospitals.

It was in Italian cities – Venice, Bologna, Florence, Naples, and Rome – that the most distinguished medieval hospitals were established. Unlike small rural foundations, hospitals in the major Italian cities often had a resident medical staff. In Italian urban centres, hospitals played a key part in caring for the poor and sick. Religious confraternities took upon themselves the duty of charity, and some administered hospitals. Severe plague outbreaks and other epidemics spurred the foundation of hospitals, so that by the fifteenth century there were thirty-three hospitals in Florence alone – roughly one for every 1,000 inhabitants. The size of these varied enormously, from under ten beds to 230 at S. Maria Nuova (founded in 1288), the largest and most eminent. These Florentine hospitals were primarily for orphans, pilgrims, widows, and the teeming poor; only seven were principally dedicated to the sick, but these did have medical staffs attached to them. At S. Maria Nuova there were six visiting physicians, a surgeon, and three junior staff members in the fourteenth century.

In England, there were about 470 'hospitals' by the close of the fourteenth century, but they were generally tiny and barely medical. Numbers of inmates varied from around two or three to about thirty, with an average of about ten. Only in London were there hospitals of any significance. The dissolution of the monasteries and chantries during the reformations of Henry VIII and

Edward VI (1536–52) brought the closure of practically all such foundations, and the Crown seized their assets. A handful were re-established, however, on a new and secular basis. St Bartholomew's (founded 1123) and St Thomas's (founded around 1215), Christ's Hospital, and Bethlem (both thirteenth-century foundations) were sold by the Crown to the corporation of the City of London. St Thomas's and St Bartholomew's expanded as hospitals for the sick poor, and Bethlem catered for the mad. Nevertheless, although Stuart London grew into a monster city – it had more than half a million people by 1700, making it, with Paris, the largest city in Europe – it had just two medical hospitals of any consequence. And beyond the capital, there were no medical hospitals at all in England in 1700.

In Catholic countries, no equivalent of the reformation of Henry VIII asset-stripped the hospitals, and in Spain, France, and Italy foundations grew in numbers in the sixteenth and seventeenth centuries in response to an increase in population. Religious and lay elements in the hospitals generally worked well together, although conflicts sometimes arose between physicians, with their medical priorities, and the nursing staff, with their pious ends. Charitable donations to hospitals played a part in local chains of protection, patronage, and family power. In France, the *hôpital général* (similar to the English poorhouse) emerged in the seventeenth century as an institution designed to shelter – or rather confine – beggars, orphans, vagabonds, prostitutes, and thieves, alongside the sick and mad. The Hôtel Dieu in Paris was more specifically designed as a healing institution; this was run by religious orders.

Perhaps the jewel amongst continental hospitals in the eighteenth century was Vienna's Allgemeines Krankenhaus (general hospital), rebuilt by the Emperor Joseph II in 1784. In the time-honoured manner, the Vienna hospital sheltered the poor as well as providing medical facilities for the sick. Planned for 1,600 patients, it was divided into six medical, four surgical, and four clinical sections; eighty-six clinical beds met the teaching needs of its medical staff. As part of Joseph II's grand design for modernizing the Habsburg Empire, provincial hospitals were also built in Olmütz (1787), Linz (1788), and Prague (1789). New infirmaries were also set up in other German-speaking territories, including the

Juliusspital at Würzburg (1789), which won praise for its operating theatre. Berlin's Charité Hospital was built in 1768, and, in the Ukraine, Catherine the Great (1762–96) erected the huge Obukhov Hospital.

Although by European standards early-modern England was exceptionally ill-endowed with hospitals – and also with sister institutions such as orphanages – this lamentable state of affairs changed rapidly in the Age of Enlightenment when philanthropy, secular and religious, raised many new foundations. The new hospitals founded in eighteenth-century England were meant for the poor (although not for parish paupers, who would be dealt with under the Poor Law). Granting free care to the respectable or deserving sick poor would, it was hoped, confirm social ties of paternalism, deference, and gratitude.

London benefited earliest. To the metropolis's two ancient hospitals, a further five were added between 1720 and 1750: the Westminster (1720), Guy's (1724), St George's (1733), the London (1740), and the Middlesex (1745). All were general hospitals. They stirred the founding of institutions in the provinces, where no genuinely medical hospitals had existed at all. The Edinburgh Royal Infirmary was set up in 1729, followed by hospitals in Winchester and Bristol (1737), York (1740), Exeter (1741), Bath (1742), Northampton (1743), and some twenty others. By 1800, all sizeable English towns had a hospital. Traditional cathedral and corporation cities came first, industrial towns, such as Sheffield and Hull, followed.

Augmenting these general foundations, humanitarians also pumped money into specialist institutions for the sick. St Luke's Hospital was opened in London in 1751, making it at that time the only large public lunatic asylum apart from Bethlem. Unlike Bethlem, criticized for its barbarity, St Luke's was launched to an optimistic fanfare, its physician, William Battie, asserting that, if handled with humanity, lunacy was no less curable than any other disease. By 1800, other great towns such as Manchester, Liverpool, and York had public lunatic asylums, philanthropically supported. Alongside lunatics, sufferers from venereal disease also became objects for charity – surely a sign of a changing climate of opinion: the harsh religious judgment that such diseases were salutary punishment for vice was evidently on the wane, being supplanted by the Enlightenment view that relief of suffering was the duty of humanity. London's Lock Hospital, exclusively for venereal cases, opened in 1746. It was paralleled by another London charitable foundation, the Magdalene Hospital for Penitent Prostitutes (1759) – less a medical hospital than a refuge where harlots wishing to go straight were taught a trade.

Another new institution was the lying-in hospital. In London, the earliest maternity hospitals were the British (1749), the City (1750), the General (1752), and the Westminster (1765). These met major needs, not least by guaranteeing bed-rest to impoverished women. They also enabled unmarried mothers, mainly servant girls, to deliver their illegitimate babies with no questions asked. Many newborns then ended up in the Foundling Hospital in Bloomsbury, opened in 1741. Unwanted children could be deposited there anonymously; they would be educated and taught a trade. The benevolent designs of lying-in hospitals were thwarted, however, by the appalling death rates of mothers and babies alike from what would later be identified as bacterial infections. Nevertheless, they served as sites where medical students could practise obstetric skills.

General hospitals provided treatment, food, shelter, and opportunities for convalescence. By 1800, London's hospitals alone were handling more than 20,000 patients a year. But, as with hospitals abroad, they restricted themselves to fairly minor complaints likely to respond to treatment, and they excluded infectious cases. Nothing useful could have been gained by allowing fevers into the hospital: they could not be cured and were sure to spread like wildfire. Separate fever hospitals were, however, set up for those with contagious diseases. London's first fever hospital (euphemistically called the House of Recovery) was opened in 1801. Another new means of healing was the outpatient department, and dispensaries were also founded.

Similar developments took place in North America. The first general hospital was founded in Philadelphia in 1751; some 20 years later the New York Hospital was established. The Massachusetts General Hospital in Boston followed in 1811. All such hospitals catered for the sick poor.

The Start of Clinical Rounds

In the eighteenth century, hospitals increasingly opened themselves to medical students, and teachers used instructive cases on their doorstep as training material. In Vienna, the hospital reforms carried through in the 1770s by Anton Stoerck led to clinical instruction on the wards. The success of the Edinburgh Medical School owed much to its links with the city's infirmary. Professor John Rutherford inaugurated clinical lecturing there in the 1740s, and from 1750 a special clinical ward was set up, whose patients served as teaching material for professorial clinical lectures. 'A number of such cases as are likely to prove instructive', noted the medical student, John Aikin, in the 1770s, 'are selected and disposed in separate rooms in the Infirmary, and attended by one of the college professors. The students go round with him every day, and mark down the state of each patient and the medicines prescribed. At certain times lectures are read upon these cases, in which all the progressive changes in the disease are traced and explained and the method of practice is accounted for.'[2] Students were expected to visit patients' bedsides on their own initiative, studying the professors' reports.

Initially, English infirmaries had little to do with teaching. The leading London surgeon-anatomist, William Cheselden, started private surgical lectures in 1711; but in 1718 he moved his lectures to St Thomas's, delivering four courses a year. Clinical instruction was set up, and students were encouraged to follow their teachers round the wards and into the operating theatre. The practice spread. The Philadelphian William Shippen attended London's hospitals in 1759, and recorded in his journal,

[4 August] saw Mr. Way surgeon to Guy's hospital amputate a leg above the knee very dexterously 8 ligatures...[23 August] attended Dr Akenside in taking in patients and prescribing for them, 58 taken in...[5 September]...saw Mr Baker perform 3 operations, a leg, breast and tumour from a girl's lower jaw inside, very well operated...[7 November] went to Bartholomew's Hospital and saw the neatest operation of bubonocele that I ever saw by Mr. Pott a very clever neat surgeon.[3]

Such accounts show that contemporaries believed that surgical treatment in hospital was improving.

Pupils became a more conspicuous presence in provincial hospitals, and student training was essential to specialist institutions such as maternity hospitals. One such, London's New General Lying-In Hospital, admitted students as pupils to the attending *accoucheurs*, as male midwives were called. As a result of all this, by 1800 London was, according to Bristol physician Thomas Beddoes, 'the best spot in Great Britain, and probably in the whole world where medicine may be taught as well as cultivated to most advantage'.[4]

Religious Nursing Orders

Hospital nursing had long been provided by religious orders as part of the Christian service ideal – and nursing remained largely the business of religious orders in Catholic Europe until recent times. All monastic orders were charged with caring for God's poor, which included the sick, and each monastery or convent had an *infirmarius* or *infirmaria* who oversaw the infirmary and, with the help of assistants, ministered to the sick. During the Crusades, the Knights of St John of Jerusalem (later called the Knights of Malta, and the progenitor of the St John Ambulance Brigade), the Teutonic Knights, the Knights Templar, and the Knights of St Lazarus were active in nursing as well as hospital building. In seventeenth-century France, a priest, Vincent de Paul, set up the Daughters of Charity primarily as a nursing order.

In the French Revolution, however, as part of the wholesale attack on the Church, religious nursing communities were abolished and charities were nationalized. Revolutionaries confiscated the coffers of religious foundations. In the event, however, political indecision, corruption, and rampant inflation led to a spectacular reduction in the welfare and hospital services being provided for the needy. By choice and necessity, Napoleon largely reverted to the *status quo ante*, with hospitals being financed by pious donations and staffed by religious orders, above all the Daughters of Charity, who flourished in the nineteenth century. Provision of nursing was much more hit-and-miss in Protestant countries. In Georgian England, the stereotypical nurse was a drunken, slovenly battle-axe.

Campaigns for Hospital Reform

If nursing left much to be desired, the hospital itself, nominally a site of recuperation, readily became a place of disease and death, spreading the maladies it was meant to relieve. The eighteenth century, however, brought campaigns for hospital reform, as part of a broad critique front of outmoded, corrupt, and unhealthy institutions. Moved by humanity, the English philanthropist John Howard turned in his last years from prison reform to the remodelling of hospitals; his extensive travels spread reform on the Continent. He was particularly insistent on the need for cleanliness and fresh air to combat the deadly miasmic effluvia that he and others blamed for sickness and shocking mortality figures in gaols and hospitals.

The medical profession itself was not indifferent to hospital reform. When Louis XVI invited the Académie des Sciences to take up hospital reform, a distinguished surgeon, Jacques Tenon, was sent to visit England. Impressed with the Royal Naval Hospital in Plymouth, and the through-ventilation permitted by its pavilion style, he returned to Paris with noble visions of new buildings. But little came of these rebuilding plans, as the Revolution distrusted hospitals, seeing them as agents of religious indoctrination and oligarchic power. The direct effect of the French Revolution on healing institutions was negative.

Surgery Rises in Status

Surgery rose in quality and status in Europe during the eighteenth century. For centuries called 'the cutter's art' and disparaged as a manual skill rather than a liberal science, surgery had been subordinate to physic in the medical pecking-order. Surgeons had normally passed not through an academic but a practical education, via apprenticeship not the university. Organized in trade guilds, surgery traditionally carried little status. It could be portrayed as demeaning and defiling; for unlike the clean-handed, bewigged, and perfumed physician, surgeons were habitually dealing with diseased and decaying flesh – tumours, wens (cysts), fractures, gangrene, syphilitic chancres, and such like. Their instruments were terrifying – the knife, cauterizing irons, the amputating saw: they were satirically compared to butchers or torturers.

Butts of satire amongst contemporaries, in the days before anaesthesia, surgeons have traditionally received a bad press from historians, who have tended to represent Old Mr Sawbones as a blundering and bloody operator. The caricature, however, tells but a partial truth, and recent studies of the surgeon's day-to-day trade in the seventeenth and eighteenth centuries have been painting a different picture. The spectacular and frequently lethal operations such as amputations or trepanning on which historians have dwelt were, in truth, the exception rather than the rule. The main business of the average surgeon was minor running-repairs: bloodletting, pulling teeth, managing whitlows, trussing ruptures, treating leg ulcers, patching up fistulas, medicating venereal infections, and so forth. The traditional surgeon had to attend to scores of external conditions requiring routine maintenance through cleansing, pus removal, ointments, and bandaging. The conditions he treated were mostly not life-threatening, nor were his interventions glamorous.

Studies of ordinary surgeons have shown low fatality rates amongst surgeons who sensibly respected their limits. The scope of internal operative surgery they undertook was narrow, because they were well aware of the risks: trauma, blood loss, and sepsis. A dextrous eighteenth-century surgeon would extract bladder stones or extirpate cancerous tumours from the breast. In 1810, the novelist Fanny Burney was cut, without anaesthetic, for cancer of the breast by the great French surgeon Dominique-Jean Larrey, and she survived – although not without experiencing excruciating pain, as this extract from her detailed account of the operation shows:

M. Dubois placed me upon the Mattress, & spread a cambric handerchief upon my face. It was transparent, however, & I saw, through it that the Bed stead was instantly surrounded by the 7 men and my nurse, I refused to be held; but when, bright through the cambric, I saw the glitter of polished steel – I closed my eyes . . .

Yet – when the dreadful steel was plunged into the breast – cutting through veins – arteries – flesh – nerves – I needed no injunctions not to restrain my cries. I began a scream that lasted unintermittingly during the whole time of the incision – & I almost marvel that it rings not in my Ears still! so excruciating was the agony. When the wound was made, & the instrument was withdrawn, the pain seemed undiminished, for the air that suddenly rushed into those delicate parts felt like a mass of minute but sharp & forked poniards, that were tearing the edges of the wound, – but when again I felt the instrument – describing a curve – cutting against the grain, if I may so say, while the flesh resisted in a manner so forcible as to oppose & tire the hand of the operator, who was forced to change from the right to the left – then, indeed, I thought I must have expired, I attempted no more to open my eyes... The instrument this second time withdrawn, I concluded the operation over – Oh no! presently the terrible cutting was renewed – & worse than ever, to separate the bottom, the foundation of this dreadful gland from the parts to which it adhered... yet again all was not over...[5]

Exploration of the abdominal cavity was strictly for the future. Malfunctions of the heart, liver, brain, and stomach were treated not by the knife but by medicines and management; major internal surgery was not contemplated before the introduction of anaesthetics and antiseptic procedures. Only after 1800 did surgeons begin to perform hysterectomies and other gynaecological surgery, and even then the more conservative members of the profession disapproved of such 'recklessness'.

Improvements were arising, however, in certain surgical fields. Take the treatment of bladder stones. A common traditional procedure, known as the 'apparatus major', had involved dilating and incising the urethra to allow the introduction of instruments to extract the stone. A superior method was introduced around 1700 by the itinerant practitioner, Jacques de Beaulieu, popularly called Frère Jacques (he wore the habit of a Franciscan friar to ensure safety on his travels). This lateral cystotomy involved cutting into the perineum and opening up both bladder and bladder neck. Frère Jacques is said to have performed some 4,500 lithotomies and 2,000 hernia operations.

Two distinguished surgeons, Johannes Rau in Amsterdam and William Cheselden in London, took up Frère Jacques's method with significant success. Cheselden won fame for performing lithotomy with exceptional rapidity – he could complete the excruciatingly painful knifework in 2 minutes flat, whereas other surgeons might take 20. As a result, he commanded huge fees, apparently up to

500 guineas a patient. This example reveals a situation common in early modern medicine: innovations first introduced by itinerants or quacks (who could afford to be daring: they had nothing to lose) in time found their way into regular practice. The same applies to hernia; traditionally the speciality of travelling itinerants, hernia was increasingly dealt with by regular surgeons, aided by truss-making improvements.

Other operations also underwent refinement. A celebrated French military surgeon, Jean-Louis Petit, developed new practices with amputations at the thigh, inventing an effective tourniquet that controlled bloodflow while the surgeon carried out ligatures as recommended by Ambroise Paré. He also demonstrated the spread of breast cancer to a woman's regional lymph glands in the armpit. Military surgery advanced, too, especially the management of gun-shot wounds. Endemic warfare and immense colonial and naval expansion created insatiable demands for junior surgeons willing to serve abroad or aboard ship. By the early eighteenth century the British fleet had 247 vessels, each carrying a surgeon and mate. For those with strong stomachs, like the surgeon-hero of Tobias Smollett's novel, *Roderick Random* (1748), naval or military service provided boundless experience and a valuable leg-up into the profession.

Specialist surgeons pioneered new techniques. By 1700 it was recognized that cataract involved a hardening of the lens. A French oculist, Jacques Daviel, discovered a method of extracting the lens of the eye once it had become opaque through cataract, performing the operation several hundred times with good results. Also skilled at the same operation was the British quack oculist, John ('Chevalier') Taylor, who practised with tremendous razzmatazz at many of the princely courts of Europe. According to his enemies, Taylor's overconfidence contributed to the blindness of Bach and Handel.

Other surgeons achieved fame for their dependable skill or innovations. A humane operator, Percivall Pott, a surgeon at St Bartholomew's Hospital in London, published on hernia, head injuries, hydrocele (swelling of the scrotum), anal fistula, fractures, and dislocations, as well as being the first to observe that chimney sweeps suffer from cancer of the scrotum. Pierre-Joseph Desault, François Bichat's teacher and founder in 1791 of the first surgical periodical, the *Journal de Chirurgie*, improved the treatment of fractures, and developed methods of ligating blood vessels in case of aneurysm. Desault insisted that surgeons should have an understanding of physiology as well as anatomy. Orthopaedics began to emerge, thanks especially to Jean-André Venel of Geneva, who designed mechanical devices to correct lateral curvature and other spinal defects.

Thanks to such improvements in surgery and changes in obstetrical practices, surgery rose in professional standing. This occurred first in France. As elsewhere, French practitioners were initially barber-surgeons – in London, the Barber-Surgeons' Company had been approved by Parliament in 1540 – but they succeeded, thanks to royal favour, in emancipating themselves from the barbers. In 1672, the Paris surgeon Pierre Dionis was honoured by being appointed to lecture in anatomy and surgery at the Jardin du Roi (the Royal Botanical Gardens). Then, in 1687, the misfortune of Louis XIV in developing anal fistula proved a golden opportunity. A successful operation on the Sun King by Charles-François Félix (he had first practised on the poor) contributed to promote surgery's prestige.

From the early eighteenth century, surgery was widely taught in Paris through lectures and demonstrations. The breakthrough came in 1731, when a royal charter established the Académie Royale de Chirurgie; 12 years later, Louis XV dissolved the link between the surgeons and barbers, and, in 1768, the convention of training surgeons by apprenticeship came to an end. Thereafter, surgeons vied with physicians in status, claiming that surgery was no mere manual art. This view of surgery as a science squared with the Enlightenment accent on practical ('empirical') rather than bookish learning. Within such a framework, it became possible to tout surgery as the most experimental and therefore the most progressive branch of medicine.

As a result of these developments, France led the world in surgery for most of the eighteenth century, drawing students from all over Europe. First in Paris and later elsewhere, the hospital became the site of surgical teaching, and the junior ranks of the surgical profession, employed as dressers, found work in hospitals as pupil teachers. The surgeon Pierre-Joseph Desault at the Hôtel

Dieu introduced bedside teaching. Moving medical education to the hospital reinforced the links that had been growing between surgery and anatomy since Andreas Vesalius in the sixteenth century, and constituted some steps towards the 'anatomico-localist' or 'patho-anatomical' perspective on disease that became so prominent in the hospitals of post-Revolutionary Paris – a view identifying diseases with specific organs and local pathological changes.

Parallel developments occurred elsewhere. It is significant that the first Alexander Monro, the first incumbent of the chair of anatomy and surgery in the Edinburgh medical school, was by profession a surgeon. Monro helped to found the Edinburgh Royal Infirmary, and made Edinburgh a major centre for medical training. His *Osteology* (1726), *Essay on Comparative Anatomy* (1744), and *Observations Anatomical and Physiological* (1758) became important anatomical texts.

Monro taught anatomy, but he also gave instruction in surgical operations, both to medical students and to surgical apprentices. The immense success of medical education as imparted in Edinburgh began to erode traditional status divisions, much more tenaciously upheld in England, between physic and surgery. From 1778, the Royal College of Surgeons of Edinburgh awarded its own diplomas, which were almost as valuable as a degree. Medical students in Edinburgh found it made sense to equip themselves to practise both skills, particularly if they expected to become general practitioners, medical jacks-of-all-trades practising all branches of healing.

The growing prominence of the hospital proved a blessing for surgeons. For one thing, the new infirmaries attracted accident and emergency cases, which were treated by surgeons rather than physicians. Moreover, hospitals afforded supplies of unclaimed dead bodies, predominantly those of the poor, whom surgeons and their students dissected postmortem. Hospitals also provided facilities for surgeons to lecture to students. Alongside hospitals, the spread of anatomy schools, first in Paris and then in London, boosted surgery's prestige.

By 1800 the surgeon had escaped the demeaning association with the traditional barber and bleeder: in London, the Company of Surgeons split from the barbers in 1745. The surgeon's status has continued to improve so that by the twentieth century the surgeon had shot up in status to become, perhaps, the most conspicuous of all the medical practitioners.

The Birth of the Clinic

Particularly with the development, around 1800, of the new medical science typified by physical examination, pathological anatomy, and statistics, the hospital gradually ceased to be primarily a site of charity, care, and convalescence; it turned into the medical power-house it has been ever since.

The new anatomical and clinical approach to medicine, pioneered in Paris, was based not on the lecture theatre but on the big, public hospital where direct hands-on experience could be gained in abundance. The 'clinic' (as this hospital medicine was to be called) became central to medicine. It made use of hospital facilities to deploy postmortems to correlate internal manifestations after death with pathology in the living. The huge numbers of patients in the public hospitals meant that diseases were identified as afflictions that beset everyone in the same way, rather than being unique to each case, and statistics were used to establish representative disease profiles. Such an approach was pioneered around 1800 by Philippe Pinel at La Salpêtrière in Paris, by René Läennec at the Hôpital Necker, and by Pierre Louis of the Hôtel Dieu. Their emphasis was not on symptoms but on lesions – that is, the objective facets of disease.

The nineteenth century brought a notable growth in hospitals, in response to population rise: London, for example, expanded from somewhat more than half a million people in the early eighteenth century to 5 million by 1900. In 1800, America's population was just more than 5 million, with only a tiny proportion of that number living in urban communities. There were, consequently, just a couple of hospitals – the Pennsylvania Hospital and the New York Hospital (founded 1771). By the early twentieth century, the USA had more than 4,000 hospitals, and few towns were without one.

New hospitals were founded to meet rising needs, and medical men started to take the initiative in setting them up – because an association with a hospital became a principal lever of professional advance. From the late eighteenth century practitioners began to found their own institutions, specializing above all in particular conditions. By 1860, London alone supported at least sixty-six special hospitals and dispensaries, designed for outpatients, including the Royal Hospital for Diseases of the Chest (1814), the Brompton Hospital (1841), the Royal Marsden Hospital (1851), the Hospital for Sick Children, Great Ormond Street (1852), and the National Hospital (for nervous diseases), Queen Square (1860).

Specialist hospitals sprang up throughout the developed world. Children's hospitals were set up in Paris in 1802, in Berlin in 1830, St Petersburg in 1934, and Vienna in 1837. The Massachusetts Eye and Ear Infirmary was established in 1824, the Boston Lying-In Hospital in 1832, the New York Hospital for Diseases of the Skin in 1836, and scores more. Women's hospitals were also instituted. Specialist hospitals had no broad caring mission; for this reason they became 'medicalized' earlier than the general hospitals, which continued to exercise a charitable role towards the ailing poor. In specialist hospitals, doctors controlled patient admission, appointments, and policy, and pioneered new therapies.

The organized teaching hospital also emerged, often associated with a university. Set up in 1828 as a non-denominational university (Oxford and Cambridge were still exclusively Church of England), University College London established its own hospital in 1834, which became linked to its medical school. King's College was the Anglican response to this development, and King's College Hospital was set up in 1839. With the evolution of the modern hospital, nursing, too, underwent transformation, becoming more professional and acquiring its own career structures.

The Age of Anaesthesia and Antisepsis

The first half of the nineteenth century brought a rise in the standing of the surgical profession, partly thanks to the image fostered by John Hunter of surgery as a progressive science. In France, two decades of war brought military surgeons to the fore, notably Dominique-Jean Larrey, a highly skilful battlefield amputator who developed the first effective ambulance, and Guillaume Dupuytren. In England, Charles Bell and the suave Astley Cooper at

Guy's Hospital gained high reputations as skilful surgeons. Cooper's *Anatomy and Surgical Treatment of Abdominal Hernia* published in two parts in 1804 and 1807 became a classic.

More daring operations were attempted, gynaecological surgery developing dramatically. American conditions proved favourable for innovation; there, the medical profession was less regulated, and, in the southern states, surgeons had slaves to practise on. In 1809, the American Ephraim McDowell performed the first successful ovariotomy (without anaesthetic) on 47-year-old Jane Todd Crawford, removing 15 pounds (nearly 7 kilograms) of a dirty gelatinous substance from her cyst. The widow not only survived but lived a further 31 years. John Attlee removed the ovaries of seventy-eight women between 1843 and 1883, with sixty-four recoveries. In 1824, the first British ovariotomy was performed by John Lizars of Edinburgh University. By mid-century the operation was being performed regularly in England by Sir Spencer Wells in London and Charles Clay in Manchester.

Another American surgeon, James Marion Sims, a South Carolinian who settled in Alabama, was responsible for successful treatment (1849) of vesico-vaginal fistula, again on a slave woman. Such operations met mixed reception: the British surgeon Robert Liston denounced them as 'belly rippers', and others argued that such operations were akin to vivisection, being carried out for the sake of scientific curiosity and surgical practice. Surgery was also put to questionable uses. From 1872 Robert Battey popularized an operation he called 'normal ovariotomy', in which normal ovaries were removed to relieve symptoms in women considered hysterical, insane, or peculiar. Unbelievable operations were also performed on 'nymphomaniacs'.

Overall, surgery's scope remained limited and its success uncertain, and comprehensive advances were hardly possible before two towering developments: anaesthesia and antisepsis. Anaesthesia – an expression coined in 1846 by an American, Oliver Wendell Holmes, to indicate the effects of ether – made surgical trauma bearable; the latter breakthrough reduced the otherwise appalling death rate from postoperative sepsis.

Anaesthesia was not entirely new, and medicine had always, of course, used certain analgesics. Early societies were aware of the pain-deadening qualities of opium, hashish or Indian hemp, and alcohol. In the first century AD, the Greek naturalist, Dioscorides, suggested the root of the mandrake, steeped in wine, should be given to patients about to undergo surgery. Yet most patients before the reign of Queen Victoria had to face serious surgery with few attempts to deaden the pain (a deeply drugged or drunk patient could be more difficult to handle than an alert one suffering acute pain).

The first gas recognized to have anaesthetic powers was nitrous oxide, the object of self-experimentation in 1795 by the Bristol physician, Thomas Beddoes, and his young assistant, Humphry Davy. After inhalation, Davy reported giddiness, relaxation of the muscles, and a tendency to laugh (hence the popular name, 'laughing gas'). In 1800, Davy published *Researches, Chemical and Philosophical, Chiefly Concerning Nitrous Oxide and its Respiration.* Yet the surgical value of nitrous oxide long went unappreciated.

In January 1842, however, William E. Clarke, a practitioner from Rochester, New York, endeavoured a tooth extraction under ether. The use of ether as a surgical anaesthetic was also developed by a Boston dentist, William T. G. Morton. Another American dentist, Horace Wells, thought of using nitrous oxide for extractions, and he had one of his own teeth painlessly pulled in December 1844, proclaiming a new era of tooth-pulling. Medical scepticism about his claims was to lead Wells to commit suicide shortly after.

Employment of ether as an anaesthetic spread to Europe. On 21 December 1846, Robert Liston, the most acclaimed London surgeon of his day (he was renowned not least for his speed), amputated the diseased thigh of a patient under ether; he called the anaesthetic method a 'Yankee dodge'. Anaesthesia gained approval although ether was soon challenged by the safer chloroform. On 19 January 1847, James Young Simpson of Edinburgh used chloroform for the first time to relieve the pains of childbirth, and it soon began to be used extensively for this purpose, even for Queen Victoria.

Acceptance of anaesthesia made more protracted surgery feasible, but it did not by itself revolutionize surgery, however, because of the severe death rate from postoperative infection. The menace of infection was well known. Working in 1848 in the first obstetrical clinic of the Vienna general hospital, Ignaz Semmelweis remonstrated against the dreadful fatality levels from puerperal fever. He observed that the first clinic (run by medical men) had a much higher rate of puerperal fever than the second obstetrical clinic, run by midwives. He became convinced that this was caused by medical staff and students going directly from the postmortem to the delivery rooms, thereby spreading infection. He instituted a strict policy of washing hands and instruments in chlorinated lime solution between autopsy work and handling patients, and the mortality rate in the first clinic was diminished to the same level as the second. Opposition to his novel views led him to quit Vienna in 1850. Resentful and frustrated, he died in a lunatic asylum.

Antagonism to Semmelweis was not mere professional closing of ranks but was consistent with the aetiological theories of the time. The leading view was that infections were caused not by contact but by miasmata in the air, emanations given off by non-human sources. Adherents of such views therefore gave priority to ventilation and prevention of overcrowding as preventive measures.

The notion of antiseptics as advocated by Semmelweis was far from unknown, however; the term 'antiseptic' means anything designed to counter putrefaction or corruption. Greek medicine used wine and vinegar in wound dressings. Alcohol gained favour, and around 1820 iodine became popular in France for treating wounds. Other substances used as antiseptics included creosote, ferric chloride, zinc chloride, and nitric acid. There was thus some interest in questions of antisepsis before the labours of Joseph Lister. It was, nevertheless, Lister who introduced effective techniques for antisepsis and who proved a vocal and effective propagandist on their behalf.

By the time Lister retired in 1892, antiseptic surgery had established itself. The carbolic spray, which saturated all concerned and was heartily disliked, came under criticism and Lister himself abandoned it. Other antiseptics came into use. As early as 1874 Louis Pasteur had suggested placing the instruments in boiling water and passing them through a flame; heat sterilization of instruments was accepted by Robert Koch in 1881. The American surgeon William S. Halsted, of Johns Hopkins Hospital, introduced rubber gloves for use in the operating theatre in 1890 – ironically, not for the patient's sake but to protect the operating-room nurse, his fiancée, whose hands were allergic to antiseptics.

By 1900, these and other prophylactic antiseptic and aseptic methods had been put into use by all surgeons. No longer did surgeons operate in blood-caked black frock-coats in dingy rooms with sawdust-covered floors. The introduction of face-masks, rubber gloves, and surgical gowns lessened the risks of infection, and clean and sterile environments were constantly being improved.

As late as 1874, Sir John Erichsen believed that the abdomen, chest, and brain would forever be closed to operations by wise and humane surgeons; and Lister rarely probed into major cavities, mainly setting fractures. But things were changing: as the result of anaesthetics and antiseptic, surgery's horizons widened dramatically. First in Zurich and then in Vienna, the celebrated Theodor Billroth made important innovations, performing the first total removal of a cancerous larynx, pioneering abdominal surgery, and developing surgery for many forms of cancer, especially of the breast. In the USA, William Halsted devised radical mastectomy, the operation in which the breast, all the lymph glands in the nearest armpit, and the muscles of the chest wall are removed. It long remained the most popular treatment for breast cancer.

Appendectomies became more common in the 1880s: in 1901, Edward VII was operated on when his appendix caused trouble just before his coronation. Removal of gallstones grew common, and cholecystectomy, the removal of the gall bladder itself, was introduced in 1882. Surgery on the small intestine, notably for cancer, was also inaugurated around the same time, and urological surgery developed, especially prostate operations. A prominent figure was Sir William MacEwen, who adopted and extended Lister's antiseptic surgical techniques and pioneered operations on the brain for tumours, abscesses, and trauma.

By 1900 a marked change had occurred in the number and type of operations surgeons were executing. Lister's notebooks record no abdominal surgery up to 1893; but the abdominal surgery practice of William Watson Cheyne at King's College Hospital in London increased steadily in the decade between 1902 and 1912, from fewer than one in twenty cases to around one in six. For so long an emergency treatment or a last resort, operative surgery had become a powerful, even a fashionable, weapon. A surgical revolution had already been wrought by the time of the First World War: conditions such as gastric ulcers became routine targets for the knife.

The new century saw the growth of surgical interventions in tubercular cases. A German, Ernst Ferdinand Sauerbruch, led the field in thoracic surgery, although it was an Italian, Carlo Forlanini, who introduced pneumothorax treatment. Two surgeons were even honoured at this time with a Nobel Prize – Theodor Kocher in 1909 for his work on the thyroid gland, and Alexis Carrel in 1911 for his techniques of suturing blood vessels and work on transplantation and tissue culture.

A professor at Berne from 1871, Kocher developed general surgical treatment of disorders of the thyroid gland, including goitre and thyroid tumours, and elucidated the workings of the thyroid gland. From the 1870s investigations had shown that the thyroid was essential to life; its malfunction was blamed for cretinism, goitre, and various other disorders. As a consequence, enlarged thyroid glands began to be surgically removed – sometimes with disastrous consequences if the thyroid tissue left behind performed inadequately. It was shown that this could be prevented by counterbalancing injections of macerated thyroid tissue. Since delayed growth and slow learning were amongst the features of cretinism, thousands of underachieving children were placed on thyroid extract, and it was recommended for sundry symptoms in adults from constipation and obesity to tiredness and depression.

In a similar way, testicular extract also became popular. On 1 June 1889, Charles-Edouard Brown-Séquard reported to a distinguished scientific society in Paris that he had rejuvenated himself through subcutaneous injections of extracts of guinea-pig and dog testicles. Rejuvenation through gland implants proved, however, a nine-day wonder.

Theodor Kocher's observations on patients suffering the consequences of surgically removing the thyroid gland (total strumectomy) helped elucidate its normal functions, and by the 1890s the isolation of active thyroid hormones made replacement therapy possible. Kocher also pioneered operations of the brain and spinal cord.

For his part, Alexis Carrel, a Frenchman from Lyons, was involved in many aspects of surgery on the blood vessels and heart, and in particular in treating aneurysm. Having migrated to the USA, he showed how parts of the aortal wall could be replaced with a piece from another artery or veins, and found ways of sewing vessels together, thereby initiating vascular surgery. Carrel's work paved the way for many later kinds of surgery dealing with aneurysms, varicose veins, and blood clots.

The 'Golden Age' of Surgery

The twentieth century was to become the century of surgery. A constellation of advances – far too many to list – followed from the crucial interlinking of pathological anatomy, anaesthesia, and asepsis. From the latter decades of the nineteenth century, surgeons directed their attention to tumours and infections leading to obstruction or stenosis (constriction of vessels), above all in the digestive, respiratory, and urogenital tracts. These could be relieved or cured by fissuring or excision. New operations of this kind included tracheotomy for tuberculosis or throat cancer, and relief of intestinal obstruction caused by cancerous tumours.

Operative surgery entered a 'golden age', when surgeons grew ever more therapeutically active. The habitual performance of operations on the gastrointestinal tract, thyroid, breasts, bones, and blood vessels made surgery safer and more reliable. Abdominal surgery advanced with new methods of extirpation of cancer of the rectum, of hernias, and with treatments for acute appendicitis and disorders of the colon. Herniotomies and appendectomies became routine after 1910. Surgery of the nervous system was almost wholly a twentieth-century advance. The first specialist in neurosurgery was Harvey Cushing, who became professor of surgery at Harvard University in 1912. All the cavities and organs of the body were conquered.

Some surgeons became positively cavalier: the Irish-born William Arbuthnot Lane advocated the removal of yards of the gut for ordinary constipation – or even as a prophylactic measure. Appendectomy not for acute but for so-called 'chronic' appendicitis became fashionable in the 1920s and 1930s, as were the many operations devised to fix abdominal organs, found by X-ray examination to be 'misplaced'. 'Hitching up the kidneys' enjoyed a great vogue.

Between 1920 and 1950 hundreds of thousands of tonsillectomies were performed, most quite unnecessary. Hysterectomies enjoyed a similar fad.

Surgical intervention was stimulated by many developments within medicine, but it was also demanded by events in the wider world. The First World War proved crucial. With war wounds occurring on hitherto unimaginable scales, debates raged once more over proper methods of wound management. Experience in the two world wars led to new methods of handling compound fractures; to the development of plastic and reconstructive surgery; and to the establishment of blood and plasma banks (the first were set up in 1935 at the Mayo Clinic in Rochester, New York State). In 1938, during the Spanish Civil War, techniques were developed of administering stored blood by indirect transfusion into the patient from a bottle; these were perfected in the Second World War. Blood transfusions, first pioneered in the seventeenth century, had finally been made safe.

By 1950, better immunological knowledge and the increased availability of drugs effective against bacterial infections had expanded possibilities of operability. Thanks to antibiotics, surgery could be performed on cases hitherto deemed too risky because of danger of infection; for example, interventions in the lung in contact with atmospheric microorganisms. With the pharmacological revolution, such patients could be treated before and after the operation with sulphonamides and later antibiotics.

Surgery entered a new phase, moving from a preoccupation with removal to a subtler concern with restoration. Surgeons developed a growing capacity to control and re-establish the functioning of the heart, lungs, and kidneys, and fluid balance. The first implantation of an artificial apparatus (prothesis) came in 1959 with the heart pacemaker, designed to adjust beat frequency by means of electrical impulses in the case of arrhythmic variations. It was developed by Rune Elmqvist and implanted by Åke Senning in Sweden. Such restorative procedures now range from eye lenses to pneumatic implants to facilitate penile erection.

A fine instance of the switch of surgical approach from excision to implantation is offered by changes in urology. Early on, emphasis lay on the cutting out of malignant tumours. This was challenged by radiotherapy as an alternative procedure: in 1906, an American, Alfred L. Gray, introduced radiotherapy for carcinoma of the bladder, and this was soon used also in the therapy of prostate cancer. Bladder cancer was then one of the first to be successfully treated with hormones (1941), thanks to the work of Charles Brenton Huggins, a Canadian-born American surgeon who undertook investigation of the physiology and biochemistry of the prostate gland. Research on dogs led Huggins to the possibility of using hormones in treating such tumours in human beings and in 1966 he shared the Nobel Prize for his discovery of hormonal treatment for prostate cancer. He also developed the use of hormones in treating breast cancer in women.

Improvements in heart surgery began with the first operation for stenosis of the mitral valve – the abnormal narrowing of the valve between the left auricle and ventricle, which slows down the blood circulation and eventually causes harm. This was performed by Henry Souttar in London in 1925, and was followed in 1947 by operations to relieve pulmonary stenosis (narrowing of the opening between the pulmonary artery and the right ventricle) by Thomas Holmes Sellors and Russell Brock, also in London. Two years later similar operations were undertaken for stenosis of the aorta itself.

In 1942, it was suggested that congenital heart disease (the so-called blue-baby syndrome) could be cured surgically. The operation, first undertaken at Johns Hopkins Hospital in Baltimore in 1944, launched modern cardiac surgery. The pioneer was Helen Brooke Taussig, an American paediatrician who was the first woman to become a full professor at Johns Hopkins University. Taussig worked on congenital heart disease in association with the cardiac surgeon Alfred Blalock. The babies were blue because of congenital anomalies that caused blood to pass directly from the right chamber of the heart to the left without being oxygenated in the lungs; this was then surgically rectified. Their joint efforts helped create a new speciality of paediatric cardiac surgery. Dramatic advances in heart surgery followed.

Operations on the mitral valves increased, but in some cases they initially produced severe brain damage by depriving the brain of oxygen. The idea was then floated of entirely removing the heart from the body, and deploying an alternative system of blood circulation.

Such 'open-heart' surgery was made possible by several key developments. One was the use of hypothermia, reducing through cold the oxygen need of the tissues. Another was the building of the heart–lung machine, maintaining artificial circulation through the great vessels while the heart was bypassed and the operation performed. The machine involved two main components: a 'lung' to oxygenate the blood and a 'heart' pump. Through experience it was discovered that the deeply cooled and bypassed heart could be stopped for up to an hour and started again without suffering damage. Open-heart surgery started in 1952 in the USA with the implantation of artificial heart valves.

A major and highly conspicuous trend has been transplantation. Successful skin grafts were described by the Swiss, Jacques Reverdin, as early as 1869. Such autografts (tissue transplantations within the same patient) were soon used to treat ulcers and burns. Skin grafting led to the rise of reconstructive surgery, first through the work of Harold Gillies on First World War casualties at Aldershot in southern England. During the Second World War, transplantation of non-vital tissue become urgent, to provide 'pacemaker' support for regeneration of connective tissues after severe injuries. The invention of the 'artificial kidney' laid the foundations for the great developments in organ transplantation in the 1950s and 1960s.

The rise of organ transplantation brought inescapable ethical and legal predicaments for medicine. Under what circumstances might living human beings ethically become donors of kidneys and other organs? Should there be a market in organs? Were the dead automatically to be assumed to have consented to the removal of organs? At what point was a person truly 'dead', permitting organ removal?

Partly in view of the demands of transplantation, the general test of death has shifted during the last generation from cessation of breathing to 'brain death', which has the convenience of permitting removal of organs from patients in whom respiration was artificially maintained right up to removal. The issues of patients queuing for organ transplantation and of sorting priorities in the allotment of organs in high demand remain difficult.

Similar moral problems surround the advances in reproductive technology made possible by the advent of the 'test-tube baby'. Here the pioneer was the British gynaecologist/obstetrician Patrick

Steptoe. He had long been interested in laparoscopy (a technique of viewing the abdominal cavity through a small incision in the umbilicus) and in problems of fertility. Together with Robert Edwards, a physiologist at Cambridge University, he worked on the problem of *in vitro* fertilization of human embryos. In July 1978, this research resulted in the birth of the first test-tube baby, Louise Brown, who was born by caesarian section in Oldham District Hospital, England, through *in vitro* fertilization and implantation in her mother's uterus.

The ethical issues surrounding test-tube babies remain controversial, but the technique has become more common, as have the related practices of sperm and egg donation and surrogate motherhood. Some of the implications of transformations in reproductive surgery and technology are considered in Chapter 10.

Organ transplants offer an illustration of the move to 'replacement surgery' during the past three decades. At the same time, prostheses such as hip joints, middle-ear bones, heart valves, and artificial organs, such as the inner ear, have become routine treatments. A key figure in replacement surgery was the British surgeon John Charnley. After serving as an orthopaedic specialist in the First World War. Charnley devoted himself to the technical problems associated with replacements for badly arthritic hip joints, above all the difficulty of finding a suitable material. Artificial joints made of polytetrafluoroethylene, known by the trade name of Teflon, proved not to wear well in the long term, but from 1962 Charnley, who was then based in Wigan in Lancashire, found that polyethylene was more effective. With scrupulous attention to aseptic techniques, he was able to perfect an operation that gave enhanced mobility to many. Not all implants have been so worthy. Cosmetic surgery has boomed with the fashion for silicon breast implants, a lucrative, if dubious, trade.

Artificial replacements illustrate the increasingly interdisciplinary character of surgery in recent decades, necessitating collaboration with such sciences as physiology, engineering, pharmacology, and immunology – to say nothing of interaction with the electronic, metal, and plastic industries.

Surveying modern surgery, it is possible to picture change in terms of three successive, overlapping, phases of development. The first stage of modern surgery involved an era of extirpation, which pioneered new ways of dealing with tumours and injuries by means of surgical excision. There followed a stage of restoration, in which stress fell on surgical physiology and pharmacology, aimed at repairing impaired or endangered function. The third age has placed greater emphasis on replacement, the introduction into the damaged body of biological or artificial organs and tissues. This last phase requires a more systemic approach to treatment that may be breaking down the time-honoured boundaries between surgery and other medical disciplines.

Surgery Becomes High-Tech

The surgical revolution would have been quite impossible without all manner of technological innovations that have come to the aid of surgery, and indeed medicine at large. The breakthrough of greatest symbolic significance was Wilhelm Röntgen's discovery of X-rays, working with vacuum tubes perfected by the English scientist William Crookes. X-rays had immediate scientific, technological, commercial, and medical reverberations. Prolonged exposure to X-rays was soon observed to have physiological effects, such as burning the skin, ulcerations, dermatitis, and hair loss. Within a year, Röntgen's discovery had been turned to therapeutic account by a Viennese physician who had used X-rays to burn off a mole from a patient. At the same time, the Danish physician Niels Finsen suggested that ultraviolet light rays were bactericidal and offered promise for treating lupus.

Hard on the heels of these wondrous developments came the discovery in 1896, by the French physicist Antoine-Henri Becquerel, of radiation, associated with heavy elements such as uranium. The husband-and-wife team of Pierre and Marie Curie joined the hunt for other radioactive elements, whose diagnostic and therapeutic implications interacted with surgical interventions in such domains as cancer therapy. By 1900, there were radium institutes, radiology journals and societies, and more than a hundred diseases for which the new miracle cures had been used, although it was for cancer that the new therapies seemed to promise most. Therapeutic enthusiasm outran caution, and the dangers of radiotherapy were only painfully realized. The martyrs to X-rays included many patients and early workers, not least Marie Curie.

In 1903, the Dutch physiologist Willem Einthoven published details of the first electrocardiograph, which picked up electrical activity from the heart, and so led to more effective monitoring of cardiac disorders. In the 1930s, the introduction of the electron microscope revealed many aspects of cell structure previously unseen. From around 1955, sonography (ultrasound) was developed in Sweden and the USA; it became surgically applicable in cardiac diagnosis. Nuclear medicine, using radioactive isotopes, became increasingly significant in measuring the functioning of endocrine glands, lungs, and kidneys. The development of catheters of various sorts enabled the investigation of heart and liver functions. Flexible endoscopes, drawing on the use of glass-fibre optics (which enabled light to be sent through a tube by total internal reflection), were developed in the 1970s. These were used not only for diagnostics but soon for therapeutic interventions, not least in connection with lasers.

In 1917, Albert Einstein unveiled the principle of the laser ('light amplification by stimulated emissions of radiation'). Its high-energy waves, capable of being focused to a microscopic point, are sterile and cause minimal bleeding and scarring. Destroying tissue rapidly by heating or by producing photochemical reactions, lasers are 'optical knives' that have proved valuable in eye surgery as well as in internal surgery. With the aid of endoscopes, they can be aimed from within the body.

Visual diagnostics leapt ahead with the introduction in 1972 of the computerized tomograph (CAT) by Godfrey Newbold Hounsfield. An electrical engineer working for the British company EMI, Hounsfield pioneered a system whereby X-ray beams could be resolved with computer assistance to produce a cross-sectional picture of the human body. The result – computer-assisted axial tomography or CAT scanning – was a major breakthrough in the non-invasive diagnosis of disease. Hounsfield shared the Nobel Prize for medicine in 1979 with Allan M. Cormack, the physicist who had established the mathematical principles on which the technique depended. A further development is magnetic resonance (MR), which also shows sections of the body but by using radio waves, and is also capable of showing metabolic organs. Positron emission topography (PET) scanners measure photons coming from radioactive decay of a radioactive tracer administered to the patient. PET scans are especially useful for examining local blood flow and the transfer of chemical information; they are beginning to play a major part in showing the biological basis of psychiatric disorders.

The Twentieth-Century Hospital

The hospital has changed its nature during the last couple of centuries, turning from little more than a poor-house into the nerve centre of modern medicine, and also becoming far more socially conspicuous. In Britain, the number of beds per thousand of the population doubled between 1860 and 1940, and then doubled again by 1980. The astounding modern growth of surgery created a huge rise in absolute and relative hospital expenditure. Vastly important were technological innovations, from the introduction of X-rays through to the electron microscope in the 1930s and the CAT and PET scanners developed in the 1970s.

The creation of tailor-made environments for surgery was equally crucial. From the late nineteenth century, the development of hygienic, well-equipped operating theatres played a major part in turning the hospital from a healing machine for the poor into an institution fit for all classes. The leap in costs began to be seriously felt by the early years of the twentieth century. Between the world wars, surgery became much more intricate, laboratory tests and other investigations were extended, medical technology grew essential, and staff costs rose. Ambulance services made the hospital the nucleus of emergency care.

With costs escalating, hospitals, traditionally funded in Britain and most other countries on a voluntary basis, ran into financial problems. In the USA, hospitals coped with funding difficulties by developing business strategies. In conjunction with insurance schemes, they enticed well-off patients on a paying basis. The absence of the American system of the underpinning of hospital budgets by insurance is one explanation (amongst many) why the post-war British government had little option but to introduce a National Health Service (NHS).

The Second World War had already led to transformations in British hospital organization. The government had made preparations for the massive civilian casualties expected from the Luftwaffe blitz. These emergency plans assigned all hospitals specific tasks, and they were to be remunerated for the beds they set aside. There were two main consequences of such an arrangement: hospitals began to count on government payments, and they became better attuned to cooperation within a state-planned scheme.

In the NHS, hospitals became by far the most significant, and costly, sector. At the time of its establishment (1948), there were more than 900 voluntary hospitals, but many were small – more than 250 had fewer than thirty beds. Most were taken into the NHS, with the ownership of buildings and land passing to the state.

Since then, hospitals have been the basic sites for therapeutic advance. By the post-war period, in the USA and Europe alike, they were seen as quintessentially part of modern medical care: high-tech, invasive, involving skilled coordinated teamwork amongst many different specialties. Yet from the 1960s critiques of hospitals grew. Particularly in the USA, medicolegal cases and third-party payment fuelled costs; tests and investigations mushroomed; and vast capital sums were spent on medical equipment.

Some critics argued that modern hospital medicine had contributed little except cost: it was public-health measures in the nineteenth century that had actually brought down mortality. In the past, hospitals might even have increased mortality. Whether the medicine of the future can afford the modern hospital remains an unsolved problem. It is conceivable that the huge hospitals of today will soon seem medicine's dinosaurs, and that they will be replaced by simpler and more varied institutions.

7. Drug Treatment and the Rise of Pharmacology

Miles Weatherall

Pharmacology, the science of drugs, became necessary when the first person to get drunk wondered what was happening to him or her. This occurred long before recorded history. There are records of grape cultivation and wine-making in Mesopotamia and Egypt at least 4,500 years ago but many fermented liquors must have been known long before then, as were other medicinal products. But how did anyone ever identify them?

The Medicines of Early Civilizations

One can only guess how the earliest drugs were discovered. Bitter experience taught people which plants were toxic, and, happier events perhaps suggested, more subtly, that some had beneficial properties. Several ancient Egyptian papyruses, dated about 1600–1500 BC, record the medical practices and drugs then in use. Prescriptions were laid out in a form that survived in Western medicine to modern times. But the hieroglyphics are difficult to interpret, and the identity of many remedies is doubtful.

Egyptians attributed medicinal virtues to various familiar fruits and vegetables. They also used tree resins, including frankincense, myrrh, and manna. Extracts of plants still sometimes used as purgatives – senna, colocynth, and castor oil – were recognized. Tannins from plant galls were used for the treatment of burns. Parts of animals were also applied therapeutically, especially fat, and more curious recipes include ox spleen, pig's brain, and tortoise gall (with honey). Antimony, copper, and some other minerals were especially favoured as astringents or antiseptics. But names of remedies must be interpreted carefully; 'ass's heads' and 'pig's teeth' may be no more what they seem than are buttercups 'cups for butter' or foxgloves 'gloves worn by foxes'.

Egyptian practices continued in the civilization of Assyria and Babylonia. Copies of herbals have survived, suggesting familiarity with hellebore, henbane, mandrake, and the opium poppy, all of which contain potent drugs well known today, but the exact purposes for which these remedies were applied are often uncertain or obscure. Other drugs may have been known and mentioned in records that have not survived.

Greek and Roman Remedies

In ancient Greece, a more critical approach developed, based on observation and experience. Much credit is given to Hippocrates of Cos and his followers. As in China, simplicity was sought by inventing a small number of basic principles, this time the four temperaments – the blood, the phlegm, the yellow bile, and the black bile, giving the sanguine, the phlegmatic, the jaundiced, and the melancholic temperaments – and in attributing disease to an excess or deficiency of the wet and dry, hot and cold humours responsible for these temperaments. Treatment gave more weight to diet and lifestyle than to drugs as a means of restoring a healthy balance. Surviving ancient Greek texts include references to books on drugs, and to suppliers of medicinal plants, but no great ancient Greek schedule of drugs is known to exist.

In the more regulated civilization of Rome, Galen of Pergamum has become the most famous, and for many centuries was probably the most influential, medical writer. Other authors sheltered under the cover of his authority, just as they had after Hippocrates, and the probably diverse medical practices of centuries became consolidated in a Galenical system, which related more to the individual patient than to the formal classification of disease. The most important record of drugs then in use came from Dioscorides, physician to the Emperor Nero (reigned AD 54–68), or at least a doctor in Nero's army.

The accumulated experience of Greece and Rome became mingled in the medieval Arabic world with that of Muslims. Among the works of this period are a systematic treatise on poisons written in the eighth century by the Arabic alchemist Jabir ibn Hayyan. The noted scientist and philosopher Ibn Sina (Avicenna) also included a book on medicaments in his *Canon on Medicine* published in the eleventh century, a text that continued to serve for 500 years. Much medical knowledge was reintroduced to Europe after Muslim conquests in North Africa and Spain, especially through the medical schools established at Salerno in Italy and at Montpellier in France in the eleventh and twelfth centuries.

Paracelsus and the Fight Against Authority

Through many centuries, thought and actions in Europe were dominated by the opinions of authority. Then came the great outburst of independence and originality in the 'rebirth of learning' or the Renaissance. In medicine, rejection of orthodoxy began gradually, and was made conspicuous by the flamboyant character Philippus Aureolus Theophrastus Bombastus von Hohenheim, who was born near Zurich and adopted the name Paracelsus in recognition of the Roman medical writer Celsus.

Martin Luther had shown his defiance of authority by burning a papal bull and a copy of canon law, and Paracelsus followed his example by burning the books of Galen and Avicenna. Appointed town physician of Basel in 1527, he also taught medical students there for a year. Later, after he had lost a lawsuit against a canon of the cathedral, he became a wandering practitioner. He treated patients, but also made chemical experiments and reported novel observations, many of which have been repeatedly confirmed.

Paracelsus noted that air was necessary for wood to burn and he claimed that without air all living things would die. He recommended various minerals as medicines, and may have introduced mercury for syphilis, as well as advising the use of antimony, arsenic, copper, iron, and lead for various purposes. His secret remedy, laudanum, probably depended mainly on opium for its benefits. Although Paracelsus was a good observer, he also was a great theorist. He sought a small number of simplifying principles, but these belonged to several sets. He invented a mystical philosophy of gnomes, sylphs, nymphs, and salamanders, which corresponded to the elementals of earth, air, water, and fire, but also related in some way to the chemical elementals of combustible sulphur, volatile mercury, and residual salt.

Paracelsus's doctrines shocked many respectable physicians of the time, who clung, sometimes with great bigotry, to Galenical doctrine in the face of Paracelsian heresy. It is so much easier to assert authority than to investigate facts, and the time was one of original ideas but not yet of their experimental evaluation. Nor was understanding of ill health sufficiently advanced to distinguish what now we call one 'disease' from another.

Injuries – broken bones, and wounds with accompanying sepsis, fevers, and tumours – were obvious enough. Certain patterns of fever could be recognized, such as tertian and quartan agues in which the fever (probably malarial) recurred on the third or fourth day. But accurate diagnosis of internal disorders was non-existent, and had little basis for developing until the elements of physiology and pathology were established in the seventeenth and eighteenth centuries by, among others, William Harvey.

The choice of drugs for treating sick patients thus depended on a mixture of authority, tradition, and philosophy (or metaphysic, or superstition). The idea of bodily humours, which caused diseases if they were out of balance, provided reasons for getting fluids out of the body, by sweating, bleeding, and purging, and led to unfounded ideas – not extinct even today – that purgation provides relief from a great many ills, even political:

> What rhubarb, senna, or what purgative drug,
> Would scour these English hence?
>
> Macbeth, 5.3

A Remedy for Every Disease

Those who believed that the world was made for humanity's benefit were inclined to think that there must be a remedy for every human disease, and that it must be labelled so that it could be recognized. Thus the doctrine of signs or signatures evolved gradually over the centuries. Yellow plants, notably saffron crocus (*Crocus sativus*) were chosen for jaundice. Red substances, such as rust or red wine, were good for bloodlessness. More subtly, the white spots on the leaves of lungwort (*Pulmonaria officinalis*) showed that the plant was good for lung disease.

Sometimes, it was argued that remedies had been put in convenient places for people to use. So, in England, the bark of the white willow (*Salix alba*) was tried for agues, because the tree grows in moist or wet soil, where agues chiefly abounded, as the Revd Edmund Stone, of Chipping Norton in Oxfordshire, observed in his report to the Royal Society of London in 1763:

the general maxim, that many natural maladies carry their cures along with them, or that their remedies lie not far from their causes, was so very apposite to this particular case, that I could not help applying it; and that this might be the intention of Providence here, I must own had some little weight with me.[1]

There are, in fact, active compounds in willow bark (one is salicin, the precursor of salicyclic acid and the basis of aspirin), which are useful in dispelling some fevers, but reliance on a helpful providence has not often been so rewarding.

Herbals, or accounts of plants and their culinary and medicinal properties, were popular sources of remedies throughout medieval Europe. As medicine became more scientific, however, they began to be supplemented and superseded by pharmacopoeias, which described how drugs in regular use should be prepared and defined what materials were acceptable. Municipal authorities in Europe started issuing such standards in the sixteenth century. In London, the Royal College of Physicians produced a pharmacopoeia in 1618; fresh editions appeared with increasing frequency until the last in 1841. After that, as a result of the Medicines Act of 1858, a *British Pharmacopoeia*, produced under the auspices of the General Medical Council, became the national standard of reference. Other nations similarly set up their own standards – Brandenburg in 1698, Russia in 1778, Portugal in 1794, and so on. The first edition of *The Pharmacopoeia of the United States of America* appeared in 1820, although its standards were not legally enforceable until an act was passed in 1906.

New Medicines from Overseas

Information about drugs was much needed, because explorers, missionaries, and colonizers were returning to Europe with unknown plants, many with supposed medicinal properties. The most notable, Peruvian or Jesuit's bark (*Cinchona officinalis*), was introduced into Europe between 1630 and 1640 and was promoted by Jesuit priests, who gave the powdered bark to those suffering from fever. Later, it was shown that it was specific for malaria, and that quinine, an alkaloid, was one of its constituents.

A legend grew up that the bark was introduced to Europe in 1641 by the Spanish viceroy of Peru, after his wife, the Countess Anna del Cinchon, was cured by it, and the remedy was called cinchona. But the story is full of inconsistencies, as are several other claims for credit, which probably belongs to the traders of the time or to Jesuit missionaries in South America. Peruvian bark is a powerful remedy for malaria and, when diagnosis was imprecise, was widely in demand for fevers of all kinds, and as a tonic. It was introduced into the *London Pharmacopoeia* in 1677. Supplies were limited, however, and the search for new sources and alternative remedies became important. No effective substitutes were found until the nineteenth century after great advances had been made in the science of chemistry.

Other introductions to Europe from the Americas included the practice of smoking the dried leaves of the tobacco plant, *Nicotiana*, brought to England by Sir Walter Raleigh in the sixteenth century, primarily as a medicine. Thus began the long history of a valuable and much-abused drug, nicotine, one of the plant's constituent alkaloids. Adventurers also brought home ipecacuanha (*Cephaelis ipecacuanha*) from Brazil, where the shrub was known as a powerful medicine. The dried root is useful against certain kinds of acute diarrhoea (such as amoebic dysentery), is an effective emetic in some cases of poisoning, and, in small doses, is used as a cough expectorant. Belief in the drug's effectiveness is emphasized by its current inclusion in many national pharmacopoeias.

In the past, ipecacuanha was famous because it was commonly prescribed in a powder with opium to provoke sweating, according to a recipe invented by a piratical physician from Warwickshire called Thomas Dover. He was second captain on the privateer *Duke* on Woodes Roger's expedition to South America in 1708–11. His powder is commemorated in this anonymous rhyme from St Bartholomew's Hospital, London, published in 1923:

> Oh, Dover was a pirate and he sailed the Spanish Main.
> A hacking cough convulsed him; he had agonising pain.
> So he mixed hisself a powder, which he liked it more and more.
> Ipecac. and opium and K_2SO_4.[2]

The First Clinical Trials

While exploration flourished abroad, scientists in Europe were starting their search for objective evidence of medicines by doing experiments. Direct evaluation of medical treatment in a scientifically respectable way began to be advocated prominently – that is, by comparing the effects of a treatment with the consequences if the treatment was not applied (either successively in the same patient, or by comparison between comparable patients). Famous trials were conducted by the English naval surgeon James Lind, who showed that lemon juice prevents scurvy, while careful analysis and enumeration of clinical records by the French physician Pierre Louis undermined the classical belief in the efficacy of bleeding. Lind and Louis were not the first to attempt the difficult practice of evaluating remedies. Although they made great advances, good practices of evaluation or re-evaluation did not become established. But the dawn of clear judgment was beginning to replace the dark night of treatment by the unquestioned authority of a priest or a physician.

The Chemical Basis of Medicines

During the eighteenth century, the science of chemistry, fundamental to understanding all living matter, began to take shape. Antoine Lavoisier, one of several men called the father of modern chemistry, thought – in part at least – of the living body as a well-knit piece of chemical machinery. Some of his experiments showed that animal heat was produced by chemical action on the food consumed – that is, there was no basic difference between bodily warmth and the production of heat by burning coal or wood. This was a most important advance, but Lavoisier's ideas could not be developed in detail until much more was known about the organization of living bodies, until the science of physiology was properly established.

Chemical methods were more immediately useful in purifying and identifying the ingredients of substances used as medicines. Clinical science was far too rudimentary to judge reliably whether a drug actually did a patient any good (or harm), but the new art of physiological experiments made it possible to show and even measure effects of potent medicines on animals in a laboratory. These investigations were immensely beneficial, because they threw new light on the way the body worked and they identified the active principles – constituents – of some important medicines. An active principle was no longer a philosopher's intellectual construct; it was there to be looked at, a crystalline substance of known chemical composition carefully preserved in a glass tube.

The great French physiologist François Magendie collaborated with an outstanding pharmacist Pierre-Joseph Pelletier in the first half of the nineteenth century in researches to isolate pure drugs. A small Indian tree called *Strychnos nux-vomica* yielded strychnine; and ipecacuanha from Brazil gave emetine. Pelletier, with his colleague Joseph Caventou, also improved the purification of morphine from opium, and isolated quinine from Peruvian bark and caffeine from coffee beans. All these substances reacted like alkalies with acids to form salts, and so were called alkaloids. Chemical analysis showed that they consisted of carbon, hydrogen, oxygen, and nitrogen and the proportions of these elements differed significantly in different alkaloids. But the structure of complex carbon compounds – the way the numerous atoms were joined to each other – was not understood until well on in the nineteenth century.

How Drugs Worked

François Magendie was primarily concerned with the normal workings of the body and drugs were his tools to separate one function from another. His one-time assistant at the Collège de France, Claude Bernard, who took over Magendie's job in 1852, did more towards explaining exactly how drugs acted. Bernard showed that certain drugs acted at strictly localized and well-defined sites, a profoundly important fact that began to displace vaguer notions that drugs had some sort of general influence throughout the body. He discovered that the poison used by South American Indians called curare (a tree resin) works where a nerve joins the muscle on which it acts, and nowhere else. It prevents the nerve impulse from making the muscle contract, and so causes paralysis as long as the curare persists. Injected into an animal – on the tip of an arrow, for instance – the poison is carried by the bloodstream to all the muscles of the body and causes paralysis and death when the muscles of respiration are made inactive.

The discovery paved the way to the chemical understanding that Antoine Lavoisier had foreshadowed a century earlier. Clearly, there was some special structure or substance that was inactivated by the curare; and similar specific points of action were recognized for other drugs. These specific structures or substances, of then unknown composition, came to be called 'receptors', and the study of drug receptors became a mainspring of fundamental pharmacology. So the reactions of drugs with bodily constituents began to be seen to be chemical events, best understood in terms of chemical knowledge.

These, however, were the ideas of the laboratory scientist, and only the wisest doctors of the time saw how important the science of chemistry was becoming to the practice of medicine. One who did was Sir William Osler, a Canadian who graduated at McGill Medical School in Montreal, became professor of medicine at Johns Hopkins University in Baltimore, and built up the first organized clinical unit in any Anglo-Saxon country. In 1905, he became regius professor of medicine at the University of Oxford. In his address to McGill University in 1894, he commented: 'the physician without physiology and chemistry flounders along in an aimless fashion, never able to gain any accurate conception of disease, practising a sort of popgun pharmacy, hitting now the malady and again the patient, he himself not knowing which.'[3]

Pharmacology Comes of Age

The initiatives of Pierre Pelletier and Joseph Caventou, and of François Magendie and Claude Bernard, spread from France to Germany, and more slowly to Britain and later the USA, and by the 1850s the experimental science called pharmacology had become widely established. It is a curiosity of history that the first chair of pharmacology was established, not in France, Germany, or Britain, but in the university at Dorpat, now called Tartu, in Estonia. Dorpat was at that time a particularly active university. It had strong links with Germany, and recruited from Leipzig an able young doctor, Rudolph Buchheim, who had already translated the classic English textbook on pharmacology – Jonathan Pereira's *The Elements of Materia Medica and Therapeutics* (1839–40). Buchheim developed the subject and was duly created a professor. His pupil, Oswald Schmiedeberg, succeeded him, and, in 1872, moved to a new department at Strasbourg. There he attracted many young doctors and scientists, who later left to develop the subject in other parts of the world.

Scottish medical schools had a strong tradition of teaching 'materia medica', largely as a branch of botany, and the departments of materia medica were well placed to take up the new science of pharmacology under the old name. These academic departments were mainly concerned with medicinal plants, and began isolating their active constituents and discovering exactly how they worked, in terms of the growing knowledge of normal physiology. Robert Christison, a medical professor in Edinburgh from 1822 to 1877, wrote a textbook on poisons and described experiments on his own heart and blood vessels with a poisonous bean from Calabar in West Africa, noting the muscular weakness or paralysis that the bean gradually induced. His successor, Thomas Fraser, isolated the bean's active constituent – an alkaloid, which he named eserine. Both researchers threw much light on the working of the autonomic nervous system. In the USA, still then a young country, developments came on similar lines, if a little later, with a profitable flow of people and ideas between the developing American universities and the established laboratories of Europe.

Spinoffs from Chemistry

Chemistry also developed rapidly in the nineteenth century, and young chemists in training had great opportunities. At the Royal College of Chemistry in London, an ambitious young student, William Henry Perkin, noted that quinine was described as $C_{20}H_{24}N_2O_2$. He thought of a simple reaction by which it could be synthesized by oxidizing allyltoluidine, a compound available to him. It looked all right on paper, but he was quite wrong. The attempt produced a coloured precipitate, certainly not quinine but exciting enough to suggest further experiments, which produced other coloured substances. Aged only 18, Perkin realized that one of them might do as a dye, and with great persistence he arranged for the material, called mauveine, to be made on a larger scale, and, finally, marketed.

Mauveine became famous as the world's first synthetic dye, and Perkin's work thus started the great dyestuff industry that developed, mainly in Germany, in the later nineteenth century. Many special chemical skills were developed in this industry, and by the end of the nineteenth century these were being applied to the manufacture of new drugs as well as dyes. Perkin's ambition to develop medicinal substances was, in a long roundabout way, fulfilled, and, after his death, on a vastly wider scale than he is likely to have foreseen.

The early history of these new substances, and especially how some came to be recognized as potential medicines, is obscure. German industrial firms worked in great secrecy, and did not reveal how they tested their new products to see if they were medicinal, or harmless, or poisonous. Some new drugs came initially from academic chemists, others from by-products of heavy chemical manufacture – pain-relievers (analgesics) and antifever drugs (antipyretics) from coal-tar distillation – and, later, from producers of fine chemicals, especially dyestuffs. Practising doctors, either on their own initiative or requested by industry, tried hitherto unknown substances on themselves, on animals, and on patients, sometimes with little more than guesswork about what the substances might do, either of benefit or of harm.

Among the most rash experiments were those with nitrous oxide, ether, and chloroform, all of which were found to cause reversible loss of consciousness. Nitrous oxide ('laughing gas'), first made by Humphry Davy about 1800, was taken up by showmen at fairgrounds to provide entertainment. Its use as an anaesthetic was inspired by observing that a man who fell and injured himself while under its influence suffered no pain at the time. Ether was more difficult to inhale, but experiments suggested that it could be more effective, and after some hesitations both substances were adopted as anaesthetics. So one horror – surgery without anaesthesia – was abolished, and new surgical procedures of all kinds became possible. Chloroform followed soon afterwards; easiest to give but more hazardous, it was for long a controversial drug.

The introduction of anaesthesia was not looked on favourably by everyone. Some thought it was unnatural and wrong to alleviate the suffering inflicted on mankind by God as a retribution for his sins. However, by the time Queen Victoria received chloroform – administered by John Snow – for the birth of Prince Leopold on 7 April 1853, the protests were medical, on the grounds of safety, rather than theological. The editor of *The Lancet* thundered, 'In no case could it be justifiable to administer chloroform in perfectly ordinary labour',[4] and went on to the special iniquity of taking risks with the Royal Sovereign. But the Queen was delighted ('The effect was soothing, quieting and delightful beyond measure', she wrote in her journal) and on the next (and last) occasion, the birth of Princess Beatrice in 1857, the critics were silent.

'Germs' and the Start of Chemotherapy

For most doctors at the end of the nineteenth century, the 'germ theory of disease' was more important than anaesthesia or any other benefits of pharmacology. The revolutionary work of Louis Pasteur and Robert Koch and their followers is described in Chapter 5; its significance cannot be overrated. The new knowledge of 'germs' started new studies of immunity and of ways in which infections could be prevented or overcome. So vaccines and antitoxins were devised. They were, by modern standards, crude and impure materials, containing complex substances far beyond the chemical knowledge of the time, and not encouraging thought on chemical lines about how they acted.

However, such thought was possible, and led the great German medical scientist Paul Ehrlich to the idea that much simpler substances might act powerfully against microbes without harming the patient. In the early part of his career, Ehrlich worked with Koch and Emil Adolf von Behring in studies of tuberculosis and diphtheria, and had an important role in the production of diphtheria antitoxin. He contracted tuberculosis himself, but recovered, and became Director of the German State Institute for Serum Research in Berlin, and later of specially endowed research laboratories. In 1908, he and the Russian Elie Metchnikoff shared a Nobel Prize for their work in immunology. By then, Ehrlich's thoughts on defence against bacteria had turned to chemical aspects, and he was investigating what he called 'chemotherapy' – the cure of bacterial infections with substances of known chemical identity.

In his student days Ehrlich had studied the staining of microbes and animal cells by dyestuffs, necessary for their observation under the microscope. It sounds an obscure subject, of purely technical interest and unrelated to the discovery of new drugs, but it was in fact fundamental. Why do dyestuffs combine with particular cells, or particular parts of cells, and not with others? Does not this question arise about any substances coloured or not, that act as drugs? Dyestuffs are convenient because they can be seen to be fixed by particular cells. But the chemical problem is the same whether the reagent is a visible dye or an invisible drug. It is the problem originally raised by Claude Bernard's studies. Ehrlich was particularly enthusiastic about the word 'receptor' for the submicroscopic structures that 'received' a dye or a drug. Developments from his lines of thought have been fundamental to pharmacology ever since.

Ehrlich looked for substances – dyes at first, other germicides later – that were fixed by microbes but not by the human or animal host of the microbe. Disinfectants and the like were effective killers but destructive also of host tissues, and he thought of modifying them chemically so that they were fixed by receptors in the microbe but not by those in the host.

The 606th compound Ehrlich studied became the famous drug called Salvarsan or arsphenamine. It was active against syphilis in rabbits, monkeys, and human beings, and was the first synthetic drug with practically useful 'chemotherapeutic' activity. It created great excitement when Ehrlich formally announced its discovery in 1910 because syphilis was at that time a socially unmentionable condition, a disease acquired immorally and ending in paralysis and insanity, and no previous remedy was curative. Ehrlich's hope that Salvarsan would kill the spirochaete bacterium that causes syphilis promptly and completely was too optimistic, but the power of the drug was undoubted and attracted the name 'magic bullet'. Salvarsan was difficult to use because it was unstable and needed to be dissolved immediately before use, and because it was active only when injected directly into the bloodstream. At that time injecting anything into a vein was unheard of except as a serious surgical procedure.

Improvements on Salvarsan were therefore looked for, and several related compounds in due course replaced it. Salvarsan and its successors attacked few other microbes, and no more magic bullets were discovered until the sulphonamides and penicillin. Ehrlich's work was followed by a period of pessimism; his success against syphilis was dismissed because the spirochaete that causes it is a very unusual organism, and many people said that antibacterial chemotherapy was an impossible dream.

The Functions of Ductless Glands

Meanwhile, physiology was making progress. From the 1830s onwards, scientists were concerned about various 'ductless' glands in different parts of the body – the thyroid and parathyroid glands in the neck, the adrenal or suprarenal glands near the kidneys, and the pituitary at the base of the brain. Some islets of tissue in the pancreas did not connect with the pancreatic ducts, and these also counted as a ductless gland. Gradually, the functions of the ductless glands were identified – by clinical observation of conditions in which the glands were enlarged or damaged or destroyed, and by seeing the results of their removal in experimental animals.

Was it possible that the glands contained materials that were essential to life? In 1891, the English physician George Murray, then in Newcastle upon Tyne, prepared extracts of the thyroid gland of sheep and fed them to a patient with myxoedema (underactivity of the thyroid). She got better, and was kept in good health for 28 years by treatment with thyroid preparations. Like the discovery of diphtheria antitoxin at about the same time, this discovery was a major advance; one of the occasions on which a completely effective treatment superseded a state in which no cure was known. Then, in 1927, material identical with the thyroid hormone was synthesized and used to treat a patient. The treatment succeeded, and no difference whatever was found between the natural and the synthetic hormone. Magical though the effect of thyroid hormone appeared to be, there was no need to attribute its benefit to any mysterious vital principle.

Other hormones presented greater difficulties. The connection between the pancreas and sugar diabetes was discovered in 1876, about the time when the thyroid was recognized as important. But feeding pancreas by mouth did not help diabetics. An injectable active pancreatic principle was sought for a long time, with several near misses. During 1921, however, Frederick G. Banting and Charles H. Best in Toronto University isolated material from the pancreases of dogs and used it to keep diabetic dogs alive. On 11 January 1922, they gave the first injections of this substance, which they named insulin, to a 14-year-old boy dying of diabetes; almost immediately his blood-sugar level fell. In 1923, with the help of a biochemist, James B. Collip, the pancreatic extracts were purified sufficiently to reduce the side-effects from the treatment. That same year, a Nobel Prize was awarded to Banting and to John J. R. Macleod, in whose physiological laboratory the research was done; Best, Banting's assistant, was overlooked. Banting was so furious at the omission of Best that he shared his half-prize with him; Macleod shared his with Collip.

Tremendous excitement was created by this discovery and there was an enormous demand for insulin, but its manufacture in sufficient quantities was far beyond the capacity of any university laboratory. Only the collaboration of the Connaught antitoxin laboratories in Toronto and the pharmaceutical business of Eli Lilly in Indianapolis made large-scale production (using pig pancreas) possible. Thereafter, diabetes in young people became no longer a death sentence but a condition entirely compatible with leading a normal life.

Hormones have been isolated from other glands, each with their own special and curious problems and consequences. The testes and ovaries were found to secrete hormones as well as producing sperm and ova, and their hormones, mostly isolated in the early 1930s, were of great value in the management of sexual and reproductive disorders. That they could also be used to control fertility was long suspected, but needed many experiments and trials to be realized practically. Twenty years later, a biologist at the Worcester Foundation for Experimental Biology in Massachusetts called Gregory Pincus, with Carl Djerassi and others, developed an oral contraceptive for women. It was not until the 1960s, however, that the 'pill' became widely available. It is interesting to speculate, but difficult to get evidence, whether discovery of oral contraceptives was an important factor in the great increase in sexual licence at the time. It is perhaps more important to appreciate their potential for allowing women to space their families and reducing world population.

Chemical or Electrical Messengers?

Hormones are not the only way in which substances secreted by certain cells influence the activity of other cells. After experiments by Luigi Galvani and others in the eighteenth century, the main controlling part of the body, the nervous system, was recognized as working by some kind of electricity. But evidence accumulated that nerves acted on other cells, and even on each other, by chemical means, by substances bridging the tiny gaps between adjacent cells.

'Of known natural processes that might pass on excitation, only two are, in my opinion, worth talking about', wrote Emil du Bois-Reymond in 1877: 'either there exists at the boundary of the contractile substance a stimulatory secretion in the form of a thin layer of ammonia, lactic acid, or some other powerful stimulatory substance; or the phenomenon is electrical in nature.'[5] Some striking resemblances between hormones and nerve transmitters (the latter were sometimes called local hormones) had been noted. The hormone adrenaline, secreted by the medullary part of the adrenal glands, acted very like the sympathetic nervous system. Could it be, physiologists wondered, that the nerves themselves released adrenaline at their endings, and that the adrenal medulla served to reinforce the effects of all the sympathetic nerves? The same question was asked about the parasympathetic nervous system, because an unstable substance called acetylcholine acted just like parasympathetic nerves. Was it the transmitter at those nerve endings? As summarized in Chapter 5, experiments by neurophysiologists such as Otto Loewi in Graz, Henry Dale and his colleagues (who included several refugees from Nazi persecution in Germany) in London, Walter B. Cannon in Cambridge, Massachusetts, and Ulf von Euler in Stockholm turned these ideas into hard fact and provided the basis on which an astonishing number of new drugs were discovered.

Chemical transmitters make muscles contract and start glands secreting, and set into train more elaborate processes. All kinds of chemical transmission (and so chemical control of particular cellular activities) can be imitated by substances that resemble the natural transmitters closely. This principle was first made to work in the USA in about 1930 in Pennsylvania, when two new drugs, carbachol and methacholine, were synthesized at the Merck laboratories and used medicinally. They imitated acetylcholine, but the effects lasted longer, so they were used for their action on the bladder to overcome postoperative retention of urine. The application was comparatively trivial, but the principle was sound and is the basis of most of the blood-pressure drugs in use today.

Vitamins

A new kind of medicine arrived with the discovery of vitamins. Although nutritional deficiency diseases had been known since the work of James Lind and others, the different chemical identities of the substances causing the diseases were not discovered until the twentieth century. The term 'vitamin' was coined in 1912 by Casimir Funk, a chemist working at the Lister Institute in London. It was partly his research that helped clarify the distinctive functions of vitamins.

When Funk started his work, it was known from clinical studies that certain human diseases were caused by a deficiency of specific vitamins: for example, beriberi for lack of thiamine (vitamin B_1); scurvy, long known to be prevented by a sufficiency of citrus fruits, for a lack of ascorbic acid (vitamin C); and so on. It was realized that where there was a lack of a particular vitamin in the diet, treatment with that vitamin was life-saving. Once this became known, there were no further doubts about how to treat specific deficiency diseases.

Regrettably, however, superstition grew fast about vitamins, and they promptly acquired a reputation as magical cure-alls. Manufacturers were quick to exploit the myth, baffled physicians were relieved to adopt it, and comfort-seeking patients were (and are) all too willing to believe it. Evidence for minor benefits from various vitamins is hard to obtain and generally of the anecdotal and unconvincing kind. But poisoning by excess, particularly of the fat-soluble vitamins, is well known: nervous disturbances and birth defects are produced by an excess of vitamin A, and excess of body calcium and kidney stones after too much vitamin D. But vitamins remain a popular and heavily promoted form of therapy, rarely (in prosperous countries) with any rational basis. They are probably more rewarding to the shareholders of manufacturing companies than to most of the people who consume them.

Whether vitamins are drugs is a matter of the use of language, and need not be pursued. The term vitamin, contracted mistakenly by Casimir Funk from 'vital amine', is misleading, because most accessory food factors are not amines, and whether they are vital, meaning essential for survival, differs from species to species. But the name has come to stay.

The way vitamins act in living cells throws much light on the ways cells work, and knowledge of this activity has been used to design drugs for specific purposes, especially antibacterial agents. The detailed biochemistry of vitamins was worked out largely in microbes – much more convenient and socially acceptable research subjects than mammals. From the knowledge so gained it was a simple step (although few saw the great possibilities) to go on to designing antibacterial drugs that interfere with the way microbes use their essential foods. Remarkable results followed.

Modern Pharmaceuticals Emerge

Before the development of such antibiotics, however, there was a discovery made on more classical lines. It took place in the laboratories of the Bayer Company in Elberfeld, Germany, in the early 1930s. A German biochemist, Gerhard Domagk, appointed to direct Bayer's research in 1927, continued Paul Ehrlich's approach of investigating dyestuffs, and presently showed that a red dye, later named Prontosil, was extraordinarily effective in curing streptococcal infections in mice. Clinical trials followed, and by 1935 the drug was used in patients with great success. One of the first to receive the new medicine was Domagk's daughter, who made a dramatic recovery from a streptococcal infection caused by a needle prick.

Prontosil proved especially effective in treating women with childbirth fever or puerperal sepsis, which is mostly streptococcal in origin and, until that time, took a sorry toll of deaths of young mothers. The discovery deserved a Nobel Prize; indeed, Domagk was nominated for one in 1939, but was forbidden by the Nazi government to accept it. When Germany was no longer at war, the Nobel rules forbade him to have the prize money after such a delay.

Meanwhile research at the Pasteur Institute in Paris showed that only a part of the molecule of Prontosil was necessary to defeat streptococci, and the active component, named sulphanilamide, soon superseded Prontosil – no doubt to the chagrin of all concerned in the Bayer Company, which held the patents for Prontosil. Sulphanilamide was a well-known substance; it was first synthesized in 1908 during studies on dyes and for nearly 30 years lay among the stores of many organic chemists, because no one knew or suspected that it could save lives.

When Gerhard Domagk and his Bayer colleagues found that sulphanilamide checked streptococcal bacteria in mice, they, and many others, naturally wondered how the drug worked. Their question was answered remarkably soon. Clinical trials with human patients showed that the drug did not work in abscesses filled with pus. Test-tube experiments showed that pus and also other materials, including yeast extracts, protected the germs against sulphanilamide. The protective principle in both pus and yeast was identified: it was a simple compound called p-aminobenzoic acid (PABA), very closely related to sulphanilamide itself. PABA was soon found to be an essential nutrient for some microbes, and these turned out to be just those species that were sensitive to sulphanilamide. Clearly, the two compounds competed. The sulphanilamide got in like PABA, but then jammed the works. The process, named 'competitive antagonism', was studied closely, and, in spite of the labyrinthine complexity of the details, provided a huge advance in understanding how drugs acted, how drugs might act, and how new and useful drugs could be invented.

The clinical trials of sulphanilamide were not elaborate by more recent standards, but the drug had dramatic effects and left little doubt about its merits. However, it also had ill-effects, altering blood pigments so that patients looked blue, and occasionally damaging the blood-forming tissues so that white blood cells disappeared. Hence the search began for better compounds, mostly from the family called sulphonamides, to which sulphanilamide belonged. Within a few years more than 5,000 sulphonamides had been examined and perhaps 50 found clinically useful against bacteria of various kinds and some other organisms. The earliest sulphonamides – sulphanilamide itself and the sulphapyridine from May and Baker (once famous as M & B 693) – were discarded when numerous safer agents were discovered.

The distinction between antibiotics and chemotherapeutic drugs is a historical accident. Several antibiotics have been prepared synthetically, and no distinction whatever has been found between these and those prepared from 'natural' fungal material. However, penicillins (there were several varieties in the materials originally extracted) are difficult to prepare synthetically, and are more economically made from cultured moulds. Nonetheless, the original penicillins have been modified chemically and with advantage for various specific purposes, and clinical practice today depends heavily on such semisynthetic materials.

Unhappily for humans, strains of bacteria resistant to drugs have emerged. Microbes pass through many generations in a matter of days or weeks, and so they evolve very rapidly. As soon as antibacterial agents were widely used, microbes that resisted them had a great advantage for survival, while their less-resistant cousins and competitors were quickly eliminated. Bacteria resistant to antibiotics such as penicillin thus steadily became more common, and so the dream faded that a few antibiotics would put an end to humanity's infectious diseases.

Some respite has been achieved by using combinations of antibacterial agents, because resistant strains have less chance of emerging if microbes are attacked by two or more drugs at the same time. Important new antibiotics are especially those that control resistant strains of familiar germs. But the conflict between humans and microbes is not resolved, nor is it likely to be, and continued research is essential if new and dangerous strains are to be kept under control.

Antiviral Agents

Finding agents against viruses has proved difficult. Most success has been obtained with vaccines, and especially the first vaccine (pioneered by Edward Jenner at the end of the eighteenth century), which made possible the elimination of a once universally feared deadly or disfiguring disease, smallpox. Vaccines against other viruses, notably that of yellow fever, have also been successful. Viruses are, however, intracellular parasites, difficult of access, and the intimate association between the metabolism of the virus and the host has for long challenged any chemical solution. Only in the past 20 years has striking progress been made, illustrated by the remarkable properties of acyclovir.

Acyclovir (Zovirax), discovered in the Wellcome laboratories in the USA and in England in the 1970s, is potent against herpes zoster (shingles), cold sores, and other herpes infections. Acyclovir is converted in cells infected with the herpes virus to a metabolic blocking agent, and so is of minimal danger to healthy tissues; the problem of toxicity to the host is largely overcome. Other viruses have been less amenable, or less intensively pursued; influenza viruses continue to be a recurrent hazard, especially the human immunodeficiency virus (HIV), which paves the way for AIDS. Zidovudine (Retrovir), a somewhat distant chemical relative of acyclovir, is the first drug to be recognized by regulatory bodies for the treatment of HIV infection.

The Chemotherapy of Cancer

A different kind of chemotherapy began with the discovery that substances called nitrogen mustards selectively kill a particular kind of cancerous cell. The story is a fine example of a trail that reached a valuable conclusion quite different from the intended objective. It began in the Second World War, when research was resumed, for obvious reasons, on chemical warfare agents. Whatever the ethics of their use, no nation could afford to be ignorant of their properties or be unprepared to treat whatever casualties might occur. In the USA, substances closely related to mustard gas were studied in depth by the pharmacologists Louis Goodman and Alfred Gilman at Yale University and found, among other properties, to destroy white blood cells (lymphocytes). When one was administered to a mouse with a lymphoma (a large solid tumour of the lymph cells) the tumour shrank dramatically, in a way never seen before. The experiment was reproducible, and so patients with lymphocyte tumours were treated with nitrogen mustards, naturally with extreme caution, but soon with considerable success.

The path was opened to the discovery of other agents for cancer chemotherapy. One promising approach was to synthesize compounds that resembled folic acid, which is used in the formation of new blood cells, including the excessive proliferation in leukaemia. Folic acid analogues were made, especially at the Lederle Laboratories. One of them (aminopterin) was shown in the 1940s to cause striking remissions in childhood leukaemia. Another approach depended on studying the pathway by which nucleic acids are synthesized. Here, too, the tactic was used of making analogues that could jam some particular part of the works without non-specific disastrous consequences. George Hitchings and Gertrude Elion at the Wellcome laboratories then in New York produced a sequence of new drugs in this way in the 1940s and 1950s. They included 6-mercaptopurine, which was also found to cause remissions in some leukaemia patients.

More fortuitous discoveries included the anthracycline antibiotic called daunorubicin, derived from a *Streptomyces* fungus and active against a variety of solid tumours as well as acute leukaemias, and the alkaloids called vincristine and vinblastine, obtained from periwinkles (*Vinca*). All of these substances are highly toxic and their use calls for specialist expertise at every stage. Many leukaemias responded well, and these conditions, once invariably fatal, now often have a prospect of recovery. But cancer cells, like microbes, become resistant to chemotherapy. Repeated courses of treatment are all too often less and less effective, and drugs, whether natural or synthetic, have, so far, proved more often palliative than curative.

Growth of the Pharmaceutical Industry

After the war of 1939–45, the pharmaceutical industry expanded greatly. By the 1980s around ten companies were usually among the top fifty major corporations in the USA, and there was similar growth in Britain and elsewhere in Europe. Research laboratories grew even faster than the companies; typically, the old-established American firm of Smith, Kline & French had a research staff of eight in 1936, which grew to hundreds in the 1950s and now is enlarged by amalgamations with other enterprises into Smith Kline Beecham.

In such laboratories millions of compounds were synthesized and tested for pharmacological and antimicrobial properties. The search was conducted in various ways, some rational, and sometimes more speculative or quite random. Many useful drugs resulted from each kind of approach; luck as well as judgment is crucial to success in research. Often, several drugs were discovered with closely similar properties, and complaints were made about the waste in such 'me-too' discoveries. However, among major series of drugs, such as sulphonamides and corticosteroids, the original agents have been completely superseded by successors widely regarded as having a better overall performance. A 'me-too' drug is not necessarily worse, and may be distinctly better than its competitor.

Does It Really Work?

It has always been much easier to believe optimistically in a remedy than to prove its worth in even a faintly scientific way. Extensive clinical research has been applied to discovering how best to use the powerful new remedies produced by the pharmaceutical laboratories, to discovering which of similar drugs is preferable, and indeed to discovering whether their use is, in the long run and in spite of superficial appearances, beneficial at all. Bedside observation of individual patients under treatment has been supplemented by collection of facts about as many as possible of the patients treated in one way or another. Sometimes it then turns out that, however excitingly some sufferers appear to recover, most of the patients being treated actually do worse than those who are left alone or receive other treatments.

Not only do new remedies need evaluating: many traditional remedies must also be questioned, as the eighteenth-century naval physician, James Lind, observed in the preface to his *Treatise on Scurvy* (1753). His wisdom remains all too true but is often forgotten:

It appeared to me a subject worthy of the strictest inquiry: and I was led upon this occasion to consult several authors who had treated of the disease; where I perceived mistakes which have been attended in practice, with dangerous and fatal consequences. There appeared to me an evident necessity of rectifying those errors, on account of the pernicious effects they have already visibly produced. But as it is no easy matter to root out old prejudices, or to overturn opinions which have acquired an establishment by time, custom, and great authorities; it became therefore requisite for this purpose, to exhibit a full and impartial view of what has hitherto been published on the scurvy; and that in a chronological order, by which the sources of those mistakes may be detected. Indeed, before this subject could be set in a clear and proper light, it was necessary to remove a great deal of rubbish.[6]

History of the use of medicines reveals, over and over again, how much trust is placed in medical beliefs that particular remedies are effective and that it is negligent or worse to withhold them. And yet, years or centuries later the remedies have fallen into disuse, if not positive disrepute, because their lack of good or their positive harm has at last been revealed by careful accumulation of evidence and refusal to be swayed by casual anecdotes.

The principles and value of good clinical trials were shown most lucidly when the efficacy of streptomycin in the treatment of tuberculosis was evaluated just after the Second World War by the British Medical Research Council, advised by Sir Austin Bradford Hill of the London School of Hygiene and Tropical Medicine. Very little of the new drug was available when the trial started in 1946 – just enough for a small proportion of the patients who might have benefited. It was therefore considered ethically justifiable to carry out a trial in which one group received streptomycin whereas a control group was treated with traditional methods. The randomized controlled clinical trial, the first of its type, provided clear evidence about which treatments were more effective than others and set a model for many subsequent studies of new drugs. It has become unacceptable to claim benefit for a new drug without clinical trials. Unfortunately, not all trials are conducted well enough to be reliable.

Unwanted Effects

The toxicity of many new agents has been discovered only after they were in regular use. The harm caused by thalidomide in the 1950s was particularly distressing and aroused powerful demands for safe drugs. Testing drugs for toxicity, however, is an insoluble problem; the number of ways in which a drug may be toxic is unlimited, and attempts to detect them all in advance have consistently been defeated, whenever new hazards have been discovered.

In recent years, the introduction of life-saving drugs has often been delayed while tests of regrettably uncertain value are done. In the 1970s, the phrase 'drug lag' became familiar, especially in the USA, to describe the delays imposed by authorities. It has been claimed that several thousand American citizens would die of heart failure between the time a drug that would prevent their death becomes available in European countries and the time it was licensed in the USA. Special procedures, sometimes called the 'fast track', were designed to overcome the lag. Gradually, it has been accepted that the most valuable safeguard rests on adequate recording of all uses of new drugs and reporting of all adverse effects.

Society and Drugs

Since the Second World War, in at least industrialized societies, people have become more preoccupied with health, illness, and medicine than ever before. Certainly, the media endlessly draw attention to medicines and drugs and arouse enthusiasm or anxiety often on very slender grounds. How far popular attitudes are fuelled by broadcasting, or by the advertising of drug manufacturers, is no part of this chapter, nor are the social processes that led to the rise and decline of the 'permissive society' and the use of 'recreational' drugs with all the hazards of toxicity, impurity, and abuse.

One may note how enthusiasm for 'science' has given place to scepticism, and particularly in medicine how the pursuit of technical improvements has got in the way of compassion and caring. There is an interesting parallel in the history of China. In about 700 BC, medical practice had become increasingly based on direct observation and was to that extent comparable to 'scientific medicine'. Then it gave way to new, or resuscitated, systems in which superstition, magic, and charms played a large part. Whether the change had any significant consequences and only time and reliable statistics will tell whether the current confusion and distaste for 'scientific medicine' is having measurable results.

As far as drugs are concerned, the important 'alternative' or 'complementary' therapies are homeopathy and herbalism. The tenets of homeopathy involve rejecting the whole basis of orthodox physics and chemistry, and the homeopathists' use of medicines does not depend on their actions as studied by pharmacologists but on an unconventional system of beliefs. Herbal remedies existed long before any evaluation of medicines was thought about. From herbs have come many important drugs, including belladonna, curare, codeine, digitalis, ipecacuanha, and nicotine. All these are potent, and the plants that produce them are recognized as poisonous. Many other herbal remedies remain of unproven worth, at least by scientific standards.

Without a demonstrable action, no active ingredient can be identified. Many herbal preparations available 'off the shelf' do not contain any potent substances and, like homeopathic medicines, give comfort if they please the patient. However, quite a number of garden plants are poisonous, and any self-treatment with such plants is dangerous. With the penchant for a 'green' way of life, accidental self-poisoning with 'natural' herbs is being recorded more frequently. Even seemingly mild herbal teas may cause harm if taken regularly for long periods of time. Also, herbal remedies are occasionally adulterated with 'chemical' drugs to achieve greater potency, regardless of safety, and the lack of control of the sale of herbal remedies is a cause for growing concern. Homeopathy and herbalism, like faith in vitamins, have been favoured chiefly for conditions in which symptoms rather than objective changes are prominent. Measurement of benefit is difficult, and evaluation by properly controlled trials is rare.

Potent drugs are as dangerous as a surgeon's sharp knife, and must be handled with equal care if they are to do good. The proper use of orthodox medicines has brought about great triumphs in prolonging life and relieving suffering, and it is silly to despise or underrate this achievement. The greater the power of the remedy, the greater the hazards of misuse.

8. Mental Illness

Roy Porter

Madness is an enigma. Being 'mad' is part of common speech. Especially in American English, 'mad' means 'angry' ('he'll get real mad!') and we speak of being 'mad about' someone, or crazy in love. In such usage, madness is a mood or feeling. Most people, medical and lay alike, also accept that madness (or mental illness, psychiatric disorder, and so forth) can be an authentic medical condition. I emphasize 'most', because leaders of the antipsychiatry movement launched in the 1960s – notably Ronald Laing in Britain and Thomas Szasz in the USA – denied the reality of mental illness in the strict sense of the term, denied that madness was a disease like measles or malaria. According to Szasz, writing in 1974, madness was a witch-hunting label pinned on 'deviants' or scapegoats for the purpose of psychiatric empire-building and to exercise social control.

The relations between being mad as extreme emotion or eccentric behaviour, and (on the other hand) madness as a medical diagnosis are complex and controversial. Even those satisfied that madness is a disease contest what it is, what causes it, and what may be done about it. To understand how madness has grown so maddeningly confusing, its history must be explored.

The Greek Tradition

Pre-Classical cultures certainly identified madness, but it is with the Greeks that madness first became an object of rational inquiry and literary depiction. In Greek myths, the heroes grow demented, driven wild with frenzy or beside themselves with rage or grief.

> DIONYSUS: The reason why I have chosen Thebes as the first place
> To raise my Bacchic shout, and clothe all who respond
> In fawnskin habits, and put my thyrsus in their hands –
> The weapon wreathed with ivy-shoots – my reason is this;
> My mother's sisters said – what they should have been the last
> To say – that I, Dionysus, was not Zeus's son;
> That Semele, being with child – they said – by some mortal,
> Obeyed her father's prompting, and ascribed to Zeus
> The loss of her virginity; and they loudly claimed
> That this lie was the sin for which Zeus took her life.
> Therefore I have driven those same sisters mad, turned them
> All frantic out of doors; their home now is the mountain;
> Their wits are gone. I have made them bear the emblem of
> My mysteries; the whole female population of Thebes,
> To the last woman, I have sent raving from their homes.
> Now, side by side with Cadmus' daughters, one and all
> Sit rootless on the rocks under the silver pines.
>
> Euripedes, *The Bacchae*

The *Iliad* reveals the remnants of archaic attitudes towards madness; it does not display insanity as later understood by medicine and philosophy, for Homer's heroes do not possess psyches or forms of consciousness comparable to that of Sophocles's Oedipus, still less to that of Hamlet or Sigmund Freud. Homer's epics give their characters no sensitive, reflective, introspective selves. Greek heroes are puppet-like, at the mercy of forces from Beyond: gods, demons, the fates, and furies. They do not have what modern authors call 'intrapsychic' existences.

The introspective mentality emerged at the height of Athenian civilization in the fifth and fourth centuries BC; and an American psychiatrist and historian, Bennett Simon, argued in his book *Mind and Madness in Ancient Greece* that the idea of the psyche then developing was to set the mould for Western reasoning about minds and madness ever since. Sigmund Freud said as much by labelling infantile psychosexual conflicts the 'Oedipus Complex', thereby paying homage to Sophocles's tragedy, *Oedipus Rex.*

Socrates, Plato, Aristotle, and other Greek thinkers of their day systematically reasoned about nature, society, and consciousness.

They probed the unknown, seeking to grasp the order of things and to depict the rational self as exemplary, creating ideals of ethical man or political man. Through self-knowledge (as in the adage 'know thyself'), reason could fathom human nature and thereby master enslaving appetites. Thus philosophy ennobled reason.

In their pursuit of reason, Greek philosophers did not deny the reality of what was not rational. On the contrary, the store they set by reason attests the dangerous power they ascribed to passions and the mysterious forces of fate, just as they were also fascinated by the transcendental 'fire' that consumed geniuses and artists. Nevertheless, Plato and his followers defined the irrational as the enemy of human dignity and freedom; and the polarity between the rational and the irrational, as with supremacy of mind over matter, became cardinal to Classical moral and medical values, remaining influential down to the present day.

If the rise of philosophy enabled the Greeks to reason on madness, how did they explain that calamity of the soul? How did they expect to prevent or cure it? There were two leading traditions through which they made sense of madness. One lay in culture, expressed in rhetoric, art, and theatre. Greek tragedians dramatized the primeval conflicts of life – the fate of the individual crushed by ineluctable destiny, the torment of divided loyalties, the rival demands of love and hatred, pity and revenge, duty and desire, mortals and deities, family and polis. And they showed these conflicts becoming (contrast Homer's puppet-like heroes) conscious objects of reflection and inner conflict, censure and guilt. Madness had become the condition and fate of minds divided against themselves. The heroes of Sophocles and Euripides were conscious of having brought madness on themselves; psychic civil war thereby became intrinsic to the human condition.

But drama also suggested resolutions, or, in Bennett Simon's phrase, theatre became therapy. As with Oedipus, desperate suffering could engender a higher wisdom, blindness could beget insight, bloodshed could purify, and public drama could stage collective catharsis. Enacting madness, forcing the unthinkable to be spoken, bringing into the open the monsters of the mental deep, reclaimed the emotional battleground for reason, all passion spent.

Thus madness could be the tormented soul, which art could capture. Yet the Greeks also developed a quite different way of grasping madness: a medical tradition. As explained in Chapter 2, the style of medical thinking expressed in the Hippocratic writings in the fifth century BC and dominant thereafter insisted that disease was natural and hence amenable to empirical and rational inquiry. Of particular relevance, a Hippocratic treatise, *On the Sacred Disease*, insisted that the falling sickness or epilepsy – heretofore regarded as a supernatural disorder – was a regular ailment like any other, a routine malady produced by normal bodily processes. So if the so-called sacred disease was natural, by implication all other abnormalities of behaviour, all madness, equally fell within medicine's bounds. Explanations of insanity should thus be couched in terms of physical causes and effects, emphasizing the heart or brain, blood, spirits, and humours; and treatments would rely on regimen and medicines. To the scientific temper, insanity was not a dilemma or a drama but a disease.

As discussed more fully in Chapters 2 and 3, mainstream Greek medicine proposed internal, constitutional causes for illness. Health hinged on the four 'humours' or body fluids. These were also the key to mental disturbance. An excess of yellow bile (*choler*) would overheat the system, causing mania or raving madness: by contrast, surplus black bile (*melancholia*) would induce dejection. Aretaeus, a contemporary of Galen active in the second half of the second century AD in Alexandria, gave particularly detailed accounts of melancholy and mania in his *On the Causes and Signs of Diseases*.[1] 'Sufferers are dull or stern: dejected or unreasonably torpid, without any manifest cause: such is the commencement of melancholy', he observed:

and they also become peevish, despirited, sleepless, and start up from a disturbed sleep. Unreasonable fears also seize them; if the disease tends to increase, when their dreams are true, terrifying and clear; for whatever, when awake, they have an aversion to as being an evil, rushes upon their visions in sleep... But if the illness become more urgent, hatred, avoidance of the haunts of men, vain lamentations are seen: they complain of life and desire to die; in many the understanding so leads to insensibility and fatuousness that they become ignorant of all things and forgetful of themselves and live the life of inferior animals.

As Aretaeus's discussion of fear, loathing, and suicidal urges makes clear, in Classical medicine melancholy was far from the delicious langour it became for eighteenth-century churchyard poets. It was a dangerous condition that bred devastating delusions. 'The patient may imagine he has taken another form than his own', commented Aretaeus:

> one believes himself a sparrow; a cock or an earthen vase; another a God, orator or actor, carrying gravely a stalk of straw and imagining himself holding a sceptre of the World; some utter cries of an infant and demand to be carried in arms, or they believe themselves a grain of mustard, and tremble continuously for fear of being eaten by a hen; some refuse to urinate for fear of causing a new deluge.

Comparable stereotypes – the man fearful of urinating, and the patient convinced he was made of glass, at any second liable to shatter – remained widespread until the eighteenth century.

Paralleling melancholia, Aretaeus depicted mania, marked by uncontrollable ferocity and visible in 'furor, excitement and euphoria'. In grave forms of mania (the Latin term was *furor*), the sick person 'sometimes kills and slaughters the servants'; in less-severe cases, he would become grandiose: 'without being cultivated he says he is a philosopher'. Rationalist by temper, Aretaeus also drew attention to manifestations of religious mania involving possession by a god (divine furor), especially among those trapped in frenzied goddess cults. In 'enthusiastic and ecstatic states', devotees of Cybele (Juno) would engage in orgiastic rituals, and occasionally 'castrate themselves and then offer their penis to the goddess'. All this, Aretaeus considered, betrayed 'an insanity . . . in an ill, drunken and confused soul'. As is evident, Aretaeus linked disturbance with the changed physical states caused by intoxication, through 'ingestion of wine, mandrake or black henbane'. Mania was typically the product of excessive heat, originating from the heart (the seat of vital heat) and sympathetically connected with the brain.

In short, through a philosophy that made man the measure of all things, Classical thinkers humanized madness. They then specified diverse schemes for explaining derangement. On the one hand, insanity might be mind at the end of its tether, tortured by the pitiless Fates, at war with itself. Or mental disorder might be somatic, a fever-like delirium, caused by bad blood or bile. The dichotomy between psychological and somatic theories of madness was left for the inheritors of the Greek legacy – and finally us – to resolve.

Medieval and Renaissance Madness

Ideas about madness in the Middle Ages and the Renaissance drew heavily on motifs inherited from antiquity. Melancholia and mania (often in English just called 'madness') provided a convenient scheme of opposites. Denys Fontanon, a professor at Montpellier, one of Europe's leading medical schools, argued in his *De Morborum Interiorum Curatione Libri Tres* (Three Books on the Cure of Internal Diseases, 1549) that mania 'arises from stinging and warm humours, such as yellow bile, attacking the brain and stimulating it along with its membranes. It sometimes even originates in incorrupt blood which may even be temperate but which harms the brain by its quantity alone'.

His younger Montpellier contemporary, Felix Plater, similarly depicted mania as a condition of excess. Maniacs, he wrote in *Praxeos Medicae Opus* (1650), would 'do everything unreasonably'. 'Sometimes they... express their mental impulse in a wild expression and in word and deed... Some of them intensely seek sexual satisfaction. I saw this happen to a certain noble matron, who was in every other way most honorable, but who invited by the basest words and gestures men and dogs to have intercourse with her.'

The contrasting models of mental alienation developed by the Greeks – madness as moral perversion, madness as disease – were assimilated within Christendom. But the Church added another conviction: religious madness as the expression of divine providence, regarded as a symptom of the warfare waged between God and Satan for the soul. Religious madness was generally viewed as a diabolical contagion, spread by witches, demoniacs, and heretics. In his celebrated *Anatomy of Melancholy* (1621), Robert Burton, an Oxford clergyman, identified Satan as the true author of depression, despair, and self-destruction. Spiritual maladies, Burton believed, had to be treated by spiritual means, especially prayer and fasting.

Although often viewed as a divine affliction – witness Herod's fate – religious madness was occasionally honoured as a wondrous revelation of holiness. A faith founded on the madness of the Cross, which celebrated the innocence of babes and sucklings, valued the spiritual reveries of hermits and mortification of the flesh, and prized faith over intellect. Such a creed could hardly avoid seeing gleams of godliness in the simplicity of the idiot or in the wild transports of mystics. Strands of medieval, Reformation, and Counter-Reformation theology therefore believed that Folly might be a medium for divine utterance and bade it be heard.

Madness in the Age of Reason

From the seventeenth century, powerful cultural forces changed attitudes towards madness. The Scientific Revolution attacked humoral medicine as part of its all-out assault on the theories of Aristotle and his followers (see Chapter 5). The fashionable view of the body as a machine promoted long-term research into its solid parts, notably the cardiovascular and the nervous systems. Anatomists laid bare the hydraulic system of pipes and the circuitry of wires coordinating the limbs, spinal cord, and cortex, and began exploring the role of the nervous system in governing sensations and motion. Within this mechanical model of the body, confused thoughts, feelings, and behaviour became attributed to some defect of the sense organs (eyes, ears, etc.) and their nervous networks. Eighteenth-century doctors popularized the term 'nerves' and coined the word 'neurosis'. For long, 'neurosis' denoted a physical lesion of the nervous system; only during the nineteenth century did 'neurosis' come to mean a mild, non-specific anxiety state, as distinct from 'psychosis'.

'I *think*, therefore I am', claimed the philosopher René Descartes in 1637; and the Enlightenment in turn endorsed the Greek faith in reason that had been poured into new bottles by the seventeenth-century Rationalists. Reformers in the age of reason set about criticizing beliefs and institutions considered unreasonable or irrational. The progress of science and technology, the development of the professions and bureaucracy, the expansion of the market economy with its laws of supply and demand, and the spread of literacy and education all contributed to the privileging of 'rationality', as understood by the right-thinking elite in the eighteenth century. Capitalist economies and centralizing states needed order, regularity, predictability, and self-discipline; abnormality provoked anxiety.

From the mid-seventeenth century, similar processes of redefinition were afoot within the Church, Catholic and Protestant alike. Traditional teachings about religious madness came under scrutiny. Popes, prelates, and preachers grew as sickened as other elites by the carnage caused by endless dogmatic faction-fighting, by witch-hunts and heresy trials. The grand apocalyptic struggles during the Reformation and Counter-Reformation between God and the Devil for the possession of souls had evidently produced only chaos; the idea of life as a spiritual Great War became repellant and was rejected. And so the reality – or at least the validity – of religious madness came into question. Especially after 1650, claims by self-styled prophets to speak with divine tongues were treated with the utmost suspicion by the authorities. Such 'Fifth Monarchists', 'Ranters', and 'Convulsionaries', it was now said, were probably nothing but blind zealots, suffering from delusion or disease, perhaps epilepsy. At the close of the 'century of revolution', John Locke found it time to reassert *The Reasonableness of Christianity* (1695). Even religion, it seemed, now had to be rational.

A similar shift applied to witches. Across Europe from the fifteenth century, authorities had treated witches as confederates with the Devil. But the witch-hunt got out of hand, creating rather than quelling anarchy. By 1650, ruling elites wanted to wash their hands of it. They argued that witchcraft was not a real Satanic plot but a gigantic delusion. So-called witches were not truly diabolically possessed but deluded, and their victims were merely prey to personal and collective hysteria. What was once attributed to Satan was increasingly seen as sickness; so-called witchcraft and demonism were (according to the fashionable physicians and philosophers who joined London's newly founded Royal Society) merely psychopathological, symptoms of mental illness. In eighteenth-century England, magistrates widely believed that the fervent excesses of Methodist converts, swooning in sermons, were fit cases for the mad-doctor. An Anglican clergyman and a healer of the sick at heart,

William Pargeter, had stronger reasons than most for denouncing Methodism as a form of mass hysteria.

> *Fanaticism* is very common cause of Madness. Most of the Maniacal cases that ever came under my observation, proceeded from religious *enthusiasm*; and I have heard it remarked by an eminent physician, that almost all the insane patients, which occurred to him at one of the largest hospitals in the *metropolis*, had been deprived of their reason, by such strange infatuation. The *doctrines* of the *Methodists* have a greater tendency than those of any other sect, to produce the most deplorable effects on the human understanding. The brain is perplexed in the mazes of mystery, and the imagination overpowered by the tremendous description of future torments.[2]

The redefinition of religious madness as essentially psychopathological widened the gulf between 'society' – those promoting polite reason – and the strange. This was a deep-seated process. In numerous ways, affluent, polite, and literate society was distancing itself from those who did not comply with its norms – criminals, vagrants, the religious 'lunatic fringe' – and was calling them irrational, crazy, or mad. Finding such outsiders disturbing it was easy to call them disturbed. Madness thus became a term of opprobrium.

But it would be glib to suggest that the notion of the irrational was simply turned into a stick with which to beat the masses. For within elite culture, fashionable eccentricity was to enjoy a long vogue. It was the done thing, throughout the eighteenth and nineteenth centuries, for certain young ladies to have fits of hysterics and for artists and poets to be morbidly oversensitive, suffering nervous breakdowns, or, like the composer Robert Schumann, going insane. Romanticism glamourized the mad genius, and nineteenth-century Bohemianism cultivated a dandified degenerateness.

Confinement of the Insane

What was the fate of the mad? In medieval and pre-modern times, most of those regarded as lunatics or idiots, mentally strange, or spiritually afflicted were taken care of – all too often a euphemism for 'neglected' – in local and familiar surroundings. In England, the immediate family was expected to shoulder responsibility for crazy relatives. The insane were generally kept at home, locked in a cellar or barn if dangerous, perhaps tended by a servant. Failing the family, the parish generally assumed control, sometimes boarding out the lunatic to a local carer. The presence in Charlotte Brontë's *Jane Eyre* (1847) of the first Mrs Rochester, raving mad and hidden away in the attic, suggests that such informal procedures continued into the nineteenth century.

Nevertheless, institutions gradually emerged for the confinement of the insane. The earliest specialized lunatic asylums had been established under religious auspices in fifteenth-century Spain – in Valencia, Zaragoza, Seville, Valladolid, Toledo, and Barcelona (Islamic models may have been influential). In London, the priory of St Mary of Bethlehem, established in 1247, was specializing in housing lunatics by the fifteenth century: it later became famous, or notorious, as Bethlem ('Bedlam'). The Netherlandish town of Geel, which had the healing shrine of St Dymphna, grew celebrated as a refuge for the mentally disturbed.

Throughout urban Europe and along the Eastern seaboard of North America, the eighteenth and nineteenth centuries brought a proliferation of schools, prisons, houses of industry and correction, workhouses, and, not least, madhouses to deal with troublesome people. The centralized state sometimes took the initiative. In 1961, the French intellectual Michel Foucault argued in *La Folie et la Déraison* that the rise of absolutism, symbolized by Louis XIV (1638–1715), inaugurated a Europe-wide 'great confinement'. Elements in society identifiable with 'unreason' found themselves at risk of being locked away. Paupers, the aged and ill, ne'er-do-wells, petty criminals, prostitutes, and vagabonds formed the bulk of this horde of 'unreason'. But their representative leaders were lunatics and imbeciles. Already by the 1660s some 6,000 undesirables – mad people included – were locked away in the Hôpital Général in Paris alone. Similar hospitals were soon set up in major French provincial cities.

Foucault argued that this 'great confinement' amounted to far more than physical sequestration. It represented a degradation of the status of madness. Hitherto, by dint of peculiarity, the mad person had possessed fascinating power: holy fools, geniuses, and jesters had uttered deep if obscure truths. Madness had spoken and society had listened. Once institutionalized, however, madness was robbed of all such allure, eerie dignity, and truth. It was reduced from a positive state ('madness') to a negative condition ('unreason'). Locked up in madhouses, lunatics resembled wild beasts caged in a zoo. It was easy to view them not as sick people but as animals.

There is a certain truth in Foucault's characterization of the age of reason 'shutting up' the mad, in every sense of the term; but it is overstated. The reign of Louis XIV saw a surge of institutionalization in Paris. Throughout the *ancien regime*, French absolutism continued to exercise a centralizing control over the insane; later, under the later Napoleonic Code, provincial prefects assumed these duties. Families could have mad relatives legally confined on obtaining a *lettre de cachet* from royal officials; such warrants deprived the lunatic of legal rights.

But elsewhere the picture is highly varied; policies differed, and often there were no policies at all. In Russia, almost no public receptacles for the insane existed before the second half of the nineteenth century. Before then, the mad, if confined at all, were kept in monasteries. Across great swathes of rural Europe – Poland, Scandinavia, or the Balkans, for instance – few people were institutionalized before 1850. At the close of the nineteenth century, two lunatic asylums sufficed for the whole of Portugal.

In spite of being densely populated and highly urbanized, even England does not easily square with Foucault's model of a 'great confinement' launched by act of state. Confinement through legislation came late. It was not until 1808 that an Act of Parliament was passed, permitting public money to be raised for county lunatic asylums, and only in 1845 – almost two centuries after Foucault's 'great confinement' supposedly began – were such asylums made compulsory. Figures are necessarily unreliable, but it appears that no more than around 5,000 people (out of a national population of some 10 million) were being held in specialized lunatic asylums in England around 1800, with perhaps as many again in workhouses and jails. In other words, there is little evidence that the English ruling elite felt insanity or 'unreason' posed a shocking threat to public order.

Indeed, in England, the rise of the lunatic asylum is better seen not as an act of state but as a service industry within a flourishing commercial society. In 1800, lunatics were mainly secured in for-profit private asylums operating within the free market economy, forming part of what contemporaries bluntly called the 'trade in lunacy'. As late as 1850, more than half the confined lunatics in England were still housed in private institutions, some good, some bad, some indifferent.

Private madhouses had taken root by the mid-seventeenth century, although evidence is scanty (owners and families alike had a vested interest in secrecy). When George Trosse, a young merchant from Exeter, went mad around 1650 (drink was probably to blame) his friends carried him off, strapped to his horse, to a fellow in Glastonbury in Somerset, who kept a house for boarding mad people. Not long after this, London newspapers begin to carry advertisements for private madhouses.

Several superior madhouses offered *de luxe* conditions for patients paying hefty fees. At Ticehurst House in Sussex, founded in 1792, the rich could live in separate houses in the grounds, install their own cooks, and ride to hounds. But most early madhouses provided at best Spartan and at worst brutal conditions for their inmates, especially the poor. Bethlem was widely criticized. But it might be unjust and anachronistic to depict institutionalization as essentially punitive. Its main role was segregation. The asylum's rationale, first and foremost, lay in the belief that sequestration was in the interests of dangerous lunatics, giving them security and maximizing prospects of cure. From the mid-eighteenth century, a new faith was emerging in psychotherapeutics. Lunatics, the argument ran, ought to be confined, because intensive treatment would restore them. As advocates of the mechanical philosophy and of a medical model of disease, eighteenth-century doctors investigated the bodily seats of insanity.

'Psychiatric' Techniques

Controlling and restoring the system through drugs and mechanical restraint loomed large in treatments of mental disorder from the eighteenth century; a rather rough-and-ready psychopharmacology remained popular on both sides of the Atlantic through the Victorian era. But the segregative environment of the asylum held out the potential of more 'psychiatric' techniques of mastering madness, ones that would directly command the mind, passions, and will. Such approaches especially appealed to critics who attacked mechanical restraint (manacles and chains) as cruel and counterproductive, provoking in the patient the frantic violence they were meant to allay. In the name of Enlightenment, new regimes were touted from the 1750s, accentuating 'moral' (or, in modern terminology, 'psychological') methods – kindness, reason, and humanity. Alienation of mind, claimed proponents of moral treatments, was not a physical disease like smallpox, but a psychological disorder, the product of wretched education, bad habits, and personal affliction – a traumatic bereavement, bankruptcy, or religious horrors like fear of hell. It needed a distinctive psychotherapeutics.

As already hinted, these new psychological approaches had deeper foundations on which to build. From Sophocles to Shakespeare, playwrights had dramatized the passions, showing the inner torments of desire and duty, guilt and grief, that tore personalities apart. In the seventeenth century, Descartes' *cogito ergo sum* ('I think, therefore I am') highlighted the role of consciousness in forging identity. His great English successor and critic, John Locke, depicted madness as the product of faulty logical processes or uncontrolled imagination (a view later underlined by Samuel Johnson). 'The defect in *Naturals*', Locke wrote in 1690,

seems to proceed from want of quickness, activity, and motion, in the intellectual Faculties, whereby they are deprived of Reason: whereas *mad Men*, on the other side, seem to suffer by the other Extream. For they do not appear to me to have lost the Faculty of Reasoning: but having joined together some *Ideas* very wrongly, they mistake them for Truths; and they err, as Men do, that argue right from wrong Principles. For by the violence of their Imaginations, having taken their Fancies for Realities, they make right deduction from them.[3]

And the *enfant terrible* of the Enlightenment, Jean-Jacques Rousseau, anticipated Sigmund Freud's *Civilization and its Discontents* (1930) by suggesting that the pressures of modern civilization alienated man from his soul, creating a divided self.

Thus emerged the building-blocks of a psychological way of reading derangement. Insanity could best be corrected, thought advocates of this model, by intense interpersonal dynamics between patient and doctor who would overcome derangement; and the right place for these close encounters was the lunatic asylum, an environment totally under the doctor's regulation. So-called moral managers made great play of reclaiming the deranged through charisma, relying on force of character and inventive psychological tactics, outwitting the wilful perversities of the disordered. First, patients had to be subdued; then they had to be motivated through manipulation of their passions – their hopes and fears, their need for esteem.

The point was to revive the dormant humanity of the mad by working on residual normal emotions still capable of being awakened and trained. Such ideas were taken several stages further around 1790 by the emancipatory visions of Vincenzio Chiarugi in Italy, Philippe Pinel in Paris, the Tukes at the York Retreat, and, perhaps more ambiguously, by Johann Reil and other Romantic psychiatrists in Germany. With their 'moral therapy', which valued kindness, calm, and rationality, such reformers aimed to treat their charges as human beings capable of regeneration. Pinel's 'French revolution' in psychiatry would free the mad from their chains, literal and figurative, and restore their rights as rational citizens.

Drawing on Locke's theory of the human understanding, such reformers stressed that the madman – unlike the idiot – was not utterly bereft of reasoning power. Madness was essentially delusion, argued the Tukes at the York Retreat, springing from error in the intellectual processes (the 'software', in a more modern jargon). Mad people were trapped in fantasy worlds, outgrowths of unbridled imagination. They needed to be treated like obstreperous children, who required rigorous mental discipline and retraining in thinking and feeling. The madhouse should thus become a reform school.

Such psychotherapeutics around 1800 were launched on a wave of noble optimism. The madhouse was not just to secure but to cure. Moral therapy led to schemes for redeeming lunatics that were implemented on a massive scale during the nineteenth century: after all, if enlightened asylums restored the insane, wasn't it society's duty to place them in such institutions? Throughout Europe and North America, the state accepted enlarged responsibilities for legislating and caring for the mad, and a new psychiatric profession emerged to manage them. The lunatic asylum became the mad person's home. Despite reformers' best intentions, all too often it proved a prison.

Nineteenth-Century Museums of Madness

The nineteenth century prided itself on being in the van of psychiatric progress. In the not-so-distant past, recalled Charles Dickens in 1852:

coercion for the outward man, and rabid physicking the inward man were . . . the specifics for lunacy. Chains, straw, filthy solitude, darkness, and starvation; jalap, syrup of buckthorn, tartarised antimony and ipecacuanha administered every spring and fall in fabulous doses to every patient, whether well or ill; spinning in whirligigs, corporal punishment, gagging, 'continued intoxication'; nothing was too wildly extravagant, nothing too monstrously cruel to be prescribed by mad-doctors.[4]

All had changed! Cruelty had been quelled, Dickens declared, kindness was the watchword. Traditional institutions like Bethlem, reminders of the bad old ways and days, were investigated and transformed. Private asylums came under strict regulation. The eighteenth-century madhouse had been a secret space, hidden from public scrutiny. Nineteenth-century reformers subjected it to the full glare of publicity. Exposés such as John Mitford's *The Crimes and Horrors in the Interior of Warburton's Private Madhouses at Hoxton and Bethnal Green* (1825) roused desires for the remedy of abuses.

Institutionalization of the mad was transformed from an *ad hoc* expedient into a system with goals and ideals. In France, for example, the reforms of Philippe Pinel and the legal stipulations of the Napoleonic Code were systematized in the epochal statute of 1838. This required each *departement* either to establish its own public asylums or to ensure provision of adequate facilities for the mad. To prevent illicit confinement, it established rules for the certification of lunatics by medical officers (although for pauper lunatics the prefect's signature remained sufficient warrant). Prefects were given powers of inspection. Similar legislation was passed in Belgium in 1850.

A comparable reform programme was enacted in England, in the teeth of opposition from vested medical interests who feared the profitability of private asylums would be threatened. Scandals revealing felonious confinement of the sane had already led to one important legislative safeguard. The Madhouses Act of 1774 had set up rudimentary licensing and certification. Under its provisions, all private madhouses had to be licensed by magistrates. Annual renewal of licenses would depend on satisfactory maintenance of admissions registers. Magistrates were empowered to carry out visitations (in London, the inspecting body was the Royal College of Physicians). Most importantly, medical certification was instituted for all but paupers. (Scotland had a different system for both the ayslums and the public administration of them.)

Further reforms in England followed after scandalous revelations led to parliamentary committees in 1807 and 1815 investigating madhouses. Evidence of gross mismanagement at Bethlem (where the recently deceased surgeon, Bryan Crowther, had himself been so deranged as to require a straitjacket) led to dismissals. The 1774 Act was strengthened by a succession of laws passed from the 1820s, which above all established the Commissioners in Lunacy, first for London (1828) and then for the whole realm (1844). The Lunacy Commissioners constituted a permanent body of inspectors (doctors, lawyers, and officials) charged to report on asylums. They had powers to prosecute and to withdraw licences. They also possessed a remit to standardize and improve conditions of care and treatment. The Commissioners ensured eradication of the worst abuses by insisting on proper patient records and the recording of all cases of physical coercion.

Safeguards against improper confinement were further tightened. Under a consolidating Act of 1890, two medical certificates were required for all patients, including paupers. In the long run, this legalistic concern to prevent asylums being abused as carceral institutions may have proved counterproductive. For, by insisting that only formally certified lunatics be quartered in asylums, it delayed the transformation of the asylum into a more flexible 'open' institution, easy of access and exit. Instead the mental hospital was confirmed as the institution of last resort; certification thus became associated with prolonged detention. The result was a failure to provide institutional care appropriate for temporary insanity, partial insanity, or mild mental disturbance.

In Europe and the USA alike, the nineteenth century witnessed a phenomenal rise in the number of mental hospitals and the patient population. In England, patient numbers rose from a few thousands in 1800 to some 100,000 in 1900 (the national population increased at less than half that rate). In the USA, similarly, there were fewer than 5,000 asylum patients in 1850 but more than 150,000 in 1904. By 1950, some 150,000 mental patients were institutionalized in Britain, half a million in the USA. Patient numbers also rocketed in the new nation states. In Italy, for example, some 18,000 were behind walls in 1881; within 35 years the number had more than doubled. Such increases are not hard to explain. Bureaucratic and utilitarian mentalities vested great faith in institutional solutions, in bricks and mortar. Reformatories, prisons, hospitals, asylums – all these, it was claimed, would solve the intensifying social problems induced by rise in population, urbanization, and industrialization.

Asylums, however, never lacked critics. From early days, Bedlam became a by-word for man's inhumanity to man. Patient protests grew, complaining of brutality and neglect, as in the dramatic *Address to Humanity, Containing a Letter to Dr. Thomas Munro: A Receipt to Make a Lunatic, and Seize his Estate; and A Sketch of a True Smiling Hyena*, issued in 1796 by a former patient, William Belcher. And a radical fringe within the medical profession always doubted the efficacy of herding the insane together. But champions long outnumbered critics, and the asylum movement was buoyed up on waves of optimism.

This was to change; in the last third of the nineteenth century, a new pessimism spread. Statistics demonstrated that expectations that asylums would prove engines of cure had been unfounded. Cure rates seemed to be dipping, and public asylums were silting up with long-stay patients. Psychiatrists had become victims of their own opinions. They had warned that society was riddled with masses of hitherto unknown psychiatric disorders – which they, and they alone, could treat. Developing such categories as 'monomania', 'kleptomania', 'dipsomania', and 'moral insanity', they had maintained that much aberrant conduct traditionally labelled vice, sin, and crime were, in truth, mental disorders that should be treated psychiatrically in the asylum. Magistrates were encouraged to divert difficult recurrent offenders from the workhouse or jail. But asylum superintendents were to discover to their cost that regeneration posed more problems than anticipated. Furthermore, the senile and the demented, along with epileptics, paralytics, sufferers from tertiary syphilis, ataxias, and neurological disorders were all increasingly warehoused in the asylum. For such conditions, the prognosis was gloomy. The asylum became a last resort for hopeless cases.

The mounting number of chronic patients gave cause for alarm. Perhaps madness was more menacing than imagined. No sooner were asylums built than they overflowed with those judged to be disturbed: alcoholics, habitual masturbators, sex maniacs, neuropaths, those suffering from general paresis of the insane, and other neurological deficits. Furthermore, bitter experience proved that the insane did not recover as predicted; the asylum was changing character, from being the retreat for regeneration to a dustbin for derelicts. Critics alleged that the asylum might be not the solution but the problem, creating the illnesses of institutionalization. Was faith in the asylum itself a form of delusion?

Defenders retorted that the true problem lay not in the asylum but in the patients. If psychiatry's best efforts didn't work cures, did this not show that many forms of mental disorder were authentically incurable? Such views encouraged the development, towards 1900, of new biomedical theories that pictured insanity as a hereditary taint, a blot on the brain. To generations of psychiatrists whose daily occupation lay in watching the living death of asylum zombies, or who pursued research into the neuropathologies of various mental disorders, sober realism pointed to 'degenerationist' theories: disorders were ingrained, they got worse over the generations. Such conclusions matched the mood of a sociopolitical elite anxious about the menace of the mass society and mass democracy.

Degeneration and Schizophrenia

Heroic efforts were made to analyse and classify mental disorders. Such nosological endeavours were stimulated by the emergence of the asylum, the rise of psychiatric specialists, and the progress of neurology. The profession needed to justify itself to society by cracking the secrets of psychosocial disorders; hence it undertook the task of psychopathologizing deviancy. Psychiatry successively staked greater territorial claims to 'discovering' mental disease where it had not been suspected before. Inordinate drinking became medicalized as alcoholism, sexual abuses such as sodomy were psychiatrized into 'homosexual neurosis', and many other erotic 'perversions' were captured by psychopathology in and after the pathbreaking *Psychopathia Sexualis* (1886) by the German psychiatrist Richard von Krafft-Ebing: bestiality, coprolagnia, exhibitionism, fetishism, flagellation, sadomasochism, transvestism, and so forth. Abnormal children, women, 'inverts' (homosexuals) and other 'perverts' were deemed mentally ill and often confined.

Degenerationist psychiatry also saw mental-disease in the decadent effusions of literary geniuses and artists such as Impressionists and Cubists, whose sensory systems, some psychiatrists suggested, must be pathologically disordered. And fears grew, above all, about the dangerous degeneracy of the rabble, who were, many psychiatrists warned, endangering civilization with mental imbecility precisely at a time when Social Darwinism was dictating that only fit societies would survive. Enlightenment optimism had peaked in the French Revolutionary aspiration that the mad could be freed from shackles and restored to reason. A century later, however, psychiatry had grown more pessimistic. A token of this lies in the formulation by the German psychiatrist Emil Kraepelin of *dementia praecox* (literally, precocious dementia), shortly to be termed schizophrenia by the Swiss doctor, Eugen Bleuler. As depicted by Kraepelin in *Einfürung in die Psychiatrische Klinik* (Lectures in Clinical Psychiatry) in 1901, the archetypal schizophrenic was not stupid; on the contrary, he might be alarmingly intelligent and astute. Yet he seemed to have renounced his humanity, abandoned all desire to participate in human society, withdrawing into an autistic world of his own. Describing schizophrenics, Kraepelin used such phrases as 'atrophy of the emotions' and 'vitiation of the will' to convey his conviction that such patients were moral perverts, sociopaths almost a species apart.

The more lurid fantasies of degenerationist psychiatry – its egregious racism, hereditarianism, and sexual prurience – were denounced by Sigmund Freud and other champions of the new dynamic psychiatries arising around the beginning of the twentieth century. And the therapeutic innovation at the heart of psychoanalysis proposed yet another optimistic new deal: the talking cure.

Modern Psychological Medicine

The twentieth century has brought efforts to fathom psychiatric diseases, establish their taxonomy, and investigate their causes. Specially significant has been the grand differentiation between psychoses (severe disturbances, involving loss of contact with reality) and neuroses (relatively mild conditions). That has been popularly seen as the grounding for distinctions between conditions with real organic aetiologies and ones that are psychological. Among the psychoses, a further cardinal contrast has been established between manic-depressive (or bipolar) conditions and schizophrenia.

Nevertheless, delineation and classification of mental illnesses remains fiercely contested. A glance at sucessive editions of the *Diagnostic and Statistical Manual* (*DSM*), the profession's diagnostic handbook produced by the American Psychiatric Association, shows just how fluid the characterization of mental illness continues to be. Requiring energetic revision every few years, and itself the subject of controversy, *DSM* reveals a proliferation of different, and often incompatible or overlapping terminologies, some disappearing and reappearing from edition to edition. A notorious postal-vote poll, held by the American Psychiatric Association in 1975, led to homosexuality being belatedly removed from its list of mental afflictions. It is not only cynics who claim that politico-cultural, racial, and gender prejudices continue to shape diagnoses of what are purportedly objective disease conditions.

Partly because of hostility to violent treatments such as insulin therapy and ECT, the new psychotropic drugs becoming available after 1950 were enthusiastically greeted. Psychopharmacology had long been burdened with worthless weapons such as bromides and croton oil (a powerful purge that put the patient out of action).

From the 1950s, neuroleptics such as chlorpromazine (Largactil), used on schizophrenics, and lithium, for manic-depressive conditions, had remarkable success in stabilizing behaviour. They made it possible for patients to leave the sheltered but numbing environment of the psychiatric hospital.

The response of patients themselves to heavy medication ('the liquid cosh') has been more ambiguous, since they can induce lethargy and mental vacancy (the 'zombie' effect). An ex-patient, Jimmie Laing, described the 'Largactil kick': 'You would see a group of men sitting in a room and all of them would be kicking their feet up involuntarily'.[5] The drugs revolution has remained incomplete. A generation ago, the British pyschiatrist William Sargant and other leading members of the profession prophesied that wonder drugs like Largactil would render mental illness a thing of the past by 1990. Such hopes have not been fulfilled.

Back to Square One?

As we have seen, the asylum movement created its own crises. Patients did not recover as promised. As early as mid-Victorian times, when the asylum-building programme was still in its infancy, even psychiatrists were prepared to admit that a gigantic asylum was a gigantic evil. A full century before the modern antipsychiatry movement, the Victorians had seen the untoward effects of institutionalization. Many psychiatric disorders were recognized to be the products of that very institution that claimed to be their cure.

Some of the most bitter critics of the asylum were its patients. There were two standard complaints: one was illegal or improper confinement – the forcible locking up of the sane, usually at family instigation, for underhand purposes, such as to overturn a will or shed an ugly wife – the other was gross brutality.

Thus mental institutions long suffered a crisis of legitimacy, but little was done. The drugs revolution, the movement for patients' rights, the terminal problems of crumbling asylums – aided by a dose of Treasury parsimony – combined, in Britain as elsewhere, to launch the 'decarceration' policies popular since the 1960s. Between 1980 and 1989, thirty mental hospitals were closed in Britain and approval was given to the closure of a further thirty-eight by 1995.

The ironies of this latest great breakthrough have become all too familiar.

For one thing, the drugs revolution was only half successful. Worse, 'community care' was introduced with little hard cash for care, and little hard thinking about community, and at a time when the British Prime Minister, Margaret Thatcher, went on record as saying 'there is no such thing as society' (a view widely taken as a symptom of a state of delusion on her part). A state of confusion remains. And that is partly because the nature of the beast remains obscure. 'Psychiatry is conventionally defined', wrote Thomas Szasz in the 1970s, 'as a medical speciality concerned with the diagnosis and treatment of mental diseases. I submit that this definition, which is still widely accepted, places psychiatry in the company of alchemy and astrology and commits it to the category of pseudoscience. The reason for this is that there is no such thing as "mental Illness".'[6]

Some find this doctrine liberating, others find it heartless; most think it exaggerated. Nevertheless, it remains true that, even amongst Szasz's critics, there is little agreement as to what mental illness truly is.

9. Medicine, Society, and the State

John Pickstone

Medicine is not just about knowledge and practice, healing and caring – it is about power: the powers of doctors and of patients, of institutions such as churches, charities, insurance companies, or pharmaceutical manufacturers, and especially governments, in peacetime or in war. This chapter explores the history of these powers in the medicine of Britain, France, Germany, and the USA during the past two centuries (regrettably for space reasons, it excludes most of Asia, Africa, and South America).

This narrative would have been easier to write in 1960, when we were more confident about the progress of medical science, the extension of medical services, and the expanding roles of government. Did anyone then foresee that the containment of costs would become the major focus of health policy, that bioethics would loom so large in public discussion, that market competition would be reintroduced into such advanced welfare bureaucracies as the British National Health Service, or that doctors would be increasingly subjected to lay managements, whether of hospitals or of insurance schemes? The progress-models common up to about 1960 now require more than a little tweaking.

We cannot, however, simply reverse the values, after the manner of some 1960s radicals, so as to present governments as increasingly oppressive and organized medicine as progressively enfeebling. That negative version seems no more plausible than its opposite number, even in the affluent West. Whether they run upwards or downwards, linear development models hardly seem adequate. Instead, we must look to the varied workings of medicine in a range of different societies over time.

At one extreme are the societies in which medicine was almost entirely a matter of free markets. For example, in the USA in the 1840s, would-be medical practitioners did not have to be licensed; if they wished to train, they could do so in a variety of competing medical schools, attached to different brands of medicine – herbal medicine and homeopathy as well as the 'heroic' forms of regular medicine. Competition depressed standards. Almost all patients then paid their individual practitioners on a fee-for-service basis. Destitute patients could be treated under a statutory welfare system (or by charity), and some doctors earned part of their salaries in this way; but most were self-employed.

At the other extreme are the societies (or segments of societies) in which most doctors were educated, regulated, and employed by government. Health services of this kind have been developed for the armed forces of many Western countries. Swedish medical services since the eighteenth century have included a substantial component of direct state employment; the former Soviet Union provided health care in this way. From 1948, UK citizens have enjoyed a National Health Service largely funded from taxation.

Between these extremes lie the intermediate institutions that have helped shape medicine in most Western countries: the associations that regulated medical practice, the agencies of 'public health', the poorhouses and hospitals for the destitute, and the friendly societies and other insurance schemes by which workers were protected against unemployment and sickness.

Medical Institutions and Politics – An Overview

In most of eighteenth-century Europe, medical education and practice were supposed to be regulated by colleges, corporations, or guilds of various kinds. Generally, their powers came to be underwritten by government, or replaced with more direct state control. In some cases, notably in German states, that transition was direct; in others, notably France and the USA, corporate forms weakened or were abolished in favour of free markets, on to which state regulation was later imposed. By about 1900, most Western states were supervising and subsidizing the education of doctors, underwriting the policing of medical conduct, and protecting the regular profession against false claims to qualifications. They did not usually prohibit unlicensed practice, but they required qualifications from the candidates for the increasing number of official medical positions, whether in direct state employment or in agencies supervised by the state.

These national histories of medical regulation corresponded to different patterns of state formation. Where states were relatively strong from the eighteenth century, as in German realms, medicine passed easily from corporate to state regulation, and was later liberalized. Where state powers were initially more restricted, as in Britain and especially the USA in the early nineteenth century, modern forms of medical regulation were developed as governments assumed responsibility for welfare services and public health. In Britain, this happened after about 1830, and the process was greatly complicated by the persistence of older corporations. In the USA, the arguments took place from about 1870, largely unencumbered by earlier institutional forms. Overall, in nineteenth-century nations, one finds a convergence from close state control on the one hand and from free markets on the other, towards the protected, restricted medical markets characteristic of twentieth-century medicine.

Shifting the focus to the politics of public health, we find rather similar cross-national comparisons. German and other strong states tried to improve the health of their populations from the eighteenth century. In France, a concern with the health of the people was central to the Revolution of 1789 and remained an obligation of nineteenth-century governments, advised by elite doctors. In eighteenth-century Britain, public health, like so much else, was a matter of local paternalism and voluntary associations. State responsibility developed in the mid-nineteenth century, as part of the effort to manage the conditions and consequences of an urban industrial economy. That programme was part of the new discipline of political economy and involved a new physiology of the social body. Both of these sciences later proved influential in continental cities and in the USA, as they, too, experienced rapid urbanization (and immigrant poverty). Towards the end of the nineteenth century, the campaigns of the elite doctors, whether for public health or professional powers, were boosted by the researches of Louis Pasteur, Robert Koch, and others; the researchers benefited in turn from the military and imperial expansions that preceded the First World War.

The politics of medical services for the destitute have a rather different history. In Catholic countries around 1750, the bulk of such services was provided by the Church; in Britain, the USA, and most German states, they were the responsibility of local government. Medicine was relatively marginal to the management of the poor, whether this was religious or secular. Doctors were more powerful in the charity hospitals of Britain that served the 'deserving poor' rather than the really destitute, but, even here, control in the eighteenth century rested with lay governors and subscribers. Since then, welfare services for the destitute have mostly come to be provided directly by governments, or at least underwritten by them. The poorhouses of France were 'nationalized' at the Revolution, but many continued to be managed by nursing sisters. In most countries, poorhouses were expanded during the nineteenth century, in line with urbanization. The power of doctors usually increased with state involvement, especially where poorhouses were used for medical teaching. Where they were not so used, medicalization was much slower: British poorhouses were marginal to medicine until the twentieth century.

In Britain and in the USA, charity hospitals rather than poorhouses became the prime site of medicalization and medical education. They were effectively run by doctors from the early nineteenth century, but their political fates diverged in the two countries. In the USA, by 1900, the 'charity' hospitals had begun to compete for patients who could pay their way; they had become part of the medical market. In Britain, this development was later and more restrained. Between the two world wars, British charity hospitals were subsidized by government, and in 1948 they were 'nationalized' as the key institutions of the National Health Service.

In discussing the increasing powers of organized medicine, the increasing powers of governments, and the ever more complex intertwinings of the two, one must beware simple trajectories or teleologies. The degree of state involvement has varied hugely between countries, and the processes of state involvement can be reversed. The government of Britain is presently trying to reduce its responsibility for medical services, as part of a 'rolling back of the state'. In the USA, the prestige of doctors appears to be declining after a century of steady advance. Western medicine seems to be entering a new political, economic, demographic, and epidemiological era; in Eastern Europe, Asia, and the less-developed countries, the future is even more uncertain. As organized medicine changes, so, too, will our understanding of its history.

Medical Markets in Enlightenment Europe

The formal organization of early modern medicine was corporate: colleges of physicians, guilds of surgeons, societies of apothecaries, or combined societies were based in regional or national capitals (see Chapters 4 and 6). One might describe the informal organization of most medicine as 'markets in hierarchical societies'. Physicians were learned men who could elicit the trust of aristocrats and supervise lower grades of doctors. 'Surgeons' were craftsmen, ranging from prestigious attendants on the powerful to local menders of the impoverished sick and wounded. Apothecaries or pharmacists sold remedies and corresponding advice. But hosts of other practitioners – men or women, settled or itinerant, full-time or part-time, trained or untrained – also sold advice, skills, or remedies. And most illnesses, then as now, were treated in the home, usually by women, with no recourse beyond family or neighbours.

All Western countries showed similar patterns of medical work, but they differed in the relative importance of corporate organization and in the links between medicine and the church, which remained strong in southern Europe. The north, and especially Britain, was becoming more secular and prosperous; more people could afford 'luxury' purchases, including medicine; communications were improving, and newspapers, which became common in the eighteenth century, carried masses of advertisements for patent medicines, often sold by itinerant vendors.

Cultural leaders were coming to be impressed by natural philosophy and by claims to the ordering of society on scientific principles.

Physicians argued that medicine might become as sure as Newtonian physics. They cultivated chemistry and natural history, and tried to classify diseases, often relating them to local conditions (Chapter 5). Surgeons took up anatomy, so establishing their claim to learning. Some apothecaries became chemical manufacturers of, for example, mineral waters; most worried about being undercut by a new breed of retailer, the chemist and druggist. In most Western countries, the growth of markets and the spread of education severely dented the various professional corporations.

In Britain and its North American colonies, medicine changed chiefly by private initiatives – sometimes commercial, sometimes through the 'voluntary' and secular associations that were conspicuous in the increasingly 'polite' society of English county towns (the world of Jane Austen's novels, and of George Eliot's *Middlemarch*). Voluntary associations built most of the hospitals that spread across England from 1720, providing respectable subscribers with a collective means to patronize the deserving poor; doctors, especially surgeons, used them to advertise major operations and to provide clinical experience for their apprentices. In London, such hospitals came to supplement the private anatomy schools newly set up by surgeons, some of whom were also men-midwives or *accoucheurs*.

University education, too, could include private enterprise. Oxford and Cambridge universities were stagnant but Edinburgh medical school boosted that city's finances by attracting students from England and North America. In Scottish universities and in the private schools of London, teaching was good business. Indeed, in a sense, education was the most dynamic aspect of the medical economy – knowledge changed much faster than therapies.

In Britain, even public health was often a 'voluntary' matter. Concern with hygiene tended to originate with army and navy doctors, worried by the loss of soldiers and sailors from disease rather than combat, as with scurvy. Such concerns were taken up by private 'reformers', who publicized the unsanitary conditions in prisons, and indeed in some of the new hospitals. Such reformers were often magistrates, driven by a desire for social discipline, fuelled by notions of scientific improvement. The best known was John Howard, who achieved a national reputation by 'exposing' conditions in prisons. Many physicians also became involved, especially in the newly industrial towns of northern England, where immigrant workers from the countryside suffered the fevers characteristic of army camps, ships, and prisons. In Manchester in 1796, local physicians joined with socially enterprising merchants to set up a fever hospital, and in the hope of supervising lodging-houses and cellar dwellings.

Few of these developments owed much to the Royal College of Physicians, the Company of Surgeons in London, or to the traditional machinery of central and local government. The physicians interested in hospitals, fever, and public welfare were mostly provincial, Scottish-educated, and religious dissenters. A campaign to open up the College of Physicians met little success: instead, reformers created new associations for discussion of medical science and philanthropy. One such scheme initiated the 'dispensary movement', through which many cities and smaller towns established charities to provide outpatient care and home-visiting for the sick poor. The new dispensaries came to serve as observatories from which honorary physicians 'discovered' the habitats of the poor. Although some physicians and many surgeons received public monies for the care of paupers in villages or parts of towns, there was little question here of statutory medical policy. British medicine was largely a matter of the free market plus the voluntary associations.

In German states, by contrast, universities and governments were much more prominent in medical matters. Local rulers sought prestige by attracting famous university teachers, who also advised on questions of public health and indeed served as personal physicians. Although some German developments in public medicine and public health were pioneered by religious groupings (as by the Lutherans in the Prussian city of Halle), most were related to 'improvements' in the management of principalities. According to contemporary theories of government, wealth would flow from fertile fields and a healthy population: so infant welfare, breastfeeding, and cleanliness were to be encouraged alongside scientific agriculture. Such German states invented *Medizinpolizei* (medical police, where the meaning of 'police' lies somewhere between 'policy' and 'police force'). Medicine, like many other occupations, was subject to considerable state control, and doctors were employed part-time to supervise public health and attend the local poor. Problems of poverty could also be subjected to scientific management – some paupers were institutionalized and set to work on scientifically minimal diets. Count Rumford (Sir Benjamin Thompson), an American adventurer who devised a scheme for the employment of paupers in Munich, was also the inventor of the soup kitchen; as a physicist he maintained that water became nutritious when boiled with bones.

The Revolution in French Medicine

Whilst medical change in Britain tended to occur outside the corporations and the state, and German reforms were often a matter of state policy, France showed both patterns – in rapid succession. Before the Revolution, France had an elaborate hierarchy of medical occupations, from elite physicians in Paris to district surgeons licensed to practise only in the countryside. But most of the physicians who took an interest in public welfare, economic improvement, and the natural history of disease, did so outside the old faculties of medicine, through new societies, sometimes under royal patronage. Elite surgeons also used royal patronage to set up a surgical academy in Paris and to advance their claims to be men of learning. After 1789, the Revolution removed the old faculties and the elaborate systems of corporate regulation of practice, but it also removed the newer institutions under royal patronage. The result was an institutional vacuum, which was indeed the preferred option of the most radical reformers of education and medicine: let patients choose doctors, let students choose teachers, let savants associate together as they wish, with neither state subsidy nor state control.

Such ultra-liberalism could hardly last in a country used to regulation, still less in a country at war. Complaints about unregulated quackery and the urgent need to supply surgeons for the conscript army of the Revolutionary wars meant that new schools of medicine were introduced in 1793. Under Napoleon they were re-ordered, and a national system of medical licensing was established in 1802. Practice was officially restricted to graduate physicians and surgeons, plus a lower order of practitioners – the *officiers de santé*, who received less training and were licensed to practise only on the poor. Thus medical education and licensing became a direct concern of the French state, unmediated by guilds or corporations, although the universities retained some autonomy. Doctors were protected by the state, but they continued to complain of unfair or unlawful competition – from the *officiers de santé*, from the mass of irregular practitioners, and from doctors, who were also pharmacists (pharmacists were subject to state education and licensing as were also midwives and some herbalists). From the Revolution onwards, hygiene was institutionalized as a concern of medicine and of the state. Doctors, especially the Paris professors, served as advisers on public-health matters; indeed, the identification of medicine with public welfare was a recurrent argument against 'ultra-liberal' schemes for the deregulation of medical practice. In nineteenth-century France, voluntary associations of doctors were late and weak compared with those in Britain or the USA.

But the chief international consequence of the French medical revolution stemmed from the re-ordering of the major Paris poorhouses, such as the Hôtel Dieu, just by the cathedral of Notre Dame. Such poorhouses had been managed by the church; they were taken over by the government. The nursing nuns were subordinated to doctors; the paupers, now unprotected by charity or religion, could be sorted out medically, used for teaching, and dissected after death. Surgeons were given parity with physicians and in these 'museums' of medicine, diseases came to be seen primarily as anatomical lesions and explored through a systematic new geography of 'tissues'; peritonitis, for example, was inflammation of the membrane lining the abdominal cavity. Clinical examinations were now applied to find evidence of tissue lesions before death and autopsy: the stethoscope came into use because there was now something to be 'looked' for in the bodies of patients.

This form of practice remained the intellectual frontier of European medicine until after 1850. It came to dominate the big state hospitals of Vienna and Berlin, which boasted of their clinical examinations and autopsies, and to some extent it penetrated the charity hospitals of Britain, where surgeons had already developed their own anatomical approaches to disease. But charity hospitals were sensitive to public opinion, their lay governors feared charges of 'experimentation', and so patients were more or less protected. In

Britain, the truly down-and-out – the paupers with no means of support – were mostly in poorhouses rather than charity hospitals. After the Anatomy Act of 1832, paupers without relatives or friends could be dissected after death; in life they were subject to mean and harsh regimes, but were not the subjects of medical teaching.

In many German states, the direct or indirect effects of the French military occupation removed older medical and scientific corporations, and strengthened the links between medicine and government. Medical education and licensing became more directly a matter of government, and cultural nationalism led to a renewal of universities, now dedicated to the advancing knowledge rather than the passing-on of professional information. This assertion of Germanic culture included medicine, usually within idealistic philosophies that were opposed to the 'analytical' knowledge then dominant in Paris. Moreover, many of the German medical schools were in small towns that did not provide the quantities of 'clinical material' essential for the development of the Paris method. For both reasons, professors in these smaller hospitals continued to teach a 'biographical medicine', which included intensive investigations of patients' histories and circumstances. From about 1850, this emphasis on the dynamics of individuals was developed into a more quantitative and physiological 'laboratory' medicine, without the intermediate stage of large-scale, Parisian, 'museum-style' analysis.

Medicine, Industry, and Liberalism

In one sense, Parisian hospital practice was a medicine of the masses – the massed paupers of the teaching hospitals; it was medical practice devised by state-salaried teachers in state institutions attended by students with state bursaries. In Britain, as we have seen, the state was marginal in the eighteenth century, both to the practice of medicine and to the maintenance of public health. But as towns grew rapidly, partly as a result of industrialization, British doctors, too, began to face the 'masses' – not just in hospitals, which became crowded and insalubrious, but in the dense, cheap housing of industrial towns and the poorer quarters of London. In the same towns, doctors experienced intense competition, a loss of traditional rank, and an entrepreneurial culture in which medicine was viewed as merely a trade.

The new industrial towns threatened disease and disorder. Their politicians prescribed remedies: the liberal panaceas of free trade and more individual responsibility. Reformers attacked 'old corruption', including the medicine of the traditional London institutions, but they also argued for new public functions to protect the nascent industrial economy from its social by-products. They campaigned for the reform of poor-relief and for public-health measures. Where possible, they believed, such functions were to be carried out by voluntary associations, or by the new municipal corporations that liberals dominated, with central government perhaps providing legislation or resources.

Questions of medical organization, public health, and poor-relief were integral to political reform as the manufacturing and professional classes exerted themselves against an older England and fought to stabilize a new order. 'Doctors' came to identify with each other. Although a doctor with a prestigious shop might still regard himself as an apothecary, most of the retail end of medicine had been lost to the chemists and druggists. A doctor who held an honorary post at the local hospital would practice as a consultant physician or consultant surgeon, advising other doctors, but he was also the doctor of first resort for richer patients. Such consultants were leaders of the local medical communities, but most doctors now saw themselves as 'general practitioners', even when they still used 'physician' or 'surgeon' as their title. There were far too many graduates in medicine for them all to be confined to the traditional routines of physicians, and most of the surgeons and apothecaries now had some formal training beyond their apprenticeships.

In the search for respectability, and to distance themselves from mere trade, British doctors established local medical societies, especially during the 1830s. There they discussed their economic grievances, but the scientific and clinical content prevented the associations from appearing as mere 'trade unions'. Rather, they resembled the new wave of scientific societies, in which doctors rubbed shoulders with lawyers and the better-educated merchants and gentlemen. Some of the local and regional medical societies attempted to produce journals. They collaborated to form a national association – the Provincial Medical and Surgical Association, which later became the British Medical Association, the voice of general practice.

The world of medicine and its interaction with political reforms was well depicted by George Eliot in *Middlemarch*, especially through the character of the young physician Dr Lydgate:

[The profession] wanted reform, and gave a man an opportunity for some indignant resolve to reject its venal decorations and other humbug, and to be the possessor of genuine though undemanded qualifications. He went to study in Paris with the determination that when he came home again he would settle in some provincial town as a general practitioner, and resist the irrational severance between medical and surgical knowledge in the interest of his own scientific pursuits, as well as of the general advance: he would keep away from the range of London intrigues, jealousies, and social truckling, and win celebrity, however slowly, as Jenner had done, by the independent value of his work. For it must be remembered that this was a dark period; and in spite of venerable colleges which used great efforts to secure purity of knowledge by making it scarce, and to exclude error by a rigid exclusiveness in relation to fees and appointments, it happened that very ignorant young gentlemen were promoted in town, and many more got a legal right to practise over large areas in the country. Also, the high standard held up to the public mind by the College of Physicians, which gave its peculiar sanction to the expensive and highly-rarified medical instruction obtained by graduates of Oxford and Cambridge, did not hinder quackery from having an excellent time of it; for since professional practice chiefly consisted in giving a great many drugs, the public inferred that it might be better off with more drugs still, if they could only be got cheaply, and hence swallowed large cubic measures of physic prescribed by unscrupulous ignorance which had taken no degrees.[1]

Local and national medical associations worried about irregular competition and conditions of poor-law employment. Many of their members wanted a single national register for all qualified medical men, and a ban on unqualified practice. Some would have liked a national licensing body on which they would have had democratic representation. A few practitioners, but only a few, even in the depressed 1840s, argued for a state medical service, 'endowed' like the Anglican church, affording a decent living even to doctors in poor areas, and with the authority to maintain public health.

For most British doctors, state medicine was a Germanic perversion, but the American example could be equally worrying. There, by the 1840s, anti-elitist politicians had removed the relatively weak forms of medical licensing set up in the decades after Independence. In the resultant free market, medical botanists and homeopaths were on a par with regulars – free to pit their herbs and small-doses against the bleeding and heroic cures of the regular profession. Medical schools in the USA also competed with each other, keeping courses short and cheap so as to attract more students. In Britain, the institutions of regular medicine proved stronger. Pushed by very public criticism – not least the scathing prose of a new medical journal, *The Lancet* – they reformed enough to survive the vitriolic debates of 1825 to 1860, maintaining control over entry to the medical elites and gaining substantial roles in the certification of general practitioners.

Campaigns for radical reform were usually met by the government extending the powers of the old corporations, especially by setting them up as national examining bodies. In 1815, the Tory government had restricted prescribing and dispensing to qualified apothecaries and so provided a framework for a national examination, and thus a major spur to the growth of the private medical schools. This Apothecaries Act increased the power of the Society of Apothecaries while maintaining the subordination of apothecaries to physicians, and excluding from 'apothecary practice' all those general practitioners who had not taken the Society's Licence, even medical graduates. Eight years later the Royal College of Surgeons established a national examination for its Membership diploma, so that LSA and MRCS became the desired dual qualification for general practitioners. The Royal College of Physicians followed, establishing an examination for its Licence, the LRCP, which outranked that of the Apothecaries.

These corporations remained the targets of radical reformers, but the politics were so complex and the interests so confused that legislation was very difficult. Not until 1858 was an Act passed to regularize medical practice in the UK. This established a single register for all doctors with recognized qualifications, but it accepted (and so helped secure) all the existing examining bodies, both university and corporate, and did not ban unqualified practitioners. It maintained the principle of 'buyer beware' as regards private practice, but it privileged 'regulars' for the increasing number of 'public' posts. The centralization of the poor law, the inauguration of public-health posts, and concern over military medicine meant that government had a growing interest in regularizing its own medical employees.

German medical reformers meanwhile were pushing simultaneously in the opposite direction. There, liberals wanted a less controlled profession, just as they wanted non-interference in other occupations. They were even ready to forego the ban on unqualified practice that was part of the existing labour laws. In 1869, an Act passed by the Prussian parliament partially deregulated medicine, so approximating the arrangements to those applying in France and developing in Britain. Medical qualifications were protected by the state, though unqualified practice was not illegal.

Interactions between the state and the profession were not limited to medical licensing. For many ordinary doctors, the arrangements for the medical care of paupers were a more pressing, everyday concern, and poor-law reforms were also central to governments' consideration of public health. Population growth had been encouraged throughout Enlightenment Europe, but by the early nineteeth century, especially in urban areas, such policies had given way to worries about the proliferation of the poor. Britain, by the 1820s, seemed to have too many people, half-employed in the countryside or crowded into the new towns. Schemes for the reduction of expenditure on poor-relief included encouragement for the emigration of 1 million paupers (from a population of 12 million). It was hardly surprising that British midwifery charities became less popular, or indeed that the middle classes began to worry about the 'abuse of medical charity', and to formulate schemes for forcing self-reliance. When workers were called 'hands', and hands were plentiful, many workers became fearful of doctors, of their hospitals, and of the official precautions against epidemics. The medical profession, not least by encouraging grave-robbing, appeared to value the poor more highly as corpses than as patients.

The answer to British worries about excessive expenditure on poor-relief in the first half of the nineteenth century was provided by a group of liberal political economists, headed by Edwin Chadwick, an unemployed lawyer and disciple of the utilitarian philosopher Jeremy Bentham. Traditional British statesmen, more used to war and foreign affairs than to social questions, were all too ready to draw on these new 'experts' and to appoint them to Royal Commissions. The exponents of political economy considered abolishing the poor law, but settled for a massive reform to amalgamate parishes into Poor-Law Unions under Boards of Guardians. Salaried overseers would now be supervised by travelling inspectors; new workhouses would be built to replace parish poorhouses. No able-bodied paupers would be supported unless they entered the workhouse; and no-one would choose to do so unless they were desperate. The system was designed to deter scroungers. In fact, most workhouse inmates were aged and infirm, or unmarried mothers with no other means of support. They received minimal medical attendance.

Some doctors felt that they, too, were victims of the same hard principles of political economy. Poor-law medical vacancies were advertised, and doctors 'tendered' for the care of a given district's paupers; the lowest tender usually won, provided it also covered the cost of medicines. If local doctors banded together to raise the remuneration, the poor-law Guardians threatened to import a newly qualified doctor, who would work for less. Similar bargaining power was sometimes exerted by the friendly societies, and from the 1820s doctors tried to organize local strikes against them. For early-Victorian doctors, 'professionalization' was often a desperate response to being treated as tradesmen. Public health would also come to serve as a 'professional' cause, linking medicine to the protective role of the state.

In Britain, the association of medicine, materialism, and radical politics is well known from such novels as *Middlemarch* – George Eliot's common-law husband was an enthusiast for Positivism, the new religion of science. The politics of most ordinary doctors, however, are unknown. To the left of the liberals, one can certainly find British doctors who identified more directly with the condition of the workers; indeed, some felt themselves proletarianized by the development of class societies and the erosion of the artisan stratum that had provided many of their own patients. Some of them gave public support to the working-class movement for political rights (Chartism) or joined the campaigns against the new poor law. However, the overall voting pattern of British doctors was probably at least as conservative as the rest of their social class: medicine was still largely a 'carriage-trade'.

Science and Morals

From the mid-nineteenth century, the threat of violent class-conflict declined. In Britain, as voting rights were extended to some working-class males, the political parties sought working-class support and consent. They extended primary education, spent money on civic monuments, and softened their attitudes to charities and poor-relief – at least where these concerned women, children, and the sick. Higher education was also encouraged (for males), not least to nurture future civil servants and teachers, whose judgment and cultivation could lend authority to government and protect against the excesses of democracy. Organized medicine benefited from these moves towards state authority and the provison of welfare.

After about 1850, the 'condition of England' became a cross-party issue to which doctors could attach themselves without discomfort. This helped their struggle for state registration and protection; in turn, the cause of public health could be projected as 'scientific', involving laboratory experiments as well as social statistics. John Simon, the first medical officer to Britain's central government, sponsored many investigations in the 1860s; he was also a key supporter of the Medical Reform Act of 1858. A cultured ex-surgeon with a background in German idealism, he helped transform 'public health' from a topic of political campaigns to a matter of incremental, executive advances – scientific, administrative, and legislative. Simon's programme suffered setbacks in the 1870s, however, when restructuring of the civil service made it subservient to the routines of poor-relief. At the same time, local sanitary programmes were boosted by smallpox epidemics that helped make the case for isolation hospitals, which local Medical Officers of Health later used for such children's diseases as diphtheria.

From the late 1860s, towns were forced to appoint Medical Officers of Health. With other doctors they preached the science of hygiene and encouraged the public understanding of 'physiology'. But their authority was not uncontested; the laws of health were also crucial to health reformers who were deeply sceptical about regular medicine, especially in its curative aspects. Hygiene in mid-century Britain was still a moral cause – a rationale for better living and a critique of industralism; many of its proponents were women.

The nursing work of Florence Nightingale, which became famous from the Crimean war in the 1850s, was in part an attempt to find useful social roles for single ladies, but it was also a campaign for hygiene and moral discipline, especially in hospitals. These were no longer to be crowded depositories for medical and surgical cases, they were to be suburban or rural, with wards designed for ventilation and surveillance – places of restorative regimes and demonstrations of the laws of health. This new view of hospitals appealed to civic authorities, especially when working men also proved ready to contribute to the maintenance of these charities. From the 1860s onwards, local hospitals emerged as key centres of 'community spirit'.

In mid-Victorian Britain, many of the hygienists were homeopaths and other opponents of regular curative practice. Many of them were religious dissenters who opposed medical monopoly as they opposed religious monopoly and state churches. Around 1870, their opposition focused on compulsory vaccination against smallpox and on government measures to force the medical examination – and, if need be, the hospitalization – of prostitutes in towns with army or navy barracks. For these reformers, medicine was a matter for the conscience; those who lived by the laws of nature and of God would have little need for cures, or indeed for the cruel experiments on animals that some doctors seemed to see as integral to scientific advance. Around 1870, vivisection was a major public issue in Britain.

Medical men were often involved in disputes about science versus religion. In Britain and Germany, the debate over evolution fuelled longstanding suspicions of 'medical materialism'. In France, especially after 1870, medical republicans, including many prominent parliamentarians, led the fight for secular education and indeed secular medicine. Republicans campaigned to set up lay nursing schools like those of England, and for municipalities to 'laicise' nursing in their local hospitals. But change was slow and uneven, not least because religious sisters were so dependable and cheap to employ.

(Britain is historically remarkable for the rarity of 'denominational' hospitals.)

Conflicts between physical and moral paradigms could also be found in discussions of lunacy. Mental diseases were increasingly differentiated and put down to physical causes, either anatomical or merely functional. No-one was cured thereby, and treatment in asylums remained largely 'moral and hygienic'. However, medicalization helped secure the right of doctors to dominate asylums, which had sometimes been questioned earlier in the century. It hid the fact that most of the medical work in asylums was general practice rather than psychiatry; it may have helped the relatives of patients by medicalizing their family's problem and so legitimating incarceration.

The growing authority of medicine and science probably owed much to the claims of experimentalism, especially the physiological experiments on animals made famous by Claude Bernard in Paris and Karl Ludwig and his associates in German universities (see Chapter 5). Their emphasis on the measurement and control of physiological processes in animals and eventually in humans was especially useful to medical educators seeking links between clinical medicine and physical sciences. Governments and large capitalists proved ready to invest in schemes that promised both social welfare and scientific authority.

'Scientific' medicine advanced fastest in Germany, in the new or reformed universities of the USA, and in the university medical schools of England (especially Cambridge and University College London). It was less successful in France and in the British schools dominated by clinicians – the hospital schools in London and the English provinces. In Britain, its progress was called into question by public campaigns against vivisection that were linked to sanitarianism, to feminism, and to other campaigns against cruelty. It could be argued that later nineteenth-century medicine benefited both from (female) sentiment and from (male) science, but not without considerable friction. Much medical rhetoric tried to combine the two appeals: doctors were tender enough to care for their patients as individuals, but tough enough to calculate what was best according to objective statistics and laboratory experiments.

Imperialism and Social Welfare

By the end of the nineteenth century, technocratic and paternalistic tendencies were becoming dominant in most Western countries. Military reformers argued that improved transport and communications required new forms of large-scale organization under the direction of a highly trained general staff; the German success in the Franco-Prussian war of 1870–1 was persuasive. Industrialists looked increasingly to corporate integration and scientific management rather than to owner-direction and small-scale competition; increasing state regulation of products and of conditions of work operated to the benefit of large companies, who saw state education and welfare as producing and protecting the skilled workforces they now required. National and imperial rivalries, together with worries about the growth of socialism and trade unions, led politicians to cultivate schemes for 'national efficiency', especially those that also secured the loyalty of the working classes. Welfare came back into fashion when fit citizens were required for the armed forces, for empire, or for factories.

In Edwardian Britain, both Conservative and Liberal politicians saw social welfare as the preferred alternative to socialism. The health of infants and school children would be monitored; old age would be cushioned by pensions that workers seemed now to deserve; health insurance, previously limited to workers in friendly societies, would be extended to all working men. In the two decades before the First World War, the foundation of the British welfare state was laid.

Many of the British schemes were borrowed from Germany, where from the 1880s social insurance had been used by Chancellor Bismarck to secure worker loyalty and limit the growth of socialism. Some were borrowed from France, where defeat by Prussia had fed fears of national degeneration and worries about the persistently low birth rate. Such worries helped qualified doctors in their campaign for protection by licensing. State medical insurance was discussed but not introduced, chiefly because organized labour was divided, and the Catholic church and the mass of small employers preferred voluntary schemes.

Some similar patterns can be seen in the USA, where a swing towards professional authority and corporate organization had begun in the 1870s, soon after the Civil War, perhaps to help overcome the sectarianism of religion and the political divides between north and south. Doctors, librarians, plumbers, and many other groups claimed to possess bodies of systematic knowledge that could be taught and used for the public good. Industrial money was laundered into trusts and given to create German-style universities. White America may not have feared industrial or imperial competition, but it did fear the rapid immigration from southern and eastern Europe that funnelled into the cities, threatening disorder and political incoherence.

Scientific Solutions to Social Problems

Scientific solutions for social problems became the mainstay of progressive politicians. Where this meant more demanding and more exclusive medical education, or more rigorous medical licensing, the aims of the progressives coincided with those of organized medicine. In all Western countries, organized medicine benefited considerably both from the extension of welfare and from the increasing acceptance of science as a source of social authority. Investment in medical education and laboratories was particularly successful after 1880, when medical men came to agree that many epidemic diseases were 'caused by' specific microorganisms. This knowledge sharpened many existing developments in sanitary management, in isolation hospitals, clean surgery, and medical diagnostics; it boosted the authority of medical science and so led to further government and charity investment; and it increased the authority of doctors as employees and advisers of the state.

In most countries, it was university medical schools that created the expertise in bacteriology – drawing on existing strengths in microscopy, pathology, and chemistry. Some new departments of public health were funded, in part, by undertaking identifications of microbes for local authorities, hospitals, or private doctors. In the USA, Johns Hopkins University in Baltimore pioneered a School of Public Health, as it had also pioneered German-style scientific medicine and the employment of clinical professors on full-time salaries (rather than honorary appointments supplementary to private practice). In Britain, the University of Liverpool developed a major programme in tropical medicine, funded by merchants persuaded that better control of disease would facilitate imperial commerce. In London, the government supported a similar school and research centre. In Germany, the new Reich helped fund Robert Koch and his collaborators: their Prussian and Imperial bacteriology was set to replace earlier, more liberal approaches to public health, not least in Hamburg, which suffered badly from cholera in the epidemic of 1892. In France, public subscriptions helped fund a research institute in Paris to honour Louis Pasteur. In the USA, the Rockefeller and Carnegie foundations channelled industrial money into medical research. The new medical science both shaped and benefited from such major end-of-century concerns as tuberculosis and infant welfare.

Sanatoria for sufferers from tuberculosis had been developed before the recognition of the causative agent, the tubercle bacillus, as extensions of nature-therapy or hygiene; but 'germs' gave them a focus, new regimes, and a link with testing agencies in hospitals and in the community. Germs were used to focus attention in public education campaigns, and governments came to see sanatoria as appropriate for state investment – as ways of restoring working men to health.

In both the voluntary and state-run sectors, sanatoria spread across Europe and North America between 1880 and 1930, and in Britain systematic state support for medical researchers developed out of the concern with tuberculosis and its costs; the Medical Research Committee (later to be renamed the Medical Research Council) was founded in 1913 partly in the hope of finding scientific solutions to tuberculosis.

Infant welfare was prominent as a political issue, especially from 1900. Mothers were to be taught about nutrition and cleanliness and health visitors were now to be employed by statutory authorities, thus coming under the control of medical officers. Midwives were to be licensed where (as in Britain) they were previously unregulated; in the USA, midwives came to be replaced by (supposedly) trained medical men. Symptoms such as infant diarrhoea, which had seemed seasonal or even humoral, were now caused by germs and their vectors. Medical officers in factory towns collected statistics on house-fly populations as their colonial colleagues, such as Ronald Ross, investigated mosquitoes.

Mental defectives were also topical. Educational developments had made them conspicuous; they were socially recalcitrant and likely to transmit their menace; they came to serve as models of biological degeneracy. What was to be done with children who could not learn? In Britain, as elsewhere, institutions begat institutions: elementary schools led to special schools for the blind, the deaf, for cripples, and for the 'stupid'. Doctors got involved, especially at the turn of the century when 'degeneration of the physical stock' became an issue in all Western countries. From about 1870, doctors had presented themselves as experts on physical constitutions and inheritance; after 1900, they could learn from the new science of genetics that stupidity resulted from a single, recessive Mendelian gene. Although few clinicians were much involved in practice with mental defectives and most public-health officers were suspicious of hereditarian arguments, many doctors took an interest in eugenics – the new science of better breeding. For some it became a great white hope – a way from urban degradation to national strength and order. Eugenic enthusiasm extended across most of the political spectrum, from those who despised the poor to those who wished them free from the burdens of excessive reproduction.

For most of these public medical programmes, support came chiefly from the state, sometimes from charitable associations (which often acted as 'pioneers'), and to a limited extent from the private market (for example, for private sanatoria). But industry, too, came to use the new medicine. Although most pharmaceutical companies (especially in Britain), continued to process traditional remedies, or manufacture 'patent remedies' sold by advertisements, a few chemical companies, first in Germany then in the USA, drew on academic chemistry to produce new synthetic drugs allied to dyes. Some of them also began to produce 'biologicals', such as vaccines and antisera, sometimes 'taking over' such production from the public laboratories in which it had been pioneered. All these new products involved extensive collaboration between companies, universities, hospitals, and the new research institutes sponsored by states and/or charity. One sees here the beginning of the modern medico-industrial complex, not least in questions of standardization, legislation, and clinical trials.

The New Medical Economy

Market effects were probably clearest for surgery, as the range and number of operative procedures increased rapidly from about 1880. These operations were needed or wanted by self-financing patients as well as by the poor, and they were often performed in patients' homes. The growth of private practice in operative surgery meant that innovative surgeons could become very rich – they thought like inventors and rubbed shoulders with financiers and major industrialists. But as surgeons came to demand elaborate antiseptic or aseptic routines, and as they undertook more and more operations, it became convenient to use private nursing homes or, where possible, public hospitals. In Britain, and especially in the USA, charity hospitals came to admit some private patients; indeed, many charity hospitals and some state hospitals began to employ almoners to ensure that all patients paid what they could towards the cost of their hospital treatment.

In as much as medical and surgical advances allowed the institutions of medicine to appeal to the self-interest of the better-off, they helped produce a fundamental transformation in the political economy of medicine, visible especially in North America, where many rapidly growing communities lacked established medical institutions. US doctors began their own hospitals, as did religious or racial groups. These hospitals, whether private or charities, competed for paying patients, who by the mid-1890s constituted most of the intake. Outside the hospitals, doctors competed by installing new equipment, such as X-ray machines; in cities, doctors often occupied suites in office buildings dedicated to medicine, where they had access to common facilities.

Public medicine grew, and so did private medicine. Indeed, the distinction between them began to blur as hospitals became more central to both kinds. In most Western countries one sees new 'professional movements' within this new medical economy. While the leading practitioners and educators – the institution men – were negotiating with governments or steering the medical aspects of welfare schemes, many other doctors, especially general practitioners, felt desperately squeezed between the advance of state medicine, the encroachments of charity medicine, and the increasing ability of organized labour to employ doctors.

Friendly societies had employed doctors from the early nineteenth century, especially in the industrial areas of Britain. By the end of the century, they were becoming a major element in medical provision for the working classes. More workers could and would pay collectively for medical care, and doctors were worried by this growth of patient-power. The entry of women into medicine – as nurses, midwives, even as women doctors – seemed an additional threat to those average general practitioners whose ideology combined patriarchy with small capitalism. The comments of one doctor sums up attitudes of many of his colleagues at the time:

Many of the most estimable members of our profession perceive in the medical education and destination of women a horrible and vicious attempt deliberately to unsex themselves – in the acquisition of anatomical and physiological knowledge the gratification of a prurient and morbid curiosity and thirst after forbidden information – and in the performance of routine medical and surgical duties the assumption of offices which Nature intended entirely for the sterner sex.[2]

To protect their income against all these threats, doctors organized medical guilds – in effect their own trade unions.

Medical syndicalism was much in evidence in Britain, France, and Germany around 1900. In Germany, the medical guilds argued for all doctors to have access to state-regulated insurance practice, and to be paid on a fee-for-service basis, rather than by capitation fees, so improving their bargaining position with the occupational insurance schemes. In Britain in 1911, the doctors reluctantly accepted National Health Insurance for working men, largely because the state scheme incorporated, and so controlled, the medical activities of friendly societies. In fact, most doctors soon found that their new relationship with the state was both more comfortable and more remunerative than their previous condition. They were represented on the local insurance committees, and, because they were paid by capitation, they no longer had to worry about the financial consequences of referring their patients to consultants in the charity hospitals. National Health Insurance thus further differentiated the general practitioner from the hospital doctor, as it also helped establish a stable relationship between the working man and his 'panel doctor'.

Medicine for Citizens, 1920–1970

The American Civil War and the Franco-Prussian War had served as models of military and medical organization. The war against the Boers in South Africa at the turn of the nineteenth century had served to worry the British state, not least because of the poor physical health of most of the young men who volunteered to fight. But the First World War of 1914–18 transcended all these in its scale, its horrors, and its duration. For a few years, the major combatant countries were forced to construct medical organizations far larger than their previous (and continuing) civilian systems. Away from the battle-lines, in the cities of Britain, colleges and mansions were taken over as hospitals. Nursing became a major sector of war-work for women, and many doctors learned to work in a large, co-ordinated system – some learned to see the advantages. In the emergencies of war, 'planners', medical specialists, and medical women found opportunities normally denied them.

Much of the system disappeared as the war ended and institutions were returned to their previous medical or non-medical functions, but some new patterns of practice could be carried over, and the expectations of many doctors were permanently changed. For example, British doctors who had specialized in orthopaedic surgery or cardiac medicine under war-time conditions may have returned to more general surgical and medical practices, but they did so with a clearer vision of specialty practice, not least from contact with colleagues from the USA, where a larger private market and more open hospitals had made specialization easier. War-time medicine had aimed to return soldiers to action, so the emphasis of specialists, whether in psychiatry or in cardiology, was on functional disabilities; civilian workers, especially in the armament factories, were the subjects for extensive researches on 'fatigue'. These functionalist attitudes, and the claims of physiologists to a role in scientific management, also carried over into post-war restructuring. For example, at the prestigious Manchester Technical College a physiologist was chosen to head a new department of industrial administration.

Medical teachers and researchers in Britain benefited considerably from war-time projects and from the conviction among higher civil servants that science could render medicine more efficient. In the 1920s, the Medical Research Council was dominated by medical scientists who had the ear of government and who tended to be scornful of mere clinicians, not least the stars of London private practice. Prestigious clinicians reacted by pulling in money for new research charities, such as the Imperial Cancer Research Fund, but they could not escape from the science/government network. Nor could they counter effectively the claims of medical scientists that disciplined research would eventually provide remedies for disease, and that meanwhile the education of doctors in scientific methods would help create a more efficient health service by eliminating ineffective, if habitual, practices.

Because the British state was now paying much of the cost of general medical care for working men, there was also a financial incentive to study common diseases and to develop a science of 'social medicine'. This broader vision of public health, incorporating social sciences and the new science of nutrition, was developed by medical 'progressives', many of whom were sympathetic to the Labour Party, then replacing the Liberals as the opposition to the Conservatives; some of them were impressed by the organization and scope of 'socialized medicine' in the Soviet Union. The lock-up surgeries run by British general practitioners, and the overcrowded outpatient departments of the charity hospitals, seemed wasteful and haphazard by comparison.

At the end of the First World War, medicine had formed part of national plans for a more collective Britain – a land fit for heroes. A new Ministry of Health was set up and a report (1921) produced by Lord Dawson, an eminent physician based in London, looked to the benefits of state organization, a rationalization of health care based on district hospitals, and primary health centres staffed by general practitioners. But this plan, like so many other hopes, faltered and faded in the economic slump of the 1920s. The decline of the old staple industries severely restricted state spending until the mid-1930s (and rearmament). Little was spent on new hospitals, and there were few major legislative initiatives compared to the 20 years before the First World War. Yet medicine did change significantly.

Partly as a result of the war, and partly as a result of successful campaigns for extension of the vote, women came to play a larger role in politics. Women's political groupings, of both left and centre, campaigned for more maternity hospitals, better midwifery, and better antenatal care. Municipalities and central government obliged, still driven by worries over the quantity and quality of the imperial population. But apart from their 'maternity benefits', most women, as 'non-workers', remained outside the state medical-insurance system, even when this was extended to cover almost all working men. Women and children were comparatively dependent on medical charities, to which working men would now be referred only for specialist or accident care. The only specialized hospital care available from the state was for tuberculosis, which remained a major concern in the interwar years.

By the late 1930s, British medicine had experienced no general reorganization, but in response to specific worries and public demands governments were building up co-ordinated services for tuberculosis, cancer, maternity, and for the care of victims of accidents. Unlike previous government concerns with environment and education, these new issues all involved hospitals; specialist hospital consultants were major protagonists and major beneficiaries. At the local level, Medical Officers of Health also became more involved with general hospitals, especially after the abolition of the poor law in 1929, when the former poor-law hospitals were turned over to mainstream local government.

These local authorities were now responsible for a huge range of health services: not just drains and rehousing schemes, but also clinics, health education, special hospitals, and most of the general hospital beds. Only the charity hospitals and general practice remained beyond the reach of local government, and these, as we have seen, were increasingly dependent on central government and subject to some local co-ordination. Hospital services, state or charity, were now for 'citizens' – paupers were no longer segregated and the richer no longer excluded themselves; they tended to use separate blocks in charity hospitals. (George Orwell's *The Road to Wigan Pier* could have featured the private patients' home built in the 1930s beside the charity hospital of that depressed industrial town.)

We might generalize that in most of the 'advanced' countries between the wars, the average man, with his wife and children, became the central focus of organized medicine. The form of the development varied according to the polity and economy concerned. Russia moved in the 1930s from a state-insurance system to a salaried medical and hospitalized service. Germany continued to operate a state-regulated insurance scheme for all the working classes. In Britain, as we have seen, state insurance covered workers for general practice but not for hospital care, for which many working-class families made voluntary contributions to the 'Saturday Funds', once a form of working-class charity, now an informal prepayment scheme. In both Britain and Germany, the insurance schemes were chiefly organized through friendly societies or employer-employee schemes. The middle classes were not covered by state systems, although some paid for private or occupational insurance schemes.

In the USA, the emphasis was on private 'consumers' rather than organized workers or citizens. During the depression of the 1930s, charity hospitals introduced voluntary insurance schemes (the Blue Cross), but commercial companies invaded the hospital-insurance market, partly by offering lower premiums to low-risk households. Doctors' organizations came to accept these insurance schemes as preferable to state intervention; around 1940 they began to organize their own schemes to cover treatment out of hospitals. Many states granted doctors a virtual monopoly for this kind of insurance and medical incomes benefited accordingly. In this way, insurance became part of the market arrangements that dominated most of American medicine. Middle-class families paid for their primary and hospital care through insurance schemes; hospitals competed with each other, and so did doctors. The indigent were covered by the low-grade 'public hospitals' and by the small proportion of 'voluntary hospital beds' that remained assigned to charity cases.

In France, the state-insurance system remunerated patients rather than doctors; there was free choice of doctor and hospital. As in the USA, the public hospitals received little investment and the average citizen now patronized the many private hospitals, often doctor-owned, which benefited from the health insurance system. There was little control on costs.

Wartime Medicine

In the First World War, thousands of doctors, nurses, and medical auxiliaries had tended the victims of trench warfare, first in the field then at base hospitals and the crowded, often improvised hospitals back home. Most of the organization was after the fact. In the Second World War, plans were laid in advance; the provision was more scientific, and so were the horrors.

It is easy to demonize the German Nazi party, the Japanese authorities who ran death camps, or the Allied commanders who ended the war by unleashing the atom bomb. But the antisemitism that culminated in the concentration camps had a long history in Germany and was evident enough in other Western countries during the 1930s. German doctors, who had seemed paragons of science, gave disproportionate support to Nazism, and many benefited from the emigration, disqualification, and persecution of their Jewish colleagues. With many honorable exceptions, German medical academics accepted the racial doctrines used to legitimate antisemitism, ranking medical researchers pursued experiments on prisoners, and experts in delousing became experts in mass murder. Medicine was central to this monstrous politics, because it depends on and so helps define the boundaries of humanity. In the case of Nazi medicine, non-Aryan races were formally defined as subhuman and thereby as expendable.

Nazi atrocities came to serve as the major reference point for postwar debates on the ethics of experimentation on humans, but we should also remember the experiments that Japanese doctors and scientists conducted on Chinese victims, not least the fact that the American government kept these atrocities secret and gave amnesty to the perpetrators so as to maintain privileged access to data on germ warfare.

During the Second World War, all the major combatant countries built up unprecedented concentrations of scientific and technical expertise. The key Anglo-American project was the creation of the atom bomb, an enterprise that shaped much military and civilian science into the 1970s. Medical men and women were marginal to this project, although the assessments of the effects of the bomb on its Japanese victims proved foundational for postwar human genetics. The obvious medical counterpart was the development of penicillin, which served as a launchpad for much of the postwar pharmaceutical industry in Britain and the USA.

Health Services after the Second World War

The success of the antibiotics and the mobilization of new physical techniques further increased popular and governmental faith in medical progress, but in most countries the effects were gradual; only in Britain was there a major postwar reorganization of peacetime medical services.

It was focused on the rationalization of hospital services, which had been funded by the state as part of the war effort and seemed financially too fragile to be returned to the voluntary sector. Liberal and Labour reformers had built on wartime social solidarity to secure promises of major extensions of welfare, including universal medical benefits and free hospital care. Doctors' representatives and most Tory politicians sought secure funding for hospitals, but were unwilling to see the prestigious charity hospitals subordinated in an extension of local authority services. Aneurin Bevan, the imaginative Minister of Health in the postwar Labour administration, nationalized charity as well as municipal hospitals.

Bevan was not an advocate of local government. He wanted the hospitals to be responsible to the Minister and to Parliament; their regional and local organization should then be functional, unimpeded by complexities of ownership. At this level he was content to follow the schemes drawn up by the medical educators and specialists, who, since the 1930s, had been interested in the rationalization of hospital services. Local authorities lost their hospitals and were left with public health services. Because of the resistance of most general practitioners to 'state employment', primary care was extended on much the same basis as had been introduced in 1911, but the whole population was now covered.

Although many reformers came to see the new system as giving too much power to doctors or to local 'philanthropists', the National Health Service proved enormously popular. It allowed considerable levelling-up of services, especially by the appointment of consultants to hospitals outside the main centres of medical teaching. The initial expense proved higher than anticipated, and hopes were soon dashed that proper treatment of the poor would lead to *reductions* in public medical expenditure, yet over the following decades the hospital system proved innovative, efficient, and relatively equitable.

The 1950s saw little investment in new hospital buildings, partly because of shortage of building materials, and partly because the 1950s government gave priority to housing and education. In the early 1960s, the Conservative government produced the first national plan for hospital building, based on the notion of full-service general hospitals in each district. In many towns, it was implemented by adding new ward blocks and technical services on the sites of the old workhouse hospitals. Much of the investment went to teaching hospitals.

In terms of medical professional organization, the NHS strengthened and extended tendencies already evident between the wars. Medical education became more integrated into the hospital regions, each of which was based on a medical school. Grants were provided for undergraduate and postgraduate medical education, and medical careers became more accessible to poor students, although male privilege declined but slowly. All hospital services were now to be supervised by consultants with specialist qualifications, including 'geriatrics', which had scarcely existed in Britain before 1940. In some regions, psychiatric patients also came under the care of consultants in general hospitals rather than in asylums.

All these developments formalized the longstanding, if previously incomplete, division between hospital consultants and general practitioners. Many of the latter had resisted the NHS, and especially the extension of general practice in 'health centres'. They chose to remain in 'small businesses' under contract to the state, and were regarded as inferior to hospital consultants. Not until the 1960s would general practice be renovated, when the threat of health centres run by local government had diminished and GPs could be encouraged to band together in group practices large enough to employ nurses and other auxiliary services.

In the 1930s, local government had loomed large in British health services, but its influence declined when the NHS took over municipal hospitals. By the 1960s it was generally accepted that clinic services would also be transferred to the NHS, leaving only environmental services in the hands of local government. By the late 1970s, after a series of clumsy re-organizations, the future structure of the NHS seemed clear. Hospitals, general practitioners, and public health were to be part of a planned, unified service, based on regions (and their medical schools); central government would decide policy, health-service professionals would manage, local politicians would be involved, and consumers would be represented. Medicine had never seemed so powerful, nor in Britain had services ever been so rationally organized.

Paradoxically, perhaps, the Western countries that were 'occupied' during or after the Second World War did not undertake major re-organization of medical services such as was seen in Britain. France continued to rely on state welfare benefits by which the patient was repaid for most of her/his medical expenditure. Most West Germans continued to use sick-funds that repaid doctors. Most Americans took out private health insurance, often through occupational schemes that were tax-deductible for employers. In the USA and in France, doctors and private hospitals competed to offer better medical care; German sick-funds were also competitive to some extent. Such competition drove expenditure upwards.

In the USA, health expenditure increased rapidly, including major capital expenditures on hospitals, often from federal funds. As standards rose, the lack of medical cover for the indigent attracted more attention and in 1965, under President Kennedy, Congress voted to make medical care a social security benefit and to provide grants towards state governments to cover the costs. The result was a massive increase in total medical expenditure.

In postwar France, dependents came to be included in the social-security schemes, which had now been nationalized. Much of the rising expenditure went to private hospitals. They continued to increase in number while 'public hospitals' (old buildings with most of the long-stay patients) languished. But as the French economy recovered, the poverty of the public sector became embarrassing, especially for the supposedly 'elite' hospitals attached to the medical schools. In 1965, the Debré Law invited the affiliation of hospitals with medical schools and offered generous full-time salaries to doctors committed to research and teaching, as well as to patient care. New blocks were added on ancient sites, often housing research laboratories, many of which worked on 'pure science' projects that in other countries would be found in universities or other 'non-clinical' institutions. More generally, the French state took powers to control the development of hospitals – partly to secure better distribution of services, partly to reduce the excess cost arising from the duplication of facilities.

In West Germany, health expenditure had begun to rise rapidly in the 1950s (15 per cent a year); the rises continued during the 1960s, funded by a buoyant economy, and in the 1970s expenditure really took off, increasing much faster than gross national product and giving rise to projections that by the year 2000 half the GNP would be devoted to health. Again, the causes of the rapid increase included hospital policy. Until 1972, the sick-funds had paid towards hospitals established by governments, religious orders, or voluntary associations, but the contributions rarely covered the full cost, so they limited expenditure and building projects. By a Federal Law of 1972, state governments assumed responsibility for hospital building, and sick-funds were required to pay the full daily costs of approved hospitals. These were expensive to run and raised standards for other hospitals. Hence an explosion in costs, so that by the later 1970s Germany, like France and the UK, was looking for ways to restrict expenditure.

In the 30 years since the Second World War, the resources of medicine had grown enormously. Infectious diseases seemed to be conquered (it was commonly, if falsely, believed that viruses as well as bacteria could be killed by antibiotics). Psychotropic drugs were used to control many mental illnesses; there was hope that transplant surgery might provide relief for at least some chronic medical conditions. Doctors, especially in elite hospitals, were oriented towards innovation and so were pharmaceutical companies, which became models of 'research-based' industry, producing a succession of new types of drugs, yet also investing heavily in minor variants within these types. But new medical procedures rarely reduced medical labour or medical costs; they usually involved elaborate tests, the proliferation of paramedical staff, and the provision of drugs – all of which could be very expensive.

Meanwhile, the power and organization of scientific medicine was under attack. From the 1950s, British and American critics of mental asylums had campaigned for 'community care'. From the 1960s, a new wave of feminists queried the increasing hospitalization of normal births: the proportion of institutional deliveries had risen rapidly as confinement times decreased, new hospitals were built, and the birth rate fell. Now feminists called for less interference in birth, and for the right to choose confinement at home. Other consumer groups developed, mobilizing patients and challenging the profession's monopoly of expertise.

The political radicalism of the 1960s tended to present science and technology as aspects of a system of domination that threatened the environment, impoverished less-developed countries, and sapped the ability of Westerners to find fulfilment in community and nature. High-tech medicine came under this criticism. The thalidomide tragedy was a powerful symbol of technical failure. Scientifically educated doctors were portrayed as lacking the human understanding characteristic of interwar GPs. Generally, the left became more critical of the costs (and profits) of high-tech medicine, more ready to argue that professionals tended to pursue private rather than public interests.

Such criticisms were perhaps most prominent in the USA, where the healthcare system was most expensive and least equitable. In Britain, a suspicion of technology and alienation from increasingly bureaucratic hospitals co-existed with public attachment to community services that represented mutual dependence.

It was the cost of high-technology medicine, however, rather than its alienating qualities, that was to determine the next phase of medical politics. From the late 1970s, in most Western countries, the politics of medicine has concentrated on cost-restraint. For 150 years, the political economy of public medicine had focused on death rates in the community; now it is becoming a branch of corporate economics, focused on the costs and benefits of medical services.

History Tomorrow?

Some economists believe in long-waves – cycles of innovative activity that last a generation or so; they give a pattern to history. Historians of the political have no such resource, unless it be the dialectics of Georg Hegel or of Karl Marx, which were very unfashionable in the 1990s. Can we say anything about the general shape of the analytical narrative in this chapter?

There is more than a suggestion in some histories, including this one, of a kind of oscillation, especially for Britain: late eighteenth-century paternalism gives way to early nineteenth-century liberalism, which gives way to late nineteenth-century corporatism and professionalism, which develops through the twentieth century until the 1970s, since when it has been increasingly challenged by a resurgence of liberalism and a return to (early) Victorian values. As a one-sentence summary, this has much to recommend it. The USA shows a similar pattern, displaced towards the liberal pole: the German oscillation takes place nearer the hierarchical, corporatist pole. But patterns are not explanations; what, beyond a dialectic of ideas, would serve to explain such patterns or elucidate the dynamic of our present?

Part of the explanation lies in the interplay of economics, military politics, and population growth. In the late eighteenth century, and again in the early twentieth century, there were strategic and economic reasons for promoting the strength of populations through health care. It seems unlikely that either the economic or the military might of the West will again depend on the aggregate of physical fitness at the level of the nation (or supernation); it is much more likely that Western businesses (and armed forces) will promote the health and welfare of their own employees, partly for reasons of physical efficiency, partly for the morale and loyalty of highly trained, expensive workforces. There is probably a general confluence, already well established in the USA, between the business as the unit of health-care insurance, and the business as the unit of medical provision. Medicine will probably appear more and more as a service industry, even within taxation-funded systems such as the British NHS. The market version of medicine may come to operate at the level of corporate suppliers and corporate purchasers, with doctors operating as skilled employees rather than as liberal professionals.

Such developments, in the affluent West, will be limited in two ways: by the considerable if diminishing powers of medical professionals, and by the need to provide adequate medicine for the poor. In Britain, the private sector is still small compared with the remaining NHS. (In 1991, 89 per cent of health-care expenditure in the UK came from the public sector compared with 79 per cent in France, 78 per cent in Germany, and 41 per cent in the USA.) Even in the USA, the key medical institutions – the big teaching hospitals – are in some sense producer cooperatives, partly because of their close links with the universities, which are state-owned or public charities and in either case directed chiefly by academics. It is hard to see this system changing rapidly. Yet, throughout the Western world, higher education is being pushed into quasi-market relations and some American firms have claimed to possess sufficient range and depth of expertise in science, teaching, and management to provide the kinds of education and research presently offered by prestige universities. One can perhaps imagine a consortium of medical-technology and medical-care companies setting up a medical school, research institute, and teaching hospital, especially if governments continued to subsidize the students and the patients.

The last point is crucial for, as we have seen, medicine is a very peculiar kind of market. State services developed in all Western countries because much of the population was unable to afford health care of a standard considered adequate by them or by governments. Costs can be spread by commercial or mutual insurance schemes, but these have always left a considerable residual population to be covered by state welfare, and usually to be served by substandard hospitals and clinics. Of course, the incomes of the poor are now much higher, relative to subsistence, than they were in mid-nineteenth-century Britain; but so are the costs of medical services. Governments will continue to support medicine for poor people, partly because of their votes, partly to reduce disaffection and infectious disease, and partly because those in authority can still be embarrassed by 'unnecessary deaths'. Life and death remain ideologically powerful, and health care, even for the poor, is a major issue, not least where the resurgence of infectious diseases, such as tuberculosis, highlights the threat posed by 'lower classes' to the rest of the population.

The key issues for Western health care continue to include equity and community. Should we allow systems that provide the poor with separate, usually inferior services? Can we not maintain equitable services such as were developed by social-democratic governments in Scandinavia and Britain? When measured in terms of health standards against cost, such systems are probably more efficient than more competitive alternatives and they have the considerable political advantage of turning equity into the positive virtue of solidarity. That the economically powerful and politically resourceful share provision with the less fortunate is the best guarantee of efficiency as well as equity.

Such arrangements are now breaking down in eastern Europe as economies decline and can no longer support former standards of service. A small proportion of the population buy Western medicines in hard currencies; the rest suffer, not just from a massive decline in the real resources of the public system but from diversion of expertise to the private sector and the loss of the social and economic co-ordination required to maintain high-technology medicine.

Some cities in Africa face rather similar problems as their economies are marginalized and the colonial and post-colonial infrastructure fails to be renewed. In addition, of course, many sub-Saharan states also face issues of subsistence and basic sanitation that most European states have considered as solved for at least a century. Old issues are presented in new forms, not least around new pandemics; the prevalence of AIDS in East Africa may have much to do with the patterns of sexual relations, but it also depends on the chronic malnutrition of much of the population, and on the prevalence of other venereal diseases that could be effectively treated.

The West keeps a horrified eye on these sufferings; it intervenes at the margins, from an attenuated conscience and a fear of global consequences. 'Tropical medicine' is no longer required by empires, any more than the former imperial powers require the fitness of their mass citizenry. Internationally, as at home, Western nations have a choice: they can tolerate the increase of inequality and worry later about the consequential threats, or they can seek a broadening of political responsibility. The infrastructure of health – decent food and water, ventilation, and drains (to which we might now add antibiotics and contraceptives) – are, however, not within the control of individuals, or even of the governments of poorer countries.

We often think of medicine as a progress running through recent history. This chapter tells a different story. Medicine is a part of the complex interplay of economic and political history. Its future, like its past, in the 'second' and 'third' worlds as well as in the West, will depend on the shifting patterns of wealth and power.

10. Looking to the Future (1996)

Geoff Watts

Modern medicine is powerful and effective, and likely to become more so. Its scientific and technological approach to ill health has yielded unrivalled benefits. Illnesses once unpreventible, symptoms once unmanageable, and conditions once incurable have succumbed to the application of knowledge about the body and its workings. Even the law of diminishing therapeutic returns has so far been offset by the growth in medical research, and the accumulation of still more understanding. For the next decade, and probably beyond, there is every reason to suppose that medicine will continue devising new therapies to combat old enemies.

This hymn of praise is not, however, the complete picture. Medicine is increasingly troubled by doubts and negative developments. While doctors have always had their critics, the past two decades have witnessed a sustained assault on the nature of professional medicine. The social polemicist Ivan Illich opened his book *Limits to Medicine* (1976) by declaring that 'The medical establishment has become a major threat to health. The disabling impact of professional control over medicine has reached the proportions of an epidemic.' Illich's criticisms were more outspoken than most; but his has not been a lone voice.

Some of medicine's most pressing problems are unintended consequences of its success. By way of example, consider a study carried out some years ago at Boston University Medical Center in Massachusetts. A group of doctors followed the progress of more than 800 patients admitted to the medical wards of their hospital. They were looking for iatrogenic complications: for illnesses induced not by nature or circumstance or the patient's own behaviour, but by the drugs and procedures used to diagnose or treat the original condition. Out of the patients admitted during the study, 290 developed one or more iatrogenic disorders – many of them drug-induced. Of these, 76 suffered major complications, and in 15 cases these contributed to their death.

Although as a specialist clinic the Boston Center receives the sickest and most difficult patients, the findings would – to a lesser extent – be true of most hospitals in most places. The discomforting fact is that modern medicine demands a price. And almost as often as it fulfills a promise, it seems to create a moral dilemma or prompt an uncomfortable question – most fundamentally about the purpose of medicine. Despite the wilder ambitions of a few Californians who have had their corpses frozen in the expectation of revival by some omnipotent physician of the future, we may assume that all of us eventually have to die. If medicine succeeded in, for example, eliminating heart disease, many more of us would live slightly longer but then die of cancer. The gain would be, to say the least, questionable. Our ignorance of the ageing process makes it impossible even now to be certain about the long-term effects of our interventions. The ideal health strategy must be to maintain the body in good physical and mental condition until shortly before death: a longer life and a healthy one. But it is just as likely that further increases in longevity will instead offer extra years plagued by degenerative disease and mental impairment. How many people would thank medicine for a gift such as this?

Small wonder, then, that public attitudes to medicine veer so disconcertingly from the laudatory to the censorious. This ambivalence seems set to continue until there is a wider agreement on the purpose of medicine. These conflicts and contradictions will form the substance of much of this chapter. First, though, a caveat.

Predictions about medicine are not new – and many have been wholly wrong. Most are simple extrapolations of present understanding. Once it had become clear that antibiotics could inhibit the growth of bacteria, it required no great insight to predict that new

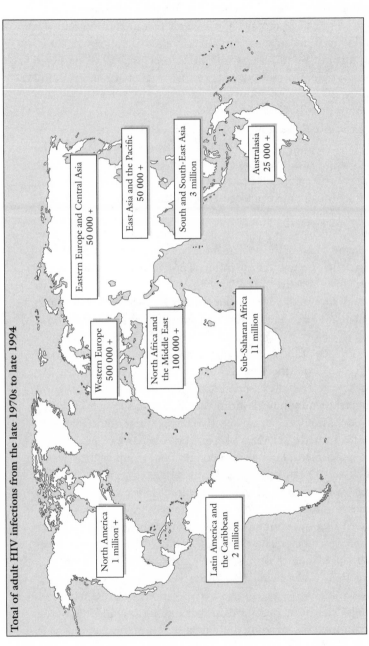

Map 6. By the end of 1994, at least 18 million adults had been infected with HIV since the late 1970s/early 1980s, 11 million of them in sub-Saharan Africa. Malaria causes many more deaths than AIDS worldwide, but whereas malaria kills mostly young children, AIDS mainly affects adults in their economically productive years and can devastate not only a family but the economics of a whole community as well. Researchers are working on a vaccine for HIV. But, even if one is developed, it may be many years before it is cheap enough for the developing world.

Total of adult HIV infections from the late 1970s to late 1994

Eastern Europe and Central Asia
50 000 +

East Asia and the Pacific
50 000 +

South and South-East Asia
3 million

Australasia
25 000 +

Western Europe
500 000 +

North Africa and
the Middle East
100 000 +

Sub-Saharan Africa
11 million

North America
1 million +

Latin America and
the Caribbean
2 million

antibiotics would be found or synthesized, and that these would improve the control of bacterial disease. But who predicted the advent of antibiotic resistance, now such a problem? And who can foresee the advent of a new microbe such as the human immuno-deficiency virus (HIV)? Likewise, on the credit side, no-one in the 1960s or 1970s could have guessed that surgery for peptic ulcers, then so common, would become a comparative rarity in the late 1980s and 1990s. To have done so would have presumed the exis-tence of a (then undiscovered) drug to stop acid secretion in the stomach. And who could have imagined the burgeoning interest in immunology, its effects on the understanding and treatment of infectious disease, and its use as a tool in almost every branch of medicine?

Neither is expertise a guarantee of exciting, imaginative, and fault-less prophecy. The results of a survey of more than twenty 'inter-national medical scientists' organized by the Bristol-Myers phar-maceutical company in 1987 were unremarkable. They suggested, among other things, that the diseases most likely to have been elim-inated by the year 2000 are AIDS and measles; that the cure rate for cancer will by that time have risen to about two-thirds (from today's half); and that most coronary bypass surgery will have been replaced by less-invasive techniques, or by drugs able to dissolve the blood clots that otherwise precipitate a heart attack. A first-year medical student would be as capable of this sort of prophecy as any 'international medical scientist'.

For a supreme misjudgment consider the words of the Nobel Prize–winning immunologist Sir Frank Macfarlane Burnet. Research at the level of cells and even molecules has already affected the practice of medicine, and will have an even greater impact in the future. Yet as recently as 1971 Macfarlane Burnet wrote this: 'I believe that biological research can provide gratifying occupation for as many people as have the necessary training, competence and motivation . . . I do not expect conventional benefits to medicine or technology from biological research to be common in the future. If they should arise they can be accepted as bonuses but need not be sought.'[1] Let this spectacular failure to predict be remembered as I review the direction of medical progress, and identify some of the hurdles and the pitfalls.

The Promise of Medicine

Before the doubts, the promises. The more that is understood of the causes of illness, the greater the potential for prevention. The decline in cigarette smoking in Western countries, for example, will eventually reduce the incidence of cancer in the developed world. Conversely, tobacco consumption in developing countries is increasing by some 2 per cent a year, so they can expect to see a corresponding increase in the disease. Preventive knowledge is effective only if acted on, and there is still little grasp of what makes people act as they do and how they can be persuaded to do otherwise. Any form of prevention that depends on behavioural change will, most likely, continue to be overshadowed by enthusiasm for cures. What follows is an outline of a few of the developments in science and technology that are now shaping the future of medicine. Nowhere is this more evident than in new approaches to inherited disease.

Many illnesses are caused by a defect in a single gene: a single segment of the hereditary material or DNA. Genetic techniques are already used to diagnose such disorders (see later). If undamaged copies of the defective gene could be introduced into the patient's body, the activity controlled by that gene would be restored to normal. This is the basis of gene therapy, itself now on the verge of entering routine practice.

In cystic fibrosis, for example, a defective gene causes patients to produce copious quantities of an abnormal mucus that makes the airways susceptible to various lethal respiratory diseases. In principle, the gene therapist might remove some cells from the lungs and breathing passages, insert normal genes into them, and then return them to the body. Such an approach is feasible for blood or bonemarrow cells; for the airways, it is impracticable. An alternative strategy is to repair the defect *in situ*.

This has already been done by exploiting a virus that colonizes the cells of the airways. Suitably doctored to render it harmless, the virus acts as a carrier for a normal version of the abnormal gene. Getting viruses into the lungs presents no problem; an inhaled aerosol will take them where they are needed. The beneficial effects of the new gene should last as long as the viral colonies continue to thrive – and in the handful of patients on whom this experiment has been tried, this is what appears to happen. An alternative way of introducing the genes is to wrap them in fatty envelopes, called liposomes, and blow them in an aerosol into the nose. The long-term benefits of both these strategies remain to be seen.

In some cases gene therapy could turn out to be far simpler, and require nothing more complicated than an injection of the normal or missing gene directly into the tissues in which it is required. This might even apply to Duchenne muscular dystrophy, an incurable disease in which certain muscles become progressively more wasted and so weaker. Muscle cells are able to absorb genetic material. If DNA containing the gene required to overcome the disease is introduced into the affected muscles, they may take it up and start to manufacture the missing protein.

Other inherited diseases – of which there are several thousand with a familiarity ranging from sickle-cell anaemia and muscular dystrophy to Tay-Sachs and Lesch-Nyan – will demand other strategies. Some are the consequence of single gene defects, whereas others are the result of several such errors. Many hitherto incurable or even untreatable illnesses will soon be candidates for gene therapy. The technique is not limited to inherited disorders. The body makes many natural products able to fight disease: substances such as interferon and interleukin. Gene therapy could be used to increase the output of these substances, or even to persuade cells that do not normally make them to do so.

The hereditary material of each human probably comprises some 100,000 genes, only a tiny proportion of which have been identified. But if – or more likely when – the ambitions of a scheme called the Human Genome Project are realized, scientists will have mapped the lot. It will then be possible to identify the defect underlying every inherited disorder and, given sufficient ingenuity and resources, correct it.

Sequencing the Genome

The remainder of the 1990s and the beginning of the new millennium will see human biology's first and perhaps only venture into 'big science'. Projects costing tens of millions of pounds and bringing together hundreds of scientists working in international groups have so far been confined to physics. Sequencing the human genome is the biological equivalent of exploring the fine structure of matter. DNA, the hereditary material, is a long, helical, double-stranded molecule built up of pairs of four types of molecular sub-units or bases. The order of these base pairs forms a code specifying the structure of all the proteins required to make and run every cell in an organism. The human genome comprises some 3,000 million base pairs, and its full analysis will be an awesome task.

The initial attempts at sequencing were carried out piecemeal, with researchers working on small sections thought to have some special significance – in causing disease, for example. It was in the mid-1980s that scientists conceived the idea of tackling the task more systematically. The Human Genome Project aims to identify the position of every gene on every chromosome, and the order of every one of the millions of base pairs. Japan, Canada, and France are among the countries collaborating in the project; but the leading laboratories are mostly in Britain (for example, at the Sanger Centre in Cambridge and the Institute of Molecular Medicine in Oxford) or in the USA (notably at the National Institutes of Health).

When this aim will be realized and at what cost are still uncertain; but 10 to 15 years, and a price of as many dollars as there are base pairs, would be realistic guesses. By early 1995, only about 5 per cent of the genome had been sequenced, so the project is still in its infancy. In spite of disagreements over patent protection (should the patenting of human genes be permitted?), division of labour, duplication of effort, and much else, the project seems certain to progress.

New Drugs – by Design

The search for new drugs has traditionally relied on trial and error. A chemist might synthesize a new molecule, which a pharmacologist would screen for evidence of useful biological action. Alternatively, a particular molecule might be known to have an action that doctors realize is useful; the chemists could then synthesize variants in the hope of making a more active version. Although this method has yielded large numbers of useful drugs, it is wasteful. Much better would be to design drugs for specific purposes. That is now becoming a reality.

The key to success lies in discovering the processes that control the body's cells, and then manipulating them. For example, much of what cells do is determined by hormones circulating in the bloodstream. These act in a lock-and-key fashion by attaching themselves to hormone-specific sites or receptors located on the membranes of cells. The attachment of the hormone serves to trigger the cell into activity; when the hormone is withdrawn, the cell switches itself off. This offers the pharmacologist several avenues of intervention. By designing a drug molecule that can stick to a receptor of just one particular type, it may be possible to mimic the action of one particular hormone. Or the drug could be made sufficiently like the hormone to attach to its receptor, but not sufficiently similar to activate the cell. Having, as it were, jammed the lock by inserting the wrong key, the cell would be effectively inactivated.

All this, of course, depends on being able to design the right drugs. It is now possible not only to know the atomic make-up of a long-chain molecule but, using a computer, to work out how the molecule will fold on itself. This understanding is vital to drug design because the three-dimensional structure of a molecule is often what determines its properties as a drug. The molecular pharmacologist can view models of drugs and receptors on computer display screens, rotate them, and even find out if one will fit snugly into the other.

The pharmacology of the future will also make greater use of natural chemicals such as interferon, interleukin, and others with less familiar names. By isolating these materials, identifying their roles in the life and control of cells, and then synthesizing them in quantity, it will be possible to manipulate the body's physiology in ways used by the body itself.

Monoclonal Antibodies

Antibodies are natural substances – proteins – made by the immune system as part of its defence against invading microbes or other foreign materials that have entered the body. Their value lies in their specificity: usually, one type of antibody molecule will attach itself only to one type of foreign material. When an antigen, as such materials are collectively described, enters the body, the immune system responds by generating large amounts of the corresponding antibody.

The body's output of antibodies is generally adequate for its needs; but to exploit their potential in new ways requires far more pure antibody than can be extracted from an intact, functioning immune system. The monoclonal antibody technique, devised at the University of Cambridge in the mid-1970s, is a way of generating a specified antibody in virtually unlimited amounts.

In principle, the technique relies on repeatedly immunizing an animal – originally mice – with the antigen complementary to the required antibody. The cells responsible for manufacturing it are found in the spleen. They can be removed and cultured, but do not survive for long. The key to the Cambridge advance lay in fusing these cells with others able to grow and divide indefinitely, and produced in a type of tumour called a myeloma. The resulting 'hybridoma' cells will grow and proliferate indefinitely, as well as make large quantities of just the one antibody. Suitably adapted, this system can produce any type of human antibody.

Monoclonal antibodies have revived interest in the field of immunotherapy. Moreover, used with ingenuity, they can do things that were previously impossible. Attached to drug molecules, for example, and injected into the bloodstream, antibodies specific for tumour cells will concentrate the drug at the site of the tumour, so minimizing remote side-effects. Alternatively, monoclonal antibodies can be used to inactivate undesirable materials. There is growing evidence that a chemical messenger, misleadingly known as tumour necrosis factor or TNF, plays a part in the sequence of events leading to and maintaining the inflammation in joints afflicted with rheumatoid arthritis. Preliminary attempts at injecting patients with an antibody that binds specifically to TNF – and so neutralizes it – offer the possibility of new biological therapies for this and similar diseases.

The range of applications will be limited only by the imagination of the scientists. For a flavour of the possibilities, consider how one Australian researcher, Warren Jones of Adelaide's Flinders Medical Centre in Australia, is developing a less-invasive method of prenatal testing for fetal abnormalities. A small number of fetal cells cross the placenta and enter the mother's bloodstream – so, in principle, it should be possible to detect abnormalities of the fetus by testing those of its cells present in the mother's blood. Using techniques that increase the amount of genetic material in a cell, it is possible to test for defective genes in a sample containing no more than a dozen or so cells. The trick is first to catch them. As there may be only one fetal cell for every 5 million maternal ones circulating in the mother's blood, this is no easy task.

One solution is to make monoclonal antibodies specific to fetal cells, and then join them to microscopic beads with a metal core. When added to a blood sample, the antibody-coated beads will attach themselves exclusively to the few fetal cells that are present. They can then be separated from the maternal cells using a magnet.

Surgery – Robots and Keyholes

The notion of robotic surgery is apt to seem not only futuristic but hazardous; the prospect of lying unconscious while an electromechanical device cuts and probes is disconcerting. But until – if ever – computer-controlled machinery can mimic the awareness, adaptability, and knowledge of a human surgeon, such a takeover in the operating theatre is unlikely. A more realistic prospect is of using robots to perform certain tasks requiring great precision.

In replacing a hip, for example, the surgeon has to remove the head of the thigh bone, excavate its interior, and then insert the shaft of the artifical joint. In practice, the area of contact between bone and prosthesis is often less than half; the space is filled out with cement. Increasing the area of contact between bone and metal makes for a more resilient and longer-lasting replacement. And this is precisely what can be achieved by having a robot excavate the interior of the bone. Similar precison is required when operating on structures inside the brain. This organ is ideally suited to robotic surgery because the surrounding skull provides fixed reference points by which to locate any particular part of the brain, and a firm base for mounting instruments.

Details of the anatomy of the bony structures can be supplied to the controlling computer in the form of pictures taken using X-rays or other imaging systems. A double control system requiring the agreement of two computer processors before any action is taken minimizes the risk of mishap – and the whole procedure can be supervised by a human surgeon.

A greater influence on surgery in the near future will be the continuing development of minimally invasive techniques. These allow surgeons to operate from outside the body, so avoiding extensive cuts in its surface. Patients need less anaesthesia, experience less postoperative pain, and can go home sooner – in many cases on the day of the surgery, or the day after.

To see inside the body cavity the surgeon uses a viewing tube or endoscope, often in conjunction with a minature TV camera. The endoscope is pushed through a small hole in the wall of the abdomen, while specially designed instruments are inserted through a further one or two holes. Keyhole procedures already in use include removal of the gallbladder, the appendix, the kidneys, and even quite large sections of bowel, the repair of hernias, the closure of the Fallopian tubes, and removal of the uterus (hysterectomy).

How much surgery will eventually be done in this way is a matter of conjecture, but enthusiasts envisage keyhole techniques becoming standard in at least half of all cases.

Transplants of Fetal Tissue

Many of the body's tissues can repair themselves; like the skin, they can regenerate if damaged. The nerve cells of the brain are not in this category. Parkinson's disease, for example, is caused by the loss of certain nerves in the part of the brain called the substantia nigra, itself resulting in a fall off of the chemical transmitter dopamine. Attempts to remedy the loss by dosing patients with one of its chemical precursors, called L-dopa, often bring a marked improvement in the symptoms of Parkinson's disease. But the treatment is far from perfect. Hence the attempts to transplant fetal material into the brains of Parkinson's patients.

Whether this will ultimately succeed is still unclear; but if it does, it will be the first of many attempts to use material from fetuses that have been spontaneously or electively aborted. Fetal cells, unlike many of their adult counterparts, can grow and divide, and seem less prone to rejection when placed in another body. Diseases for which this approach might be suitable include Alzheimer's, Huntington's, and diabetes. It might even be possible to use fetal material to repair the damage after a heart attack. The closure of one of the coronary arteries deprives part of the muscular wall of the heart of the oxygen it needs, and so kills it. The muscle cannot repair itself; but if the surgeon could introduce sufficient fetal material, it is possible that the new cells might grow and divide and replace the damaged tissue.

Computers in Medicine

In medicine as elsewhere, computers will radically alter the way in which medical staff work. The traditional means of storing patient records – a thick wadge of papers bearing semi-legible handwriting, and all too frequently lost – will soon be replaced by a computer memory. Doctors, whether in primary care or in hospitals, will call up the information they require on desktop visual display units. Many case notes are already handled in this way, and it is only a matter of time before X-rays, body scans, and other visual data are similarly stored. All this information would then be instantly available on a display unit in whatever hospital department a patient happened to be visiting.

Diagnosis is also being computerized. Simple tests for blood constituents such as glucose and cholesterol are already available in kits for home use. The development of electronic biosensors will enable many more body fluids to be monitored for the signs of impending ill health.

Some people are prepared to go to any lengths to engage in do-it-yourself diagnosis. Some Japanese researchers foresee the age of the intelligent toilet, equipped to monitor urine and faeces for the presence of blood, sugar, certain proteins, and any other chemicals that might offer clues to an individual's health. Data obtained in this way could be dispatched, down a telephone line, to a central computerized health-monitoring station. On detection of any abnormality, the individual concerned would be contacted and told to visit the doctor.

Benefits to the Poor

To see medicine's most spectacular achievements you should look to the poor: to the effects of preventive and public health medicine in developing countries. In this century, they have witnessed the dramatic impact of scientific principles on high infant mortality and endemic infections. In due course, patterns of mortality in developing countries will begin to resemble those of the industrial nations, with cancer and cardiovascular disease displacing infections as the main causes of illness and death. Many of these liberated peoples, either through the absence of means or the lack of inclination, have so far failed to limit the growth in their numbers – a catastrophe in the making.

The triumph of death control in the absence of compensating birth control has long been, and remains, socially and ideologically contentious. Countless attempts at planning have been subverted by religious, political, economic, and other vested interests that variously portray population increase as acceptable or even desirable, and all attempts to limit it as conspiratorial or oppressive. Does population increase matter? And in so far as medicine has fuelled it, what role can or should the medicine of the future have in dealing with it?

Only the wildest optimist can believe that population increase represents no conceivable threat. In 1995, there were around 5,700 million of us, and the end of the twenty-first century may see a doubling or even a trebling of this number. More than 90 per cent of the increase will be in developing countries: the have-nots of the planet.

Optimists count on the poor countries of the southern hemisphere undergoing the kind of demographic transition that Europe experienced in the nineteenth century. Before that transition, high birth rates were balanced by high death rates; so the population grew slowly if at all. In the first stage of the transition, health and living standards improved and death rates fell; but because the birth rate remained high, the population began to increase. Only in the third stage did the gains of economic development allow the birth rate to fall; birth and death rates were once more in alignment.

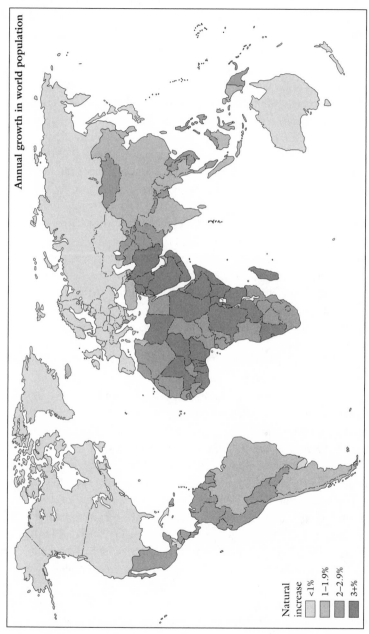

Annual growth in world population

Natural increase
<1%
1–1.9%
2–2.9%
3+%

Map 7. Population growth rates are highest in Africa and the Middle East. By 2010, the world's population of around 5,700 million (mid-1995 figure) is expected to have grown to around 7,000 million and, by 2025, to around 8,000 million. Data from Population Reference Bureau, 1995.

The fact that many countries have already made this transition, however, cannot be taken to indicate that all others can or will. Circumstances in Africa and much of Asia are vastly different from those prevailing in Europe when it went through its demographic transition. Many poor countries are at risk of the negative feedback loop – the 'demographic trap'. It happens when a population entering the first stage of the transition lives in a country with an already overstretched ecosystem – as in the horn of Africa. In these circumstances, a rising population can all too easily precipitate famine. Preventive medicine and public health have tipped many developing countries into the transition before their fragile economies can feed, house, and otherwise sustain the consequent increase in numbers. The next phase of the transition – a lower birth rate – simply isn't happening as rapidly as is needed. In a few cases, it isn't happening at all.

Having contributed so much to the problem, medicine can hardly wash its hands of the matter. It is agreed that there is a vast unmet demand for contraception in developing countries. Although the provision of birth control – depending on the method – is not exclusively or even mainly a medical affair, the cooperation of medicine is vital. Some doctors, notably Maurice King of the Department of Public Health Medicine at the University of Leeds, feel that more radical action may become inevitable.

In 1990, Dr King set out the health problems of the poor, and put them in the context of global ecology.[2] He argued that the celebrated World Health Organization's definition of health as 'a state of complete physical, mental and social well-being, and not merely the absence of disease' should be amended to include the word 'sustainable' in front of 'state'. He also wrote of the need for the rich countries to modify their lifestyles, of the importance of devising more equal ways of distributing the world's resources, and of the global initiatives that might set these changes in motion. All this, though, was familiar; much less so was the extent to which Maurice King confronted some of the more nightmarish consequences of his dire predictions.

The first hint that he was about to think the unthinkable was an oblique one. 'The reduction of human death rates has always been seen as an absolute good in public health, and unease about

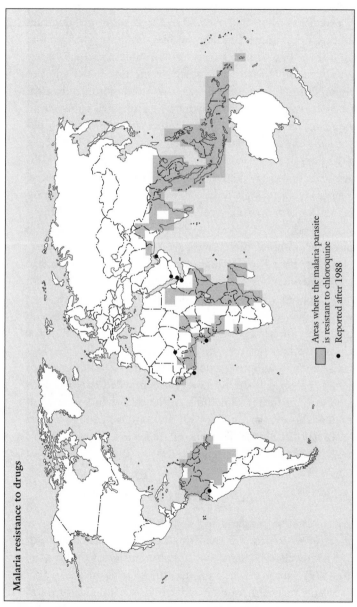

Map 8. Mosquitoes that carry the malaria parasite have become resistant to insecticides and the parasite itself has developed resistance to anti-malarial drugs. If the insect vector re-establishes itself in areas from which it was once eliminated, and, as a result of global warming, expands into temperate latitudes currently free of the disease, we could see widespread epidemics of malaria in the future. The need for a successful vaccine has never been so acute.

In the map legend:

Areas where the malaria parasite is resistant to chloroquine

● Reported after 1988

Malaria resistance to drugs

population increase has never been an accepted constraint on any public health measure. Will visions of the ultimate effects of population expansion alter this view? Are there some programmes that, although they are technically feasible, should not be initiated because of their long-term population-increasing consequences?'

By way of example Maurice King chose the oral rehydration of children suffering from severe diarrhoea. Although an individual doctor may be duty bound to rehydrate an individual child within his or her care, Dr King questioned whether there is an equal obligation to set up programmes of oral rehydration in the first place. Such measures, he suggested, 'should not be introduced on a public health scale since they increase the man-years of human misery, ultimately from starvation'. In effect, what's the point of denying infants a quick death now when all they face is a lingering and more painful one as adults?

From some authors, these views would have been unacceptable. From Maurice King, a man with a distinguished career in medicine in Africa, they could be repudiated but not dismissed. The article aroused much debate, with critics arguing that Dr King was variously neglecting the unfulfilled desire of many women in poor countries for better (or any) birth control, overstating the strength of the link between birth rate and economic development, and generally adopting a defeatist stance. What is significant is that Dr King himself should have felt compelled to voice such an argument; it indicates something of the despair now felt by at least some of those most familiar with the condition and prospects of the poorest of the poor. To make matters worse, there is global warming.

Fears of the Rich

The expectations of people living in rich industrial countries are altogether more demanding than those of the poor. The politician Enoch Powell, who served as British minister of health from 1960 to 1963, famously declared that 'there is virtually no limit to the amount of health care an individual is capable of absorbing'. Although this claim is much debated, it is true to say that never before have so many people had their suffering so effectively minimized. Yet far from growing more contented with what they have, many of the citizens of these privileged nations view both present and future with apprehension.

First there is the matter of cost. For decades, developed nations have been accustomed to a rising expenditure on health. At first, this seemed appropriate. But as the proportion of each nation's wealth so deployed has crept steadily upwards, doubts have began to crystallize, especially in the USA where spending on medicine – fuelled by private health insurance and unhindered by the controls operating in state-funded systems – accounts for more than 13 per cent of gross national product (relatively the highest of any Western nation). Although it may be difficult to identify the optimum level of spending on health care, most Americans sense that benefits are not keeping pace with outgoings. Something, they know, will have to be done to limit the flow of dollars. In the absence of a lead from the federal government, some states are trying their own schemes – of which the most draconian and thought-provoking has been devised by Oregon.

The Oregon State Legislature instructed its Health Services Commission to arrange all publicly funded (Medicaid) medical services in order of priority, taking account of the views of the public. The commission then worked out the annual cost of providing each of these services. Once the state's annual Medicaid budget had been decided, it would be possible to say how far the money would go. Given x million dollars, items one to n would be paid for; anything below that cutoff point would not.

Public consultation took several forms. Telephone surveys were used to rank twenty-six states of disability. At meetings held throughout Oregon the public was asked to rate the importance of various categories of activity such as 'the treatment of fatal conditions which can't be cured and won't extend life more than five years'. The commission also held public hearings at which special interest groups were able to plead their case. The priority list that finally emerged comprised just over 700 items. In fact, the state's first Medicaid budget under the new system stretched as far as item number 587: treatment for contact dermatitis and other eczema. Item 588, not to be funded, was medical and surgical treatment for acne. Among other items below the cut-off point were infertility services and the treatment of infections in the later stages of HIV disease.

Even its sympathizers recognize the crudity of the Oregon experiment; but it does provide some pointers for anyone contemplating the future of health-care financing. Commentators have pointed out that the Oregon commissioners were simply making explicit a process that happens anyway. All health care is rationed. In a wholly free market it is rationed by the purchaser's capacity to pay for it; in a state-funded system such as Britain's National Health Service it is rationed by the willingness of the government to pay the bills, and by the waiting lists that form when demand for a particular procedure outstrips supply. The Oregon approach defines the choices that have to made, and offers a system for making them. Elsewhere, these decisions are made *ad hoc*, according to political expediency, and in line with professional interests. The means used in Oregon may be deficient; but their end – explicit decisions on what to make available – will surely become a feature of all collectively funded health systems.

Another feature of the Oregon approach was that the commissioners weighted their decisions according to the quality of the patients' lives after treatment. Although this makes the calculations more onerous, it will soon become a regular part of all calculations of medical costs. Finally, there is public consultation. Slavishly following public opinion in making complex technical decisions is foolish; but so is a total neglect of the popular view of what is worth doing. Here, too, Oregon has pointed the way forwards.

The high cost of scientific medicine is not simply a consequence of people seeking and getting more of the same. Many of the diagnostic and treatment innovations devised by medical researchers depend on new and expensive gadgetry. A few decades ago, for example, nothing could be done about blocked coronary arteries. Then came bypass surgery in which small blood vessels taken from the leg are used to fashion a new blood supply to the heart muscle. More recently surgeons have developed a technique called angioplasty, in which, using X-ray guidance, a small balloon on the end of a fine tube is threaded though the blood vessels and into the blocked coronary artery. Pumping up the balloon restores the artery to its normal diameter. Small coiled springs can be placed in the expanded vessel to keep it open. Other researchers are developing lasers with which to unblock the coronary artery from inside. So it has gone on, and so it seems set to continue. With technology, what was once a death sentence can now be repealed. The same is true of most other branches of medicine from kidney transplantation to artificial hips.

New drugs are subject to close scrutiny of their safety and effectiveness, but control over new instruments and procedures is much less rigorous. Although the body scanner – a system for obtaining X-ray pictures of soft as well as bony tissues – was invented in Britain, it was in the USA that the instruments themselves began to proliferate. This rapid spread, however, owed little to good evidence that they improved the outcome of the patients' treatment. They were popular because they were glamorous and they offered physicians another profitable investigation. Proper technology assessment would prevent such excesses. But even when thoroughly applied – which, so far, is seldom – it cannot prevent the extra cost arising through genuinely valuable additions to the doctor's hardware. Short of banning most research and development it is hard to see how the growth of costly advances in medicine can be contained. In this respect, of course, state-financed health systems are in a stronger position; even when a new gadget or procedure is available, they can simply refuse to pay for it. Private expenditure is more difficult to limit.

Optimists see hope in some of the genetic and molecular techniques described earlier. They suggest that costly procedures such as bypass surgery are 'half-way technologies', which will eventually be replaced by cheaper molecular-based approaches for preventing disease or dealing with it at an earlier stage of its development. Their argument is plausible, but not proven. There are, however, some new and improved treatments derived from biomedical research that have already proved to be money savers. For example, the US National Institutes of Health spent 20 million dollars developing a treatment for the chronic skin disease psoriasis. It relies on giving patients the chemical precursor of a drug that is then activated by exposing diseased areas of skin to ultraviolet light. The annual savings through use of this technique are estimated at almost 60 million dollars. This is a healthy return on research investment; but whether it is typical remains a matter for debate.

Another and deeper disquiet about the future is rooted in the very thing that underpins medicine's success: science. Along with ortho-dox medicine goes a machine model of the human body. Where kidney disease might once have been considered the consequence of evil spirits, wicked deeds, a malicious deity or some other such influ-ence, it is now viewed as a material problem: a failure of the biolog-ical equipment that should be filtering, cleaning, and adjusting the chemical make up of the body's fluids. The renal physician is neither a priest nor a shaman but the physiological equivalent of a domestic plumber. And so it is with most other branches of medicine from gastroenterology to gynaecology; doctors are trained, primarily, as technicians skilled at diagnosing and fixing failed body mechanisms.

To pursue this demanding trade they need sophisticated equip-ment such as brain scanners, fetal monitors, endoscopes, lasers, radioactive chemicals, artificial hearts, and computers. Learning to handle these things may take months or years; to use them safely often absorbs much of the doctor's attention. It is understandable that patients may feel alienated, and begin to wonder if the doctor has forgotten that they are not merely malfunctioning biological mechanisms, but people with problems that go beyond the biolog-ical. The doctor as a healer has been replaced, to a varying extent, by the doctor as a body technician. Although grateful to receive this form of assistance, most people do not find it sufficient. They need someone prepared to relate to them on a spiritual and human level, and able to appreciate their distress. Sympathy of the kind that a garage mechanic might express when reporting a broken crankshaft is not enough.

One of the first commentators to give clear public expression to these doubts was the London University lawyer Ian Kennedy. In the book based on his 1980 BBC Reith Lectures, he wrote: 'Modern medicine has taken the wrong path. . . an education which demands high skills in scientific subjects before going to medical school, and involves years of breathing the heady air of one field after another of scientific endeavour once there, produces what it is intended to produce: a doctor who sees himself as a scientist. It may not produce what is so often needed: someone who can care.'[3]

Medicine thus faces a challenge: to make full use of technol-ogy without losing the human contact that has to be part of any

satisfactory system of health care. There are many possible remedies. Teaching medical students how to communicate with their
eventual patients has become a priority. Some medical schools use
actors to play the part of patients as students practise their first fum-
bling attempts to explain difficult ideas or break bad news. The aim
is to make the patient rather than the illness the focus of the consultation. Other doctors are turning to complementary medicine,
seeking to retain their scientific approach to disease while recognizing that science by itself does not answer all medical needs. There
are movements to bring art into hospitals, to reconsider their architecture, to fashion new relationships in which the wishes and feelings of patients are taken into consideration. The success of these
and other moves will decide whether the public sees medicine as in
broad sympathy with their needs, or as an enterprise from which it
feels evermore alienated.

The Flight from Science

The doctors' dilemma is made no easier by a widespread suspicion
of science and technology in general. In spite of their impact on the
way we live, ignorance about them is common. Science is thought
of as antithetical to human values; technology is associated with
pollution, weaponry, and all manner of environmental destruction.
Medical science suffers by association and, of course, by its own
tragedies and misapplications: thalidomide; the overzealous use of
life-support systems; the exploitation of unwitting patients as experimental subjects, and so on.

One response has been to seek alternative forms of health care
based on other philosophies. To the extent that this is a rejection of
what is wrong with orthodox medicine it is sensible and desirable.
But in so far as it represents another facet of the flight from science into irrationality, it bodes ill. Some of the bewildering variety
of complementary therapies now available – radionics, for example, or the alleged benefits of wearing a crystal or sitting inside any
pyramidal structure – can appeal only to the credulous. They dis-
card the exacting framework by which science has so painstakingly
attempted to know the world, and replace it with a bogus, back-of-
the-envelope mysticism.

The sheer ingenuity of scientific medicine has also created a raft of new ethical dilemmas, which are especially apparent in reproductive medicine.

More Reproductive Dilemmas

In vitro fertilization (IVF) has already produced its own crop of ethical issues: the ownership of eggs that have been fertilized and frozen for storage, for example. Still more exotically, surrogate motherhood is now feasible. A couple able to produce healthy sperm and eggs but not to have a child in the normal way can now donate eggs and sperm to be fertilized in the test-tube. The resulting embryo can then be implanted in the womb of another woman. Genetically speaking, the baby to which she gives birth will be the child of the donor couple. Most societies feel uneasy about the prospect of this 'womb renting', and many countries have made it illegal. But simply because it is technically feasible, attitudes may change; womb renting may one day be no more controversial than adoption or artificial insemination.

IVF has also added another twist to the eugenics story. Prenatal screening for inherited disease requires a willingness to contemplate termination. With IVF, it is possible to fertilize several eggs, allow them to develop to a multicell stage, and then remove from each a single cell for genetic testing. Up to a certain stage of development, all the cells of a dividing egg remain identical, so the loss has no effect on the resulting embryo. In the light of the test results, it is possible to select and implant only defect-free embryos.

The possibility of treating as opposed to merely detecting genetic disorders – gene therapy – has been described already. It continues to provoke public disquiet, some of which actually stems from a misconception. The use of the word 'gene' seems to imply that whatever is done to alter its function – or, in the case of a missing gene, to replace it – will be transmitted to later generations. If this were so, any ill-judged tampering could have adverse consequences for later generations. In fact, this will be the case only if the cells altered are those of the germline that give rise to eggs and sperm. This more ambitious project would indeed rid an individual's progeny of an unwanted gene; but if the potential gains are greater, so, too, are the risks. In the long run, however, it seems likely that this kind of gene therapy will be contemplated.

Moving from the beginning of life to its end, here medical advances are creating additional new dilemmas. When the English poet Arthur Hugh Clough wrote of doctors, 'Thou shalt not kill; but need'st not strive officiously to keep alive', he meant it as a sneer. But he was writing in the nineteenth century, well before the development of life-support systems that can maintain the life of a body whose higher brain centres are no longer functioning: the persistent vegetative state. Strangely, Clough's mocking couplet has become a cherished aphorism used by many doctors to emphasize their awareness of the cruelty of artifically extending the lives of certain seriously ill patients. There is, though, much disagreement about the interpretation of 'officiously'. In 1975, for example, fearful of the power vacuum that would follow the demise of the Spanish dictator Franco, his doctors contrived most horribly to delay his death while the politicians agonized about the succession. Grotesque examples of this kind are, fortunately, rare. But the injudicious use of antibiotics to pull an elderly person through an episode of pneumonia ('old man's friend') when all have agreed that death would be appropriate is not uncommon.

The development of effective life-support systems has opened up another clutch of moral dilemmas related to transplant surgery. Subject to the agreement of relatives, the crucial issue nowadays in timing the withdrawal of life support may be the availability of a would-be recipient of that person's organs. Such arrangements need strict codes of behaviour to ensure that it is the physician supervising the donor patient – as against the doctor in charge of the recipient – who decides that the patient has nothing further to gain from life support.

Reactions to medical practice and innovation vary, as they always have done, from place to place. Religious and social attitudes influence the use of abortion, contraception, artificial insemination, IVF, euthanasia, the use of cadavers to teach anatomy, and much else; and future developments, particularly in reproductive technology and genetic engineering, will continue to startle if not frighten many people.

Some countries are toying with the idea of national bioethics commissions to which these matters could be referred, and from which would come suggestions about legislation and guidelines or codes of professional conduct. A few countries have already set up bodies of this kind; France, for example, has had one for more than a decade. There is also something of the kind in Denmark, this organization making particular efforts to inform the public about bioethics, and to seek its views. This approach is less cumbersome than creating a series of *ad hoc* committees to consider individual issues. A standing bioethics commission, already familiar with the territory, should be able to respond without delay. To suggest that developments in medicine merit public scrutiny is not to question the judgment or probity of doctors and medical researchers. Many, already weary of a succession of horror stories and false alarms, would welcome a body in which they, as well as the public, could place confidence. The one certainty is that some branches of medical research have become altogether too ingenious to leave solely in the hands of the researchers.

The Future of Research

The belief that medicine will go on devising new methods of diagnosis and treatment assumes that medical research will continue to flourish. This seems likely; no researcher need lack a project while there are still uncertainties about, for example, the relative importance of environmental as opposed to inherited factors in common diseases from cancer to arthritis. But certain public policy decisions – notably the balance of spending on basic as against targeted or goal-oriented research – could affect the success of attempts to find out. To take cancer as an example, should researchers be given a grant and instructed to find a cure, or should they be funded to carry out whatever studies they think might reveal something about the nature of all cells, malignant and otherwise? This kind of question will increasingly exercise the trustees of charitable research foundations; why should such bodies give their money to scientists who work on cell division in multicellular green algae – organisms not greatly troubled by cancer or any other human disease? In the

1970s, two American doctors made an impressive effort to answer this and similar questions.

Julius Comroe and Robert Dripps of the universities of California and Pennsylvania, respectively, had become troubled by the increasing popularity of targeted research, and the growing doubt that scientists left to their own devices could be counted on to produce useful findings. Anecdotal evidence on this issue is unhelpful. Louis Pasteur was commissioned by the French government to find ways of preventing wine from turning into vinegar, and to stop sheep dying of anthrax. In solving these and other practical problems he effectively created the science of bacteriology: a good advertisement for targeted research. But Wilhelm Röntgen stumbled upon – and saw the medical potential of – X-rays while studying the emissions from a certain type of vacuum tube. His work was basic physics, and had no practical end in view, let alone one to do with medicine.

Comroe and Dripps set themselves the hugely ambitious task of tracking down the sources of the knowledge that underpinned a series of important medical advances. They chose heart, blood vessel, and lung diseases – these being the branches of medicine in which they themselves worked. With the help of other specialists they compiled a list of significant advances, and then asked forty or fifty experts to vote on their relative importance. For each of the top ten on their lists they identified the bodies of knowledge that had made them possible. In total, they picked out 137 such bodies of knowledge: things such as the development of anticoagulant drugs, the invention of electrocardiography, the identification of blood types, and the management of infection.

Next they identified some 2,500 reports published in the scientific literature that were important in the creation of these bodies of knowledge. With the help of no fewer than 140 consultants they chose 529 key reports for close analysis. In the case of electrocardiography, for example, the chronicle of relevant findings stretches back several hundred years to the first, faltering attempts to understand electricity. Key articles in the chain of events leading to the modern electrocardiogram include Luigi Galvani's 1794 report that the discharge of an electric eel could cause heart muscle to contract, and Carlo Matteucci's 1842 observation that a muscle contracts if its nerves are laid across another contracting muscle. When Willem Einthoven first measured a human electrocardiogram in 1901, he was relying on knowledge garnered by people who knew nothing of the existence let alone the significance of electrical rhythms within the heart.

What the stupendous and time-consuming effort of Comroe and Dripps revealed was that 61 per cent of all the knowledge judged to be essential for later clinical advance were reports of basic research findings. They concluded that clinical research requires different types of research and development, and not one to the exclusion of the other. As far as basic research is concerned, their data revealed a powerful case for the long-term support of 'creative scientists whose main goal is to learn how living organisms function, without regard to the immediate relation of their research to specific human diseases'.[4] In short, basic research pays off.

A contemporary illustration of the extent to which basic research findings can accelerate the understanding of a new malady is HIV disease. AIDS was first recognized as an illness in 1981. In 1983, the American researcher Robert Gallo suggested that it was caused by a retrovirus, a type of virus that carries its genetic information in the form of a molecule of RNA. The following year Luc Montagnier of the Pasteur Institute in Paris succeeded in isolating the virus. By 1986 there was a drug, AZT; preliminary vaccine testing began around the same time. Despite repeated claims that governments have been less than wholehearted in their support for AIDS research, it would be difficult to name any other disease in which understanding has progressed more rapidly. The researchers were able to build on research projects carried out in the late 1960s and 1970s. Much of this went on under the banner of cancer research; but most of it was, in truth, basic cell biology and immunology. The lessons for the future are obvious.

The years since the pioneering work of Julius Comroe and Robert Dripps have seen many attempts at analysing the sources of useful knowledge – and, by extension, the best way of acquiring it. This research has led to the development of technology foresight, an enterprise devoted to the identification and promotion of those areas of strategic research that are likely to yield to the greatest economic and social benefits. Its advocates, arguing that there is not one but many possible futures, seek partly to predict the likely direction of research, and partly also to shape it. The value of technology foresight in medicine, and elsewhere, remains controversial.

Change and Adaptation

Some fear that scientific medicine, driven by its own imperatives and enthusiasms, will continue to plough ahead irrespective of the needs and fears of its recipients. But this is a bleak view, and there are reasons to reject it. While medicine's attachment to scientific models of disease and healing may have created some of the problems, science itself fosters the very scepticism that makes for change and adaptation.

Doctors no longer bow to the authority of long-departed gurus. The idea of relying on the past in the way that physicians for so long viewed the works of Galen as holy writ is now unthinkable. All scientific knowledge is provisional: to be treated not as ultimate truth, but as an understanding that may have to be revised in the light of future discoveries. The very essence of science lies not only in creating hypotheses about the world, but in testing them and, when they fail, replacing them with better ones. It is true that doctors are not scientists as such, and that much supposedly scientific medicine is not as scientific as its practitioners like to suggest. But for all such legitimate carping, medicine does have the kind of mindset in which change is acceptable. So where is the evidence that medicine might be confronting some of the doubts raised earlier, and might even adapt to them?

Of the many hopeful signs that could be offered in evidence, I will pick just three: medicine's renewed interest in the quality of life; its changing attitude towards complementary medicine; and the rise in numbers and importance of patient self-help groups.

Quality of Life

Consideration of the quality of patients' lives is not a new phenomenon in medicine. But the doctors' burgeoning interest in curing illness encouraged them to measure their achievements in the most tangible ways. Has the infection been eliminated, the disease process halted, and, ultimately, death prevented? These questions can be succinctly and quantifiably answered. That treatments may successfully halt the disease but cause pain and distress, or that a surviving patient would really rather be dead are matters all but eclipsed by the grand imperative to treat and to save life at all costs.

It is hardly surprising that doctors' enthusiasm for using their power to intervene sometimes carries them beyond the wishes of their patients; centuries of medical impotence in the face of illness are still being exorcised. Only when the profession's love affair with its new-found potency had at last begun to cool did it become aware that patients were not always grateful to be kept alive, and were not always convinced that this operation or that course of drugs was really worth having if the price of a longer life was extra years of pain or discomfort.

A concern for quality of life began, formally, to edge its way back on to the agenda. But how to quantify it? Many solutions have been attempted, but most rely on scales of some kind ('On a scale of one to ten, how bad is this pain?') or on comparative rating of various disabilities ('Is it worse to lose an arm or a leg?'). One particularly ingenious attempt at combining quality and quantity of life in a single measurement is the quality-adjusted life year or QALY. This assumes that one year of healthy life is worth as much as two, three, or however many years spent in a state of disease or disability. The value to the patient and to the community of performing a particular medical procedure can then be judged in terms not of the extra years of life it yields, but of the extra number of QALYs. The difficulty, of course, is to establish the appropriate mathematical relationship between a calendar year and a QALY.

This has been done by asking people to rate, on a scale from 0 to 100, the extent to which a range of disabilities would reduce their quality of life. Although this sounds disturbingly hit and miss, there are sophisticated methodologies for helping people to establish preferences among dozens or even hundreds of alternatives. The scores that have emerged provide the conversion factors required to translate calendar years into QALYs for a wide range of physical and mental disabilities.

QALYs are most obviously beneficial in evaluating treatment options for an individual: this is what you'll gain from procedure A, this from procedure B. When used by health planners to give priority to treatments they become more controversial. Critics claim, for example, that QALYs discriminate against the elderly. Advocates deny this, and argue that some kind of systematic approach to measuring quality of life is essential if health-care systems are to spend their money wisely.

As the need to curb rising health costs grows more pressing, it seems likely that explicit attempts will be made to take quality of life into account in decision-making. Either way, it is certain that quality of life will become an increasingly important concern in the medicine of the future.

Complementary Medicine

Something similar will also be true of complementary medicine. The suspicion of science and of scientific medicine already referred to, and doctors' increasing preoccupation with the technology of their trade, have driven many patients in rich countries to search for methods of healing that they regard as more 'natural'. Doctors, proud of their high-tech gadgetry and their scientific interventions, are now reluctant to see themselves as healers. Yet healers – individuals who offer more than technical solutions to biological problems – are what many people obviously want. The advent of science offered a new and firmer boundary in the traditional antagonism between approved and non-approved ways of practising medicine. Henceforth, anything scientifically acceptable became 'orthodox', anything not became 'unorthodox'. As the people of many Western countries became more and more enamoured of unorthodox therapies, so the medical establishment mounted periodic offensives designed to fend off the challenge. In great measure they have failed. Indeed, increasing numbers of doctors with an entirely orthodox training have begun to go over to the 'enemy', and to sympathize with the aspirations if not always the methods of the fringe.

Complementary medicine shows no signs of diminishing in public esteem, not least because one of its concerns is for the quality of patients' lives. Looking to the future, how is the rise of unorthodoxy to be regarded? In so far as it relies on unproven methods used by people with little training and less theory, and panders to irrational beliefs, it is to be deplored. And this, of course, is precisely how the medical establishment has chosen to portray it. In fact, this is only part of the truth, and probably a small part.

Some techniques – acupuncture, osteopathy, and chiropractic, for example – have come in from the fringe, and now command the respect of many doctors. Some practitioners of complementary medicine have come to see the logic of trying to establish the efficacy of their methods according to the standards of proof routinely demanded (in theory, at least) by orthodox medicine. The role of healer is one which many unorthodox practitioners are happy to adopt. And in assuming it they sometimes prove better than orthodox medicine at offering comfort in chronic illness, and solace when no treatment is effective. Enlightened doctors know this. And while it would be wrong to suggest that all tensions between the mainstream and the fringe have been or are likely to be overcome, naked antagonism is withering away. So here, too, orthodox medicine, albeit reluctantly, is showing itself able to accept the demands being made by the patients, and adapt accordingly.

Self-Help

A third development now helping to shape the future is the advent of patient self-help and support groups. All decisions about health and disease were once regarded by doctors as matters for them alone. Patients had a passive role; having been told what was the matter with them (and sometimes not even that) their only task was to obey whatever instructions the doctor thought fit to issue. But while denied autonomy in strictly medical decisions, they then had to cope alone with the everyday non-medical problems created by their illnesses. Attitudes towards doctors, at least in most developed countries, have changed much in the past few decades. Authoritarianism in medicine has been much eroded; many patients now expect to be advised rather than instructed on their treatment, and to be given an opportunity to express their own preferences when there is more than one possible course of action.

This climate did much to boost the creation of patient self-help groups. There are now hundreds of these bodies offering practical advice and emotional support to people with all manner of chronic and/or debilitating illnesses from agoraphobia and AIDS to vitiligo and vaccine damage. Often set up with the active assistance of doctors, they provide a forum through which patients can meet and pass on to each other the kind of practical tips that make the difference between coping with an illness and being defeated by it. These groups will continue to flourish, and become an ever more central part of the response to illness.

Universal Medicine

Scientific medicine, like the rest of science and technology, has proved itself the most international of all our practical and cultural achievements. The skill, the equipment, and the buildings in which doctors work vary greatly from place to place; but from Bombay to Bloemfontein to Buenos Aires the medicine they practise is recognizably the same. Go to China and you find an elaborate system of traditional medicine; go to India and you find Unani, Ayurveda, and many lesser known brands of healing; go to any developing country and you find systems of herbal medicine. But while all these practices co-exist with scientific medicine, it alone is ubiquitous.

Could there come a time when scientific medicine no longer occupies this dominant position, and some other system commands the global orthodoxy? This seems as improbable as science itself losing its central role as the way in which we interpret the material world. Once science had emerged, it was soon impossible for medicine to do anything but throw in its lot with this new vision. And as long as science holds its current position, medicine will surely stay with it. Not bounded by it; that is one of its current weaknesses. But rooted, practically and intellectually, within it.

Looking to the Future Revisited

Geoff Watts

A lthough the phrase 'rewriting history' often comes loaded with pejorative overtones, there is nothing intrinsically dishonourable about it. When new facts come to light, new interpretations are made, and not to rewrite history would be a disservice to our understanding. But the pace of such reinterpretation tends to be leisurely. So when Cambridge University Press decided, a decade after the original publication of this history of medicine, to reissue it in a new format, they did not anticipate that major textual revisions would be required. And so it seems to have been with nine of the ten chapters.

The tenth, 'Looking to the future', was another matter. I had been asked by the book's editor, the late Roy Porter, to review what I thought might happen in medicine in the medium term. By my definition that was 10 to 15 years. I agreed to do it with the condition that the text include some (admittedly self-protective) caveat that most predictions about the future course and likely outcome of any enterprise involving science turn out to be wrong. How wise I was to get my defence in early! The one prediction in which I had real confidence – that predictions in medicine seldom hit the bull's eye – was indeed accurate.

Rather than amend the original text I have added a brief commentary that roughly follows the original topics and their ordering. It identifies some of the developments I'd failed to spot or which I'd underemphasised. Any further predictions will be as precise as those in the first edition of this book. . . .

Two things that have not changed over the past decade are medicine's capacity to devise new and more costly remedies and the uncertainty with which so many of us view the entire enterprise. Indeed both phenomena have become more pronounced over the years. Never have so many people had such immediate access to so many treatments; yet, paradoxically, never have so many people worried so much about their health. There is nothing to suggest that this tension will not continue, and possibly even intensify.

In one important respect I feel more cautiously optimistic than I did ten years ago: the future prospects for life in old age. Fears that increased longevity will reward us only with extra years spent in decrepitude and dependency are not, according to geriatricians and age researchers, being realised. Considering its importance to us all, the evidence remains surprisingly sparse. But it seems to show that gains in overall life expectancy are being at least matched by those in active life expectancy. There is also a continuing trend towards lower rates of chronic disability and institutionalisation among older people. In short, old age morbidity is being proportionately compressed, not stretched.

In its attempts to influence our behaviour and encourage us all to live more wisely, public health medicine has made only modest advances. Tobacco consumption in most developed countries has gone down, but use of other drugs has increased. This limited success should be no surprise; ingenious technical fixes are invariably easier to devise and implement than anything requiring large numbers of humans to alter their habits and their lifestyle.

Not that technical fixes are always a rapid success. Gene therapy, for example, has signally failed to begin delivering what it promised a decade ago. My airy comments on the ease with which new genes can be delivered to the point at which they are required were altogether wide of the mark. Even if the genes can be successfully conveyed to the cells that need them, encouraging those genes to insert themselves correctly and permanently within the host genome has proved something of an obstacle. While the technique remains as attractive as ever in principle, in practice it's currently marking time.

Much more attention is now being paid to what is sometimes called 'gene-based' therapy: the attempt not to introduce new genes into the body, but to take more control over those we already have.

The development that gave this enterprise its big lift-off was the publication in 2002 of the first working draft of the makeup of the human genome. We may have turned out to possess roughly half as many genes as had been supposed, but the findings have already had a galvanising effect on attempts to apply molecular understanding in just about every branch of medicine. Of course, the knowledge that a particular gene, or variant of a gene, is linked to this or that disease is only the first step on the road to a treatment. Achieving this goal depends on working out the gene product: the protein for which the gene carries the formula and which acts as the molecular signal to stop, start, or otherwise modulate some component of the cell's metabolic machinery.

Applying insights of this kind therapeutically still requires finding a way to block (or enhance) the effect of the chemical signal. Not surprisingly, biologists have grasped this challenge with enthusiasm, especially in cancer. But translating what they learn into drugs suitable for the clinic is a long, demanding, and expensive process. As a consequence, ingenious ideas are running ahead of the system's resources for testing them.

Our burgeoning grasp of which gene does what offers two other significant promises. One has come to be known as 'personalised' medicine. It has long been apparent that some people respond well to a drug, others indifferently, and still others not at all. At least some of this difference is inherited. If the relevant genes or gene variants could be identified, and patients tested to establish which versions they have, doctors could predict whether a drug (or which of possibly several drugs) would most likely be effective. This, it is argued, would save money – and in the long run it might. But it could also have two other effects: it could make drug development more expensive because of the need to test groups of people with different gene variants; and it could prove discriminatory if pharmaceutical companies devoted all their efforts to developing drugs for the most common variants. No-one, at this stage, is sure if personalised medicine is a dream, a nightmare, or a fantasy.

Much the same is true of the other promise of our knowledge of genes. If a disease is caused principally by a single gene – Huntington's chorea is the classic but extreme example – a gene test allows doctors to make a certain prediction of the patient's likelihood of developing it. But most diseases are not like this. They are caused by the interaction of heredity and environment; and to the extent that heredity plays a role, it may be through the combined effect of 2 or 10 or 20 different genes interacting with one another. Despite the enthusiasm of biotechnology entrepreneurs and the fears of the insurance industry, gene testing to predict our future likelihood of developing the most common killers, such as diseases of the heart and blood vessels, may be limited. The prospect of a battery of predictive and life-defining genetic tests is remote.

The idea though, even in its milder forms, remains seductive. This is no doubt why the British Government asked its advisory body the Human Genetics Commission (HGC) about the value of creating a complete gene profile of every baby at birth. The HGC gave it the thumbs down. For the present, cost alone rules out the idea of 'bar-coding babies', as the idea is facetiously known. Any future utility it may have remains unproven and unlikely – if not outright unethical.

Treatments based on monoclonal antibodies have, as predicted, continued to make progress. One example, a drug called beva-cizumab, will serve to give a taste of what has happened. To grow to any significant size, tumours must trigger the formation of new blood vessels to supply them with oxygen and nutrients. Bevacizumab interferes specifically with the chemical messages that would prompt such growth. So long as the drug is present, tumours should be inhibited from reaching the size at which they would pose a threat. The cancer is not killed, but it is rendered harmless.

In surgery, the use of robotic instrumentation has not yet made dramatic leaps. This may be due to a continuing enthusiasm for broadening the range of procedures that can be carried out using keyhole surgical techniques. These continue to make conventional surgery through a large open wound appear more outdated than ever. Maybe it's through the keyhole that robotic surgery will even-tually find its place.

Do-it-yourself diagnosis has moved from pregnancy and choles-terol into genetics. A simple mouth swab posted to one of the several companies that offer the service will reveal which variants of several genes you possess, and so your alleged risk of developing certain disorders. For reasons already alluded to, the value of such testing – certainly at this stage of the art – is minimal.

Remarkably, the intelligent toilet that can check the chemistry of your urine has gone into commercial production. However, it costs $3,000 to $5,000 more than a conventional toilet, and it seems not to have made much progress beyond Japan, its home country.

One enterprise that did seem set to flourish in the middle 1990s was the use of transplants of foetal tissue to repair injury or disease in various parts of the body. But during the past decade another source of transplantable material – one that many doctors believe has far greater potential – has begun to loom large on the biomedical research landscape: stem cells. Although their existence in embryos and in some adult organs had been known for a long time, only stem cells in the bone marrow were being exploited ten years ago. Intensive laboratory work has shown how to harvest them from adult tissues, including the brain, how to extract them from embryos, how to grow them in the lab, and how then to influence their destiny.

Stem cells are the source from which the body's tissues replenish themselves. By repeated division, those found in adult tissues are programmed to give rise to more adult cells of a particular kind – skin, bone, blood, or whatever. Many stem cells are inaccessible or difficult to culture and, in any case, generate adult cells of one type. Embryonic stem cells, by contrast, have the capacity to give rise to every type of cell in the body. Microscopic manipulation techniques allow stem cells to be removed from embryos. Embryonic stem cells from animals and, more recently, humans, have been grown in culture and even persuaded to differentiate into cells of various adult varieties. Laboratories around the world are competing to prove that stem cells of this kind will be able to, for example, repair injuries to the central nervous system or help a damaged heart to repair itself. As with gene therapy, translating the endeavour into clinical practice could run into unforeseen difficulties. Right now, though, all the signs look encouraging, and even cautious clinicians are optimistic.

Although Britain is unique in having specifically legalised research on human embryos up to the age of 14 days, the work continues to arouse controversy on ethical grounds. Opponents of this work back an alternative approach. They argue that it may be possible to reprogramme adult stem cells to provide the range of tissue types that clinicians might need. Therefore, they say, work on embryos is unnecessary. They may be right; but until this becomes clear, most researchers prefer to back both runners.

It took no great insight to prophesy that in medicine, as in every other area of life, computing would continue to play an evermore central role. The NHS, for example, has embarked on what is probably the world's largest non-military information technology project. The ambition is threefold: to digitise and store all patient records on computer, with access as appropriate to any doctor requiring them; second, to allow primary care physicians to book their patients' hospital appointments; and third, to create electronic prescriptions that can be e-mailed to a community pharmacist of the patient's choosing. Whether this hugely ambitious scheme will be delivered on time and on budget – indeed whether it will actually function as intended – remains at the time of writing a topic of much discussion.

Computer technology also underpins the growth of imaging in medicine. The falling cost and rising power of computers have made it possible to record scans of a resolution and detail that were unimaginable ten years ago. Most impressive is the development of serial imaging of the body: the scanning equivalent of slicing a loaf of bread and then examining each of the cut surfaces. And just as a whole loaf can be reconstructed from its component slices, so too can the computer reassemble successive images to create the three-dimensional appearance of the body's internal organs. Instead of, for example, examining the interior of the large bowel with a flexible viewing tube, the doctor can now take a virtual journey through it on the computer screen – and see just as much, with no discomfort to the patient.

The development of magnetic resonance imaging (MRI) has made it possible to perform such scans without recourse to X-rays, and so with no known damaging effects to the body. Soft tissue can be scanned as readily as bone. And the speed with which the machines work allows doctors to record a sequence of images in rapid succession. This has opened the way to 'functional' MRI, a method of scanning that allows the operator to follow changes in the flow of blood in various regions of the brain – and therefore, by inference, changes in the activity of those regions – in real time. It is now possible to look for differences in brain activity associated with various tasks, with particular states of mind, or even with clinical conditions such as depression or schizophrenia. Brain activity can be closely correlated with behaviour.

All of this is, of course, very expensive – and politicians are no more adept at dealing with the cost of medicine than they were ten years ago. According to one analysis of Oregon's attempt at cost containment, the way the plan actually worked during its first five years was far from straightforward. The cut-off line between what would be paid for and what would not proved to be fuzzy, and administrators sometimes shifted procedures into the 'paid-for' category to satisfy constituency pressures or the federal government. No other state or country has followed the Oregon model.

That said, one of Oregon's aims was to ensure that decisions on what would and would not be available were made openly and explicitly and, as I suggested, this has become an increasingly common feature of medical systems – with the UK's National Institute for Clinical Excellence (NICE) being a case in point. The NHS will only pay for new drugs and certain other forms of treatment once NICE has given its approval on grounds of cost-effectiveness. This has not ended pleas from worried patients and frustrated clinicians, but it has brought some unity and order to what were previously a bewildering variety of *ad hoc* and contradictory decisions; previously, what patients could expect depended on where they lived.

The public attitude towards science in medicine remains as ambivalent as it was in the middle 1990s. In Britain in particular, the outbreak of BSE followed by the mass slaughter of cattle along with unfounded assurances about there being no risk to human health undermined peoples' trust. Later, when unsubstantiated claims that the triple mumps/measles/rubella vaccine could be a cause of autism were widely publicised, parents ignored the denials of more orthodox medical science and deserted the vaccine in droves. Britain's experience may have been an extreme manifestation of the suspicion of science, but to some degree it haunts nearly all Western nations. Nor is it clear how this shifting and uneasy conflict will resolve itself.

That said, human attitudes are nothing if not flexible. The debate in Britain over the use of embryonic stems cells was, by and large, conducted quietly and intelligently. A significant minority were unhappy about the change in the law that allows research on embryos; but its passage was entirely civilised. In medicine, the ethically unthinkable has a way of becoming acceptable when its implementation is manifestly to the benefit of individuals and the community. Ten years ago you would have been hard-pressed to find many people, professional or lay, willing to countenance the desirability of germ-line gene therapy: that is, making gene alterations to the cells which give rise to the gametes, thus ensuring that the change is passed to future generations. Now this too is gradually coming up for discussion. Likewise with voluntary euthanasia: even the medical profession, still deeply antagonistic to it in many countries, shows signs of softening its opposition.

When originally considering scientific medicine's capacity to adapt to changing circumstances, I picked three indicators that I found encouraging. One was medicine's formal recognition of the importance of the patient's qualify of life. This view is now firmly entrenched – and, in principle if not always in practice, few doctors continue to pursue patient survival to the exclusion of all else.

Another indicator was the rise of patient self-help groups and doctors' recognition that people already suffering from an illness were better-placed than medical professionals to offer practical advice on how to live with it. The past decade has seen this patient involvement continue to grow, and even extend into research. The pioneers were American AIDS patients and other activists who took to lobbying – or, in some cases, disrupting – the grant-awarding committees that decide what research should be carried out and how. With the researchers' acceptance that patients actually had something to contribute to these decisions, confrontation gave way to co-operation. There are now instances – the UK's Alzheimer's Disease Society, for one – in which patient and/or carer members have the majority say on which research projects to fund. It seems to work.

The third of my three indicators was the tolerance – or even acceptance – by the orthodox medical establishment of complementary medicine. This process continues – but there are grounds for some nervousness about the future. Ten years ago doctors had begun to recognise that complementary practitioners were particularly good at what I referred to as the 'healing' component of good medicine. In some rather ill-defined and perhaps naïve way I envisaged a growth in co-operation whereby the two groups' activities would, literally, complement each other. Doctors would provide the specific remedies that work, principally, by bringing about direct physiological changes to the body, while complementary practitioners would continue to mobilise patients' capacity for self-healing and generally help them feel better about themselves and their disease. I fear that the erstwhile intellectual arrogance of scientific medicine is in danger of swinging too far in the opposite direction. Confronted with popular demand for arrant nonsense, too many orthodox practitioners now seem inclined to take an unduly relativistic view, or to even give up and adopt a posture of intellectual submission. Perhaps the relationship between orthodoxy and the fringe is one that will continue to see-saw indefinitely.

I originally suggested that scientific medicine's most dramatic benefits were to be seen in its effects on morbidity and mortality among the poor. I stand by that – with the proviso that this is not to say that the world's poor see enough of medicine, or of its most effective fruits. TB has not undergone the decline that it should, not least because of the emergence of resistance to the drugs for treating it. As TB is predominantly a disease of the underprivileged, there is little incentive for drug companies to spend money developing new and more effective agents. Governments and private foundations, working with the pharmaceutical industry, have now devised various non-profit collaborations to develop more drugs for tackling the illnesses of the poor. Their initial experience is encouraging – but there is still a great distance to go.

In rich developed countries, mortality from HIV has fallen spectacularly – but the cost of the drugs required to achieve this still puts them beyond the reach of the poor. The long-term remedy has to be a vaccine: something which has so far defeated the best efforts of the researchers. The same is true of a vaccine against malaria. In both cases researchers understand the problems to be overcome, and are confident that they will do so. They are less confident about when. The risk of being sued by patients who, rightly or wrongly, believe their children to have been injured by vaccines has made the field less attractive for commercial investment. Only a handful of drug companies remain active in vaccine development.

Nor is there any reason for us to feel confident that rising wealth brings automatic protection against infectious disease. If AIDS has not yet shattered such complacency, another influenza pandemic might. The outbreak of 'Spanish flu' in 1918 killed approximately 50 million people, and virologists claim that further episodes of this kind are inevitable. At the time of writing, an outbreak of bird flu in the Far East shows some of the warning signs. And in the twenty-first century, with its larger and more crowded cities and the frequency of long-distance travel, the rate of spread would be proportionately greater than in the outbreaks of last century.

More encouragingly, the WHO remains moderately optimistic about its chances of success in the attempt to eliminate polio. By the end of 2003, the disease had vanished from all but six countries, and the world is now well into a four-year strategic plan designed to interrupt transmission of the polio virus and open the way to eradication by the end of this decade or soon after. In the meantime, the guinea worm still looks to be a better bet in the eradication stakes. In 1986 there were 3.5 million cases worldwide; by 2004 this had fallen to 15,500, all in Sudan and West Africa.

Overshadowing all these achievements is the prospect of global warming. In the short run the poor – as usual – will suffer most, in large part due to the increased incidence of infectious disease it will usher in. In the longer run all bets are off – except one. None of us will escape its wider consequences.

REFERENCE GUIDE TO
THE CAMBRIDGE HISTORY OF
MEDICINE

CHRONOLOGY

MAJOR HUMAN DISEASES

NOTES

FURTHER READING

INDEX OF MEDICAL PERSONALITIES

GENERAL INDEX

Chronology

Selected non-medical events appear in bold

BC

c.9000	**Early domestication of plants and animals – rise of new human diseases**
c.4000	**First urban centres (Mesopotamia)**
c.3000	**Writing invented**
c.650	Epilepsy described in Babylonian text
585	Thales of Miletus active; beginnings of Greek philosophy
430	'Plague' of Athens (to 427 BC)
428	**Birth of Plato**
420	Hippocrates of Cos active
399	**Death of Socrates**
384	Birth of Aristotle of Stagira
310	Praxagoras of Cos active
300	Alexandrian Museum and Library founded
c.200	Chinese herbal *Pen T'sao*

AD

23	Birth of Pliny the Elder, Roman writer on natural history
40	Celsus's *On Medicine*
60	Dioscorides active
c.110	Rufus and Soranus (both of Ephesus) active
129	Birth of Galen of Pergamum
140	Asclepieion of Pergamum rebuilt
165	Antonine 'plague' begins (to 169)

Chronology

313	**Christianity legalized in Roman Empire**
330	**Constantinople founded as eastern capital of Roman Empire**
350	First hospitals in Eastern Roman Empire
390	Fabiola founds a hospital in Rome
512	Illustrated edition of Dioscorides's *De Materia Medica*
541	First plague pandemic (to 749) and Plague of Justinian (to 544)
610	**Byzantine Empire established**
618	**T'ang dynasty founded in China**
632	**Death of Mohammed**
650	Paul of Aegina active
700	Japan's 'age of plagues' begins
710	**Muslim invasion of Spain**
750	**Abbasid caliphate established in Baghdad**
800	**Charlemagne crowned Holy Roman Emperor**
c.850	Hunain ibn Ishaq's *More Questions and Answers*
900	ar-Razi (Rhazes) active
929	**Caliphate established at Córdoba**
979	**Sung dynasty reunites China**
1000	al-Zahrawi (Albucasis) active
1037	Death of Ibn Sina (Avicenna), author of *Canon of Medicine*
1066	**Norman conquest of England**
1080	School of Salerno (to 1200)
1095	**The Crusades (to 1278)**
1123	St Bartholomew's Hospital founded in London
1136	Pantokrator Hospital founded in Constantinople
1187	Death of Gerard of Cremona, translator of Ibn Sina's *Canon*
c.1200	Universities of Paris and Oxford founded
1204	**Latin crusaders sack Constantinople**
c.1250	First Islamic medical schools in Turkey; anatomy demonstrations at Salerno
1258	**Mongols sack Baghdad; end of Abbasid caliphate**
1275	**Marco Polo arrives in China**
1280	Death of Albertus Magnus ('Doctor universalis')
1284	Mansuri Hospital founded in Cairo

Chronology

1288	S. Maria Nuova Hospital founded in Florence; death of Ibn an-Nafis, describer of the pulmonary circulation of blood
c.1315	First dissection of human corpse by Mondino dei Liuzzi in Bologna
1321	**Death of Dante**
1337	**Hundred Years' War between England and France begins (to 1453)**
1347	Black Death begins (ends 1352)
1363	Guy de Chauliac's *Grande Chirurgie*
1368	**Ming dynasty founded in China**
c.1400	Milan institutes a permanent health board
1415	**Portuguese capture Ceuta – beginning of European Expansion**
1424	First recorded regulations for midwives, Brussels
1453	**Ottoman Turks capture Constantinople; end of Byzantine Empire**
c.1455	**Gutenberg's Bible printed at Mainz**
1490	Galen's works first printed in Latin
1492	**Fall of Granada; Arabs and Jews expelled from Spain; Christopher Columbus crosses the Atlantic**
1495	Charles VIII's army infected with syphilis during the siege of Naples
1498	**Vasco da Gama sails to India via the Cape of Good Hope**
1500	**Pedro Alvares Cabral claims Brazil for Portugal**
c.1510	**African slaves first taken to the New World**
1519	**Magellan begins his circumnavigation of the world (to 1522); death of Leonardo da Vinci**; Thomas Linacre's translation of Galen's *Method of Healing*
1521	**Cortés leads Spanish overthrow of Aztec Empire**
1525	*Hippocratic Corpus* printed in Latin
1526	**Mughal dynasty founded in India**
1534	**Henry VIII of England breaks with Rome**
1540	The companies of Barbers and Surgeons unite in London
1541	Death of Paracelsus
1543	**Nicolaus Copernicus writes of a Sun-centred planetary system**; Andreas Vesalius publishes his great work on human anatomy, *De Humani Corporis Fabrica*
1546	Girolamo Fracastoro's *De Contagione et Contagiosis Morbis* – an early version of the germ theory of disease

Chronology

1553	Michael Servetus, Spanish physician and theologian, burnt at the stake in Geneva
1559	Realdo Colombo's *De Re Anatomica*
1571	**Portuguese create colony in Angola**
1577	**Francis Drake sets out on his circumnavigation**
1584	**Sir Walter Raleigh sends first of three expeditions to the Americas**
1588	**Spanish Armada defeated**
1590	Death of French surgeon Ambroise Paré
1600	**English Dutch East Indies Company founded**
1601	**English Poor Law system established**
1602	**Japanese dynasty of Tokugawa shoguns begins rule (to 1868)**
1603	**Dutch East Indies Company founded**; Girolamo Fabrizio's study of veins
1607	**First permanent English settlement in America – at Jamestown, Virginia**
1608	**French colonists found Quebec**
1610	First well-documented Caesarian section (in Germany)
1611	**Authorized 'King James' version of the Bible**
1616	**Death of Shakespeare**
1618	**Pilgrim Fathers leave for the New World in the *Mayflower***
1621	Robert Burton's *The Anatomy of Melancholy*
1628	William Harvey writes on the circulation of the blood
c.1630	Obstetrical forceps invented by Peter Chamberlen
1633	French clergyman, Vincent de Paul, founds the Daughters of Charity
1636	First American university, Harvard College, founded
1641	René Descartes' *Meditationes de Prima Philosophia*
1642	**Abel Tasman discovers Tasmania and New Zealand; death of Galileo**
1644	**End of Ming Dynasty in China and founding of Qing dynasty by the Manchus**
1647	First New World epidemic of yellow fever begins in Barbados
1648	Johannes Baptiste van Helmont's *Ortus Medicinae*
1653	Francis Glisson describes the liver
1658	**Aurangzeb, Moghul Emperor, begins rule in India**

1660	Robert Boyle's law on the relation between gas pressure and volume; Royal Society of London founded
1663	Marcello Malpighi writes on the lung
1665	Great Plague of London
1666	Thomas Sydenham writes on treating fevers; Acadèmie des Sciences founded in Paris
1672	Regnier de Graaf discovers structures in the ovary, called Graafian follicles after him
1677	Cinchona bark included in the *London Pharmacopocia* as a fever treatment
1687	**Isaac Newton's *Principia Mathematica***
1690	John Locke's *Essay Concerning Human Understanding*
1701	In Constantinople, Giacomo Pylarini inoculates with smallpox; Yale University founded
1704	**Newton's *Opticks***
1705	Raymond Vieussens describes left ventricle of heart and course of coronary blood vessels
1707	**Death of Aurangzeb and decline of Moghul power in India**; pulse watch introduced by John Floyer
1708	Herman Boerhaave's *Institutiones Medicae*
1709	Great plague in Russia
1714	Gabriel David Fahrenheit constructs the mercury thermometer
1717	Giovanni Maria Lancisi suggests that malaria can be transmitted by mosquitoes; Lady Mary Wortley Montagu brings Turkish practice of smallpox inoculation to England
1721	Obstetrical forceps used by Jean Palfyn
1726	Stephen Hales measures blood pressure of the horse Edinburgh University Medical School founded
1728	Pierre Fauchard describes how to fill a tooth
1729	**First performance of J. S. Bach's *St Matthew Passion***
1730	First tracheotomy for treatment of diphtheria performed by George Martine
1733	Stephen Hales in *Haemostaticks* describes his measurements of blood pressure; William Cheselden's *Osteographia*
1735	***Systema Naturae* published by Linnaeus**
1736	First successful appendectomy performed by Claudius Amyand in France; American physician William Douglass describes scarlet fever
1741	Foundling Hospital in London opens

1745	The Company of Surgeons splits from the Barbers in London
1747	First textbook on physiology – Albrecht von Haller's *Primae Lineae Physiologiae;* James Lind discovers that citrus fruits cure scurvy
1748	John Fothergill describes diphtheria in his *Account of the Putrid Sore Throat*
1751	Large public mental institution (St Luke's) opens in London; Robert Whytt demonstrates that pupil contraction in response to light is a reflex motion
1752	William Smellie's *Theory and Practice or Treatise on Midwifery* – first scientific approach to obstetrics; René-Antoine Ferchault de Réaumur discovers that digestion is a chemical process
1753	James Lind's *Treatise of the Scurvy*
1754	First female medical doctor graduates from the University of Halle
1756	First description of casting models for false teeth by Philipp Pfaff
1759	Caspar Friedrich Wolff shows that specialized organs develop out of unspecialized tissue
1761	Leopold Auenbrugger develops percussion technique for diagnosing chest disorders
1763	First American medical society founded in New London. Connecticut
1765	John Morgan founds first American medical school at the College of Pennsylvania, Philadelphia
1766	Albrecht von Haller shows that nervous stimulation controls muscular action
1768	**James Cook charts coast of New Zealand and explores east coast of Australia (returns to England in 1771);** Robert Whytt's *Observations on the Dropsy of the Brain* – first description of tuberculosis meningitis in children
1771	John Hunter's *The Natural History of the Human Teeth*
1772	**James Cook circumnavigates the southern oceans (to 1775);** Antonio Scarpa discovers labyrinth of the ear
1773	Lazzaro Spallanzani discovers digestive action of saliva
1774	Joseph Priestley discovers oxygen; William Hunter's *Anatomy of the Human Gravid Uterus;* Franz Mesmer uses hypnosis as a medical treatment
1775	**American Declaration of Independence;** Percivall Pott suggests that environmental factors can cause cancer

Chronology

1776	**Adam Smith's *The Wealth of Nations*;** Matthew Dobson shows that the sweetness of diabetics' urine is caused by sugar; John Fothergill gives first clinical description of trigeminal neuralgia
1780	Luigi Galvani experiments with muscles and electricity
1781	Henry Cavendish determines the composition of water
1784	Goethe, the German poet, discovers human intermaxillary bone
1785	William Withering introduces digitalis (from the foxglove) to cure dropsy
1789	**George Washington becomes first President of the USA; French Revolution begins;** Antoine-Laurent Lavoisier's *Traité elementaire de Chimie*
1793	Epidemic of yellow fever in Philadelphia; Matthew Baillie describes the appearance of each organ in the first English text on morbid anatomy
1794	Lavoisier guillotined
1795	Thomas Beddoes and Humphry Davy experiment with nitrous oxide, or 'laughing gas'; Sir Gilbert Blane makes use of lime juice mandatory in the British navy
1796	First vaccination against smallpox by Edward Jenner; C. W. Hufeland's *Macrobiotics, or the Art to Prolong One's Life*
1798	Thomas Malthus's *Essay on the Principles of Population*
1800	François Bichat studies postmortem changes in human organs; chlorine used to purify water; Davy makes nitrous oxide in quantity and suggests its use as an anaesthetic; Benjamin Waterhouse is first US physician to use smallpox vaccine
1801	Philippe Pinel advocates a more humane treatment of the insane; Thomas Young discovers the cause of astigmatism
1804	**Napoleon Bonaparte crowned Emperor of France; black republic established in Haiti**
1805	**Battle of Trafalgar;** morphine isolated by Frederick Sertürner
1807	**Slave trade abolished within the British Empire**
1809	First successful ovariotomy (without anaesthetic)
1810	Samuel Hahnemann introduces homeopathy
1811	Charles Bell's *New Anatomy of the Brain*
1812	Benjamin Rush's *Medical Inquiries and Observations upon the Diseases of the Mind*

Chronology

1815	**Battle of Waterloo; giant eruption of Tambora volcano in Indonesia in April kills thousands of people and causes two cold summers in Europe and N. America**
1816	Stethoscope invented by René Laënnec
1817	First cholera pandemic begins; James Parkinson's *Essay on the shaking palsy*
1818	**Mary Shelley's *Frankenstein***
1821	Charles Bell describes facial paralysis
1822	**Liberia founded as colony for freed slaves**
1823	William Prout discovers hydrochloric acid in stomach secretions; *The Lancet* started
1824	Henry Hickman uses carbon dioxide on animals as a general anaesthetic; second cholera pandemic begins; Justus von Liebig appointed professor of chemistry at Giessen aged 21
1825	**First railway, from Stockton to Darlington**; Pierre Bretonneau performs first tracheotomy
1826	Bretonneau describes symptoms of diphtheria
1827	Richard Bright describes kidney disease
1828	Friedrich Wöhler synthesizes urea
1829	Johann Schönlein describes haemophilia; scandal of William Burke and William Hare, who murdered to supply bodies for dissection
1830	Charles Bell distinguishes different types of nerves
1831	**Charles Darwin joins crew of HMS *Beagle***; cholera epidemic starts in Europe; American chemist, Samuel Guthrie, discovers chloroform
1832	**Reform Bill in England**; Pierre-Jean Robiquet isolates codeine; Warburton Anatomy Act legalizes sale of bodies for dissection in England; Thomas Hodgkin describes cancer of the lymph nodes
1834	**New Poor Law in England**; amalgam used for filling teeth; Pierre Louis' *Essay on Clinical Instruction*
1837	**Victoria accedes to British throne**
1838	Registration Act (births, deaths, and marriages) in England
1839	Third cholera pandemic begins; Theodor Schwann defines the cell as the basic unit of animal structure
1840	**First Opium War between China and Britain**; the English quaker Elizabeth Fry founds the Institute of Nursing in London

Chronology

1841	F. G. J. Henle publishes treatise on microscopic anatomy
1842	Edwin Chadwick's *Report on the Sanitary Conditions of the Labouring Population of Great Britain*
1844	Horace Wells uses nitrous oxide to pull one of his own teeth painlessly
1845	**First failure of Irish potato crop**
1846	**Smithsonian Institution established in Washington, DC (opened in 1855)**; William Morton uses ether as an anaesthetic at the Massachusetts General Hospital
1847	James Young Simpson uses chloroform to relieve the pain of childbirth; Karl Ludwig invents the kymograph
1848	First Public Health Act sets up General Board of Health in Britain, leading to local medical officers of health; Ignaz Semmelweis introduces antiseptic methods in Vienna
1849	In USA, Elizabeth Blackwell becomes first woman to qualify as a doctor in modern times; Thomas Addison describes anaemia
1851	Hermann von Helmholtz introduces the ophthalmoscope
1853	**David Livingstone's explorations in Africa begin**; smallpox vaccination made compulsory in England; John Snow administers chloroform to Queen Victoria for the birth of Prince Leopold
1854	**Crimean War begins (ends 1856)**; John Snow breaks the Broad Street pump in London
1855	Thomas Addison describes the hormone-deficiency disease that results from malfunctioning adrenal glands
1856	First synthetic dye – mauvine – made by William Perkin
1858	Medical Reform Act sets up Medical Register and General Medical Council in Britain; first edition of *Gray's Anatomy*; Rudolf Virchow's *Cellularpathologie* demonstrates that every cell is a product of another cell
1859	**Charles Darwin's *The Origin of Species***
1860	Nightingale Nursing School founded at St Thomas's Hospital, London
1861	**Outbreak of American Civil War**; Louis Pasteur discovers anaerobic bacteria
1863	Etienne-Jules Marey invents the sphygmograph; fourth cholera pandemic begins
1864	International Red Cross founded

1865	**End of American Civil War and of slavery in USA; Gregor Mendel's** *Plant Hybridity*; Joseph Lister introduces phenol as a disinfectant in surgery
1866	Thomas Allbutt develops the clinical thermometer
1867	**Russia sells Alaska to USA; Dominion of Canada established**; first international medical congress in Paris
1869	**Suez Canal opens**; Jacques Reverdin describes skin-grafting; Sophia Jex-Blake matriculates in medicine at Edinburgh University (but university reverses decision in 1873)
1871	**Darwin's** *Descent of Man*
1873	William Osler writes on blood platelets
1874	Louis Pasteur suggests placing instruments in boiling water to sterilize them; London School of Medicine for Women (later the Royal Free Hospital) opened by Sophia Jex-Blake
1875	Public Health Act passed in Britain
1876	**Alexander Graham Bell patents the telephone**: Robert Koch identifies the anthrax bacillus; Cruelty to Animals Act passed in Britain; connection between the pancreas and sugar diabetes discovered
1879	Patrick Manson discovers that mosquitoes transmit filariasis
1880	Charles Laveran isolates blood parasite that causes malaria
1881	Fifth cholera pandemic begins; Institute of Midwives established in London; Louis Pasteur devises a vaccine for anthrax
1882	**Eruption of Krakatoa in the Sunda Straits**; Robert Koch isolates the tubercle bacillus; operation for the removal of the gall bladder introduced
1883	Robert Koch discovers the cholera vibrio
1884	Elie Metchnikoff describes phagocytosis
1885	Louis Pasteur develops a rabies vaccine
1886	**Gold discovered in the Witwatersrand, South Africa**
1889	**Brazil ends Portuguese rule**; Johns Hopkins Hospital opens in Baltimore
1890	Emil von Behring and Shibasabura Kitasato develop vaccines against tetanus and diphtheria; William Halsted introduces surgical gloves
1893	Jean Charcot writes on the use of hypnotism; Daniel Williams performs first open-heart surgery in Chicago; Johns Hopkins Medical School founded

Chronology

1894	**Nicholas II becomes last Tsar of Russia**; first use of diphtheria antitoxin in Britain, by Charles Sherrington
1895	Wilhelm Röntgen discovers X-rays; Elie Metchnikoff succeeds Louis Pasteur as director of Pasteur Institute in Paris
1896	Antoine Becquerel discovers radiation; Scipione Riva-Rocci invents device for measuring blood pressure
1897	Ronald Ross locates the malaria parasite in the *Anopheles* mosquito; first of seven volumes of Havelock Ellis's *Studies in the Psychology of Sex*
1898	Patrick Manson's *Tropical Diseases*; Pierre and Marie Curie obtain radium from pitchblende
1899	**Boer War begins (ends 1902)**; sixth cholera pandemic; London School of Hygiene and Tropical Medicine founded; aspirin introduced
1900	Sigmund Freud's *The Interpretation of Dreams*; Karl Landsteiner identifies four major human blood groups (A. O. B. and AB); US Army Yellow Fever Commission founded
1901	**Death of Queen Victoria**; first Nobel Prizes
1902	William Bayliss and Ernest Starling discover the hormone secretin; Registration of Midwives Act passed in Britain
1903	**Wright Brothers fly in petrol-powered aircraft**; Willem Einthoven describes the first electrocardiograph
1904	Rockefeller Institute for Medical Research founded in New York
1905	George Washington Crile performs first direct blood transfusion; J. B. Murphy develops first artificial hip joints
1906	Frederick Gowland Hopkins starts experiments on 'accessory food factors' (vitamins); Charles Sherrington's *The Integrative Action of the Nervous System*, a classic of neurology
1907	John Scott Haldane develops method for bringing divers to the surface safely
1908	Sulphanilamide first synthesized
1909	**Industrial production of plastics begins after Bakelite developed; Robert Peary and Matthew Hensen reach the North Pole**; Archibald Edward Garrod's *Inborn Errors of Metabolism*
1910	Paul Ehrlich announces his discovery of Salvarsan for syphilis – the beginning of modern chemotherapy

1911	**Roald Amundsen reaches the South Pole**; National Insurance Act sets up first state medical insurance scheme in Britain; William Hill develops the first gastroscope
1912	**The _Titanic_ sinks on maiden voyage**; Harvey Cushing's _The Pituitary Gland and Its Disorders_; Casimir Funk coins the term 'vitamin'
1913	John Jacob Abel develops first artificial kidney; establishment of Medical Research Committee (Council from 1920) in Britain
1914	**Outbreak of First World War; Panama Canal opens**; Alexis Carrel performs first successful heart surgery on a dog; Henry Dale discovers the neurotransmitter acetycholine in ergot
1916	**Albert Einstein's _General Theory of Relativity_**; Walter Gaskell names the involuntary nervous system; Margaret Sanger founds first American birth-control clinic in Brooklyn, New York; Mary Stopes's _Married Love_
1917	Carl Jung's _Psychology of the Unconscious_
1918	**End of First World War**; start of influenza pandemic
1919	**Ernest Rutherford splits the atom; first crossing of the Atlantic by air**
1920	**League of Nations set up**; establishment of Tavistock Clinic, first UK centre for the teaching and deployment of Freud's psychoanalytical ideas
1921	Marie Stopes opens her first birth-control clinic in London; F. G. Banting and C. H. Best isolate insulin
1922	**USSR established**
1923	**Turkish republic formed – end of Ottoman Empire**; Albert Calmette and Camille Guérin develop the BCG vaccine for tuberculosis
1926	First enzyme (urease) crystallized by American biochemist James B. Sumner
1927	Philip Drinker and Louis Shaw develop the 'iron lung'
1928	Alexander Fleming discovers penicillin in a mould: Albert Szent-Györgyi isolates vitamin C
1929	**Wall Street Crash**: Henry Dale and H. W. Dudley demonstrate chemical transmission of nerve impulses; Werner Forssmann develops cardiac catheter
1932	Armand Quick introduces a test to measure the clotting ability of blood; Gerhard Domagk discovers the first sulpha drug, Prontosil

Chronology

1935	Development of prefrontal lobotomy to treat mental illness; first blood bank set up – in the USA at the Mayo Clinic, Rochester; Hans Zinsser's *Rats, Lice, and History*
1936	Ugo Cerletti describes electroconvulsive therapy
1937	Development of vaccine against yellow fever by Max Theiler and of first antihistamine by Daniel Bovet; Charles Dodds discovers a synthetic oestrogen (stilboestrol)
1938	New Zealand Social Security Act provides pioneering state medical service; John Wiles develops the first total artificial hip replacement, using stainless steel
1939	**Outbreak of Second World War**
1940	Howard Florey and Ernst Chain develop penicillin as an antibiotic; Karl Landsteiner discovers the Rhesus factor in blood
1941	Norman Gregg links rubella (German measles) in pregnancy and cataract and other abnormalities in children
1942	Report by William Beveridge paves way for the idea of a National Health Service in Britain
1943	Wilhelm Kolff develops first kidney dialysis machine; Selman Waksman discovers the antibiotic streptomycin
1944	Alfred Blalock performs first blue-baby operation
1945	**End of Second World War; beginning of Cold War**; fluoridation of water introduced in the USA to prevent tooth decay
1946	**First meeting of United Nations General Assembly in New York**; start of first randomized clinical trials of streptomycin for TB treatment
1948	World Health Organization (WHO) formed within the UN; National Health Service formed in Britain and National Institutes of Health in the USA; Philip Hench discovers that cortisone can be used for rheumatoid arthritis
1951	John Gibbon develops heart–lung machine and operates (1953) successfully using it
1952	Douglas Bevis develops amniocentesis; open-heart surgery begins with implantation of artificial heart valves
1953	E. A. Graham and E. L. Wynder show that tobacco tars cause cancer in mice; James Watson and Francis Crick determine the double-helical structure of DNA
1954	First successful kidney transplant; plastic contact lenses produced

1957	**Treaty of Rome, leading to the establishment (1958) of the European Economic Community**; Albert Sabin develops a live polio vaccine; Clarence Lillehei devises first compact heart pacemaker
1958	Ian Donald uses ultrasound to diagnosis disorders of the foetus
1961	Seventh cholera pandemic begins
1962	**Cuban missile crisis**; lasers first used in eye surgery; thalidomide withdrawn
1963	Measles vaccine licensed for general use in USA; Thomas Starzl's first human liver transplant; the tranquilizer valium introduced
1964	**Outbreak of Vietnam War between N. Vietnam and USA (to 1973)**; home kidney dialysis introduced in the UK and USA
1966	**Cultural Revolution begins in China**
1967	Mammography for detecting breast cancer introduced; Christiaan Barnard performs human heart transplant; Rene Favaloro develops coronary bypass operation; Marburg virus disease recognized
1969	**Neil Armstrong lands on the Moon**; first attempt to use an artificial heart in a human; Patrick Steptoe and Robert Edwards announce the fertilization of human eggs outside the body
1972	Computerized axial tomography (CAT) introduced commercially for medical imaging; first showing of TV hospital drama, *MASH*, based in Korea
1976	Epidemics of Ebola virus disease in Sudan and Zaire
1978	First 'test-tube' baby born in England
1979	World declared free of smallpox
1980	Experimental vaccine against hepatitis B developed
1981	AIDS first recognized by US Centers for Disease Control
1983	First successful human embryo transfers
1986	Human Genome Project set up; gene for duchenne muscular dystrophy discovered
1991	**Collapse of USSR**
1994	The Americas are declared a polio-free zone
1995	WHO given licence to develop and distribute Manual Patarroyo's malaria vaccine

Major Human Diseases

Disease	Cause	Means of transmission
acquired immunodeficiency syndrome (AIDS)	viruses (HIV-1 and HIV-2)	sexual intercourse; blood products; intravenous drug use; mother to child in the uterus
amoebic dysentery	amoeba (*Enteramoeba histolytica*)	ingestion in contaminated food and water
Argentine haemorrhagic fever	virus	disease of rodents; probably infects humans through direct contact, or food contaminated with rodent excreta
ascariasis	roundworm (*Ascaris*)	consumption of mature eggs in food or water contaminated with human faeces
beriberi	deficiency of thiamine	historically has affected those with diets centred on rice

(cont.)

Major Human Diseases

Disease	Cause	Means of transmission
Bolivian haemorrhagic fever	virus	disease of rodents that probably infects humans through contaminated food, water, and air
brucellosis	bacterium (*Brucella*)	contact with infected animals
Carrión's disease	bacterium (*Bartonella*)	bloodsucking sandflies
Chagas' disease (American trypanosomiasis)	protozoan (*Trypanosoma cruzi*)	harboured by animals; transmitted to humans by infected bugs
chickenpox (varicella)	virus	human to human
cholera	bacterium (*Vibrio cholerae*)	faecal–oral route, especially in contaminated water
dengue	arbovirus	infected female *Aedes* mosquitoes
diphtheria	bacillus (*Corynebacterium diphtheriae*)	human to human
dracunculiasis (Guineaworm infection)	nematode worm (*Dracunculus medinensis*)	ingested in contaminated water
Ebola virus disease	virus	unsterilized needles and syringes, and other unknown routes
encephalitis lethargica (sleepy sickness)	virus	seems to accompany and follow epidemic influenza
ergotism	ergot fungus (*Claviceps purpurea*)	consumption of ergot-infected grain or grain products
erysipelas (St Anthony's fire)	bacterium (*Streptococcus*)	passed by infected humans through surgical instruments, wounds, and contact
filariasis (includes elephantiasis)	filarial nematode worms	infected mosquitoes

Major Human Diseases

Disease	Cause	Means of transmission
hepatitis A and B	virus	A by ingestion of infected food and water; B through infected blood
hookworm disease (anycylostomiasis)	nematode worms	penetration of the body, typically through the skin of the feet from infected soil
influenza (grippe)	virus	human to human (reservoirs in animals)
Lassa fever	virus	urine from rodents, then human to human
leishmaniasis	protozoan (*Leishmania*)	bloodsucking sandflies
leprosy	bacillus (*Mycobacterium leprae*)	human to human after prolonged contact
leptospirosis (Weil's disease)	spirochaete bacteria (*Leptospira*)	contact with infected animals, especially their urine
malaria	protozoans (*Plasmodium*)	bite of infected female mosquitoes, especially *Anopheles*
Marburg virus disease	virus	apparently through the blood of infected monkeys or humans
measles (rubeola)	virus	human to human
mumps	virus	human to human
onchocerciasis (river blindness)	filarial nematode worms (*Onchocerca*)	blood-feeding flies
pellagra	deficiency of niacin (vitamin B_3)	historically has affected those with diets centred on maize
pinta	spirochaete bacteria (*Treponema*)	skin-to-skin contact
plague	bacterium (*Yersinia pestis*)	bite of a flea from an infected host, usually a rat
poliomyelitis (polio)	virus	faecal–oral route

(cont.)

Major Human Diseases

Disease	Cause	Means of transmission
protein-energy malnutrition	usually weaning to low-protein diet	mostly affects children in the developing world; worsened by infection
relapsing fever	spirochaete bacteria (*Borrelia*)	lice and ticks
Rift Valley fever	viruses	bloodsucking sandflies
Rocky Mountain spotted fever	rickettsia	ticks
rubella (German measles)	virus	human to human
scarlet fever	bacteria (*Streptococcus*)	close human contact
schistosomiasis (bilharziasis)	trematode worm (*Schistosoma*)	penetration of the skin in contaminated water
scurvy	deficiency of ascorbic acid (vitamin C)	affects those on diets lacking fresh fruits and vegetables, such as sailors
sleeping sickness (African trypanosomiasis)	protozoan (*Trypanosoma brucei*)	bite of a tsetse fly
smallpox (variola)	pox virus	airborne droplets, human to human
syphilis (venereal)	spirochaete bacteria (*Treponema*)	sexual intercourse or from mother to child in the uterus
syphilis (non-venereal)	(same as above)	human (usually children) to human through mucous membranes
tetanus (lockjaw)	bacterium (*Clostridum*)	through wounds
trachoma	bacterium (*Chlamydia trachomatis*)	from eye to eye via the fingers; by eye-seeking flies; from mother to baby
trichinosis	nematode worm (*Trichinella spiralis*)	consumption of under-cooked meat, usually pork
tuberculosis	bacillus (*Mycobacterium*)	human to human
tularaemia (rabbit fever)	bacterium (*Francisella tularensis*)	contact with infected animals

Major Human Diseases

Disease	Cause	Means of transmission
typhoid and paratyphoid	bacteria (*Salmonella*)	faecal–oral route
typhus (ship fever, prison fever)	rickettsia	bite of fleas, lice, and mites
whooping cough	bacterium (*Bordetella pertussis*)	mainly airborne
yellow fever	virus	bite of infected mosquitoes, especially *Aedes*

Notes

Introduction

1 Lord Horder, 'Whither medicine', *British Medical Journal* vol. i (1949), pp. 557–60 (quote p. 558). 2 Lewis Thomas, 'Biomedical science and human health – the long-range prospects'. Paper presented at a Festschrift in honour of Dr Otto Westphal, Freiberg, 1 February 1978.

Chapter 2. The Rise of Medicine

1 Quoted in J. V. Kinnier Wilson and E. H. Reynolds, 'A Babylonian treatise on epilepsy, *Medical History* vol. 34 (1990), p. 192. 2 Quoted in H. E. Sigerist, *A History of Medicine I: Primitive and Archaic Medicine* (New York, Oxford University Press, 1951), p. 324. 3 Ibid., p. 334. 4 Margery Kempe, *The Book of Margery Kempe* (Penguin Books, 1985); quoted by R. Porter, *A Social History of Medicine* (London, Weidenfeld & Nicolson, 1987), p. 108.

Chapter 3. What Is Disease?

1 Quoted in Timothy P. Weber, 'The Baptist tradition', in Ronald L. Numbers and D. W. Amundsen (eds), *Caring and Curing: Health and Medicine in the Western Religious Tradition* (New York, Macmillan, 1986), p. 291. 2 Quoted in Richard Palmer, 'The Church, leprosy and the plague in Medieval and Early Modern Europe', in W. J. Sheils (ed.), *The Church and Healing* (Oxford, Basil Blackwell, for the Ecclesiastical History Society, 1982), pp. 79–100 (quote p. 97). 3 W. H. S. Jones (transl.), 'The sacred disease', in *Hippocrates* (London, Heinemann, 1923), vol. 2, p. 141. 4 N. D. Jewson, 'The disappearance of the sick man from medical cosmology, 1770–1870', *Sociology* vol. 10 (1976), pp. 225–44. 5 Michaela Reid, *Ask Sir James* (London, Hodder & Stoughton, 1987), p. 201. 6 E. L. Griggs (ed.), *Collected Papers of Samuel Taylor Coleridge*, vol. 1 (Oxford, Clarendon Press, 1965), p. 256: Coleridge to Charles Lloyd, Sr., 14 November 1796. 7 Gustav Broun, 'The amputation of the clitoris and labia minora: a contribution to the treatment of vaginismus'; transl. from the German by Jeffrey Moussaieff Masson in *A Dark Science: Women, Sexuality, and Psychiatry in the Nineteenth Century* (New York,

The Noonday Press, 1988), pp. 128–38. **8** Thomas Beddoes, *Essay on the Causes, Early Signs, and Prevention of Pulmonary Consumption for the Use of Parents and Preceptors* (Bristol, 1799), p. 6. **9** Quoted in Susan Sontag, *Illness as Metaphor* (London, Allen Lane, 1979), p. 29. **10** Quoted in W. S. Lewis (ed.), *The Yale Edition of Horace Walpole's Correspondence*, 48 vols (New Haven, Yale University Press, 1937–83), vol. 25, p. 402. **11** Quoted in R. W. Chapman (ed.), *The Letters of Samuel Johnson*, 3 vols (Oxford, Clarendon Press, 1952), letter 891, vol. 3, p. 81. **12** Quoted in J. W. Warter (ed.), *Southey's Common-Place Book* (London, Longman, 1831), p. 551. **13** 'Bec's birthday', in Harold Williams (ed.), *The Poems of Jonathan Swift*, 3 vols (Oxford, Clarendon Press, 1937), vol. 2, p. 761. **14** Edward Shorter, *From Paralysis to Fatigue: A History of Psychosomatic Illness in the Modern Era* (New York, Free Press, 1992). **15** W. H. Helfand, 'James Morison and his pills', *Transactions of the British Society of the History of Pharmacy* vol. 1 (1974), pp. 101–35. **16** Charles E. Rosenberg and Janet Golden (eds.), *Framing Disease: Studies in Cultural History* (New Brunswick, NJ, Rutgers University Press, 1992).

Chapter 4. Primary Care

1 [George] Bernard Shaw, Preface (1911) to *The Doctor's Dilemma: A Tragedy* (Harmondsworth, Penguin, 1946), p. 76. **2** William Buchan, *Domestic Medicine: Or, A Treatise on the Prevention and Cure of Disease*, 10th edn (London, 1788; first published 1769), pp. 162–3. **3** Adolf Kussmaul, *Jugenderinnerungen* (Stuttgart, 1922), pp. 222–3. **4** W. Brockbank and F. Kenworthy (eds.), *The Diary of Richard Kay, 1716–51, of Baldingstone, near Bury: A Lancashire Doctor* (Manchester, Chetham Society, 1968), pp. 162–4. **5** Arthur E. Hertzler, *The Horse and Buggy Doctor* (New York, 1938), p. 117. **6** James B. Herrick, *Memoirs of Eighty Years* (Chicago, University of Chicago Press, 1949), pp. 100–1. **7** Edward Sutleffe, *Medical and Surgical Cases: Selected During a Practice of Thirty-eight Years* (London, 1824), pp. 409–10. **8** Benjamin Rush, 'Observations and reasoning in medicine' (1791), in Dagobert D. Runes (ed.), *The Selected Writings of Benjamin Rush* (New York, Philosophical Library, 1947). p. 249. **9** William Douglass, *A Summary, Historical and Political, of the... Present State of the British Settlements in North America*, 2 vols (Boston, 1755), vol. 2, pp. 351–2. **10** *The Spectator in Four Volumes* (London, Dent, 1945), vol. 1 (24 March 1711), pp. 64–5. **11** D[aniel] W. Cathell, *The Physician Himself and What He Should Add to the Strictly Scientific* (Baltimore, 1882), p. 139. **12** Q. J. C. Yeatman, quoted in I. S. L. Loudon, 'The origin of the general practitioner', *Journal of the Royal College of General Practitioners* vol. 33 (1933), pp. 13–18. **13** Karl Stern, *The Pillar of Fire* (New York, Harcourt, 1951), pp. 102–3. **14** Hertzler, *Horse and Buggy Doctor* (1938), op. cit. (note 5), pp. 101–10. **15** D[aniel] W. Cathell, *Book on the Physician Himself from Graduation to Old Age*, Crowning edn (Philadelphia, 1924), p. 132. **16** Hertzler, *Horse and Buggy Doctor* (1938), op. cit. (note 5), p. 9. **17** William Victor Johnston, *Before the Age of Miracles: Memoirs of a Country Doctor* (Toronto, Fitzhenry and Whiteside, 1972), p. 58. **18** Quoted in Walter Rivington, *The Medical Profession* (London, 1879), pp. 338–9. **19** Anon, 'St Bartholomew's Hospital: Casualty Department', *The Lancet* vol. i (11 January 1879), pp. 59–60 (quote p. 60). **20** Joseph McDowell Mathews, *How to Succeed in the Practice of Medicine* (Philadelphia, 1905),

p. 133. **21** George T. Welch, 'Therapeutical superstition', *Medical Record* vol. 44 (8 July 1893), pp. 33–8 (quote p. 35). **22** A. Conan Doyle, *The Stark Munro Letters* (London, 1895), p. 208. **23** Robert I. Lee and Lewis Webster Jones, *The Fundamentals of Good Medical Care* (Chicago, 1922, Publications of the Committee on the Costs of Medical Care, no. 22), p. 244. **24** James Mackenzie, *The Future of Medicine* (London, 1919), p. 171. **25** Quoted in Erna Lesky, *Die Wiener Medizinische Schule im 19. Jahrhundert* (Graz: Böhlau, 1978), pp. 146–7. **26** Bernhard Naunyn, *Erinnerungen, Gedanken und Meinungen* (Munich, 1925), p. 516. **27** Jacob Bigelow, 'On the medical profession and quackery' (1844), in Bigelow, *Modern Inquiries: Classical, Professional, and Miscellaneous* (Boston, 1867), pp. 199–215 (quote p. 214). **28** Oliver Wendell Holmes, 'Currents and counter-currents in medical science' (1860), in Holmes, *Medical Essays, 1842–1882* (Boston, 1911), pp. 173–208 (quotes pp. 184, 203–4). **29** William Osler, *The Principles and Practice of Medicine* (New York, 1892), p. 75. **30** Hertzler, *Horse and Buggy Doctor* (1938), op. cit. (note 5), pp. 99–100. **31** Max Neuburger, *Hermann Nothnagel: Leben und Wirken eines deutschen Klinikers* (Vienna, 1922), pp. 146, 159, 162, 406, n. 20. **32** [Autobiography] *Barney Sachs, 1854–1944* (New York: privately printed, 1949), p. 48. **33** Quoted in C[larence] B. Farrar, 'The four doctors', in *Proceedings of the Seventh Annual Psychiatric Institute, September 16, 1959* (Princeton, New Jersey, 1959), pp. 105–16 (quote p. 110). **34** C.B.F. [Clarence B. Farrar], 'I remember Osler, Psychotherapist', *American Journal of Psychiatry* vol. 121 (1965), pp. 761–2 (quote p. 762). **35** Lewellys F. Barker, *Time and the Physician* (New York, 1942), p. 270. **36** G[eorge] Canby Robinson, *The Patient as a Person: A Study of the Social Aspects of Illness* (New York, 1939), pp. 9–10, 410–14. **37** Francis Weld Peabody, *The Care of the Patient* (Cambridge, 1927), p. 34. **38** William R. Houston, *The Art of Treatment* (New York, 1936), pp. 72, 74. **39** Cathell, *Book on the Physician Himself* (1924), op. cit. (note 19), pp. 63–4. **40** Guy de Maupassant, *Mont-Oriol* (Paris, Gallimard, 1976; first publ. 1887), p. 238. **41** Joseph S. Collings, 'General practice in England today: a reconnaissance', *The Lancet* vol. i (25 March 1950), pp. 555–85 (quote p. 577). **42** Rivington, *The Medical Profession* (1879), op. cit. (note 23), p. 54. **43** Wilmot Herringham, 'The consultant', *British Medical Journal* vol. 2 (10 July 1920), pp. 36–8 (quote p. 36). **44** John Brotherston, 'Evolution of medical practice', in Gordon McLachlan and Thomas McKeown (eds.), *Medical History and Medical Care* (London, Oxford University Press, 1971), pp. 87–125 (quote p. 108). **45** Cathell, *Book on the Physician Himself* (1924), op. cit. (note 19), p. 33. **46** Naunyn, *Erinnerungen* (1925), op. cit. (note 38), pp. 164–5. **47** Ralph W. Tuttle, 'The other side of country practice', *New England Journal of Medicine* vol. 199 (1 November 1928), pp. 874–7 (quote p. 876). **48** W. Stanley Sykes, *A Manual of General Medical Practice* (London, 1927), pp. 54–5. **49** Keith Hodgkin, *Towards Earlier Diagnosis in Primary Care* (1963), 4th edn (Edinburgh, Churchill Livingstone, 1978), p. ix. **50** J. M. Last, 'The iceberg: "Completing the clinical picture" in general practice', *The Lancet* vol. ii (6 July 1963), pp. 28–31 (quote p. 30). **51** Sykes, *A Manual of General Medical Practice* (1927), op. cit. (note 61), p. 2. **52** John H. Budd, 'Art vs. science in medicine: a look at public perception of physicians', *Postgraduate Medicine*, vol. 69 (1981), pp. 13–19 (quote p. 15). **53** Herrick, *Memoirs of Eighty Years* (1949), op. cit. (note 9), p. 103. Herrick was present at the scene, involving an unnamed family physician.

Chapter 5. Medical Science

1 Friedrich Hoffmann, *Fundamenta Medicinae*, transl. and introduced by Lester S. King (London, MacDonald, 1971; first published 1695), p. 5. 2 Quoted in A. C. Corcoran, *A Mirror up to Medicine* (Philadelphia, J. B. Lippincott, 1961), p. 60. 3 Quoted in W. F. Bynum, *Science and the Practice of Medicine in the Nineteenth Century* (New York, Cambridge University Press, 1994), p. 98. 4 Quoted in Corcoran, *A Mirror up to Medicine* (1961), op. cit. (note 4), p. 261. 5 Thomas Lewis, 'The Huxley Lecture on clinical science within the university', *British Medical Journal* vol. 1 (1935), pp. 631–6.

Chapter 6. Hospitals and Surgery

1 Jerome, *The Principal Works of Jerome*, transl. by the Hon. W. H. Freemantle (Oxford, James Parker; New York, The Christian Literature Co., 1893), p. 190. 2 Quoted in W. B. Howie, 'Medical education in eighteenth-century hospitals', *Scottish Society for the History of Medicine, Report Proceedings* (1969–70), pp. 27–46 (quote pp. 41–2). 3 Quoted in Toby Gelfand, ' "Invite the philosopher, as well as the charitable"; hospital teaching as private enterprise in Hunterian London', in W. F. Bynum and R. Porter (eds.), *William Hunter and the Eighteenth-Century Medical World* (Cambridge, Cambridge University Press, 1985), pp. 129–52 (quote p. 146). 4 Quoted in R. Porter, *Doctor of Society: Thomas Beddoes and the Sick Trade in Late Enlightenment England* (London, Routledge, 1991), p. 77. 5 J. Hemlow (ed.). *The Journals and Letters of Fanny Burney (Madame D'Arblay)*, 12 vols (Oxford, Clarendon Press, 1972–84), vol. 6, p. 598f.

Chapter 7. Drug Treatment and the Rise of Pharmacology

1 E. Stone, 'An account of the success of the bark of the willow in the cure of Agues', *Philosophical Transactions of the Royal Society* vol. 53 (1763), pp. 195–200. 2 Anonymous, 'Yo-Ho-Ho. Pulv. Ipecac. Co. (Dover's Powder)', in *Round the Fountain* (London, St Bartholomew's Hospital Medical Journal, 1923). 3 Sir William Osler, 'Teaching and thinking'; address given at McGill Medical School in 1894, reprinted in *Aequanimatas*, 3rd edn (London, H. K. Lewis, 1941), pp. 119–29 (quote p. 121). 4 *The Lancet* vol. i (1853), p. 453. 5 Quoted by H. H. Dale, in 'Acetylcholine as a chemical transmitter of the effects of nerve impulses', *Journal of the Mount Sinai Hospital* vol. 4 (1937–8), pp. 401–29. 6 James Lind, Preface to *A Treatise on the Scurvy* (London, 1753).

Chapter 8. Mental Illness

1 Aretaeus the Cappadocian, *The Extant Works*, ed. and transl. by Francis Adams (London, The Sydenham Society, 1856). 2 William Pargeter, *Observations on Maniacal Disorders* (Reading, for the author, 1792), p. 31. 3 John Locke, *An Essay Concerning Human Understanding*, ed. by P. H. Nidditch (Oxford, Clarendon Press, 1975), pp. 160–1. 4 C. Dickens and W. H. Wills, *A Curious Dance Around a Curious Tree* (1852); reprinted in *Charles Dickens' Uncollected Writings from Household Words* (Bloomington, Indiana University Press, 1968), vol. 2, pp. 281–91. 5 Jimmie Laing and Dermot McQuarrie, *Fifty Years in the System* (Edinburgh, Mainstream,

1989), p. 89. **6** Thomas S. Szasz, *The Myth of Mental Illness: Foundations of a Theory of Personal Conduct*, rev. edn (New York, Harper and Row, 1974), p. 1.

Chapter 9. Medicine, Society, and the State

1 George Eliot, *Middlemarch: A Study of Provincial Life* (London, Dent in Everyman's Library; first published 1871–2), pp. 149–50. **2** W. Rivington, *The Medical Profession* (Dublin and London, 1879), pp. 135–6.

Chapter 10. Looking to the Future

1 Frank Macfarlane Burnet, *Genes, Dreams and Realities* (Aylesbury, Medical & Technical Publishing, 1971). **2** Maurice King, 'Health is a sustainable state', *The Lancet* vol. 336, pp. 664–7 (1990). **3** Ian Kennedy, *The Unmasking of Medicine* (London: Allen & Unwin, 1981), p. 26. **4** Julius Comroe and Robert Dripps, 'Scientific basis for the support of biomedical science', *Science* vol. 192, pp. 105–11 (1976).

Further Reading

General and Reference Works

Ackerknecht, E. H., *A Short History of Medicine* (Baltimore, Johns Hopkins University Press, 1968). Probably the best brief history.

Ackerknecht, E. H., *Therapeutics from the Primitives to the Twentieth Century* (New York, Hafner, 1973).

Brieger, Gert H., 'History of medicine', in Paul T. Durbin (ed.), *A Guide to the Culture of Science, Technology and Medicine* (New York, Free Press, 1980), pp. 121–96.

Bynum, W. F., 'Health, disease and medical care', in G. S. Rousseau and R. Porter (eds.), *The Ferment of Knowledge* (Cambridge, Cambridge University Press, 1980), pp. 211–54.

Bynum, W. F., and Porter, Roy (eds.), *Companion Encyclopedia of the History of Medicine*, 2 vols (London, Routledge, 1993). The most up-to-date work of reference.

Castiglioni, Arturo, *A History of Medicine*, transl. and edited by E. B. Krumbhaar (New York, Alfred A. Knopf, 1941).

Clarke, Edwin, *Modern Methods in the History of Medicine* (London, Athlone Press, 1971).

Conrad, Lawrence *et al.*, *The Western Medical Tradition: 800 BC to AD 1800* (Cambridge, Cambridge University Press, 1995).

Garrison, Fielding H., *An Introduction to the History of Medicine* (Philadelphia, Saunders, 1960; first published 1917).

Howells, John G., and Osborn, M. Livia, *A Reference Companion to the History of Abnormal Psychology*, 2 vols (London, Greenwood Press, 1984).

Illich, I., *Limits to Medicine: The Expropriation of Health* (London, Marion Boyars, 1976; paperback edition, Penguin, 1977).

Jordanova, L. J. 'The social sciences and history of science and medicine', in P. Corsi and P. Weindling (eds.), *Information Sources in the History of Science and Medicine* (London, Butterworth Scientific, 1983), pp. 81–98.

Kiple, Kenneth F. (ed.) *The Cambridge World History of Human Diseases* (Cambridge, Cambridge University Press, 1993).

Magner, Lois N., *A History of Medicine* (New York, Marcel Dekker, 1992).

McGrew, Roderick E., *Encyclopedia of Medical History* (New York, McGraw-Hill, 1985). An extremely useful work of reference.

McKeown, T., *The Role of Medicine: Dream, Mirage or Nemesis?* (London, Nuffield Provincial Hospitals Trust, 1976; Princeton, Princeton University Press, 1979; Oxford, Blackwell, 1979).

Morton, L. T., *A Medical Bibliography (Garrison and Morton): An Annotated Checklist of Texts Illustrating the History of Medicine*, 4th edn (Aldershot, Hants, Gower, 1983).

Neuburger, Max, *History of Medicine*, transl. by Ernest Playfair, 2 vols (London, H. Frowde, 1910–25).

Olby, R. C., Cantor, G. N., Christie, J. R. R., and Hodge, M. J. S. (eds.), *Companion to the History of Modern Science* (London, Routledge, 1989).

Payer, Lynn, *Disease-Mongers: How Doctors, Drug Companies, and Insurers are Making You Feel Sick* (New York, Wiley, 1992).

Pelling, Margaret, 'Medicine since 1500', in P. Corsi and Paul Weindling (eds.), *Information Sources in the History of Science and Medicine* (London, Butterworth Scientific, 1983), pp. 379–407.

Shryock, Richard H., *The Development of Modern Medicine: An Interpretation of the Social and Scientific Factors*, 2nd edn (New York, Alfred A. Knopf, 1947; reprinted Madison, University of Wisconsin Press, 1980). A dated but highly stimulating work.

Sigerist, Henry E., *Civilization and Disease* (Ithaca, Cornell University Press, 1943; reprinted Chicago, University of Chicago Press, 1962).

Sigerist, Henry E., *A History of Medicine I: Primitive and Archaic Medicine* (New York, Oxford University Press, 1951).

Sigerist, Henry E., *A History of Medicine II: Early Greek, Hindu and Persian Medicine* (New York, Oxford University Press, 1961).

Singer, Charles, and Underwood, E. Ashworth, *A Short History of Medicine* (Oxford, Clarendon Press, 1928; 2nd edn, New York, Oxford University Press, 1962).

Sournia, Jean-Charles, *The Illustrated History of Medicine* (London, Harold Starke, 1992). Very finely illustrated.

Temkin, O., *The Double Face of Janus and Other Essays in the History of Medicine* (Baltimore, Johns Hopkins University Press, 1977).

Walton, John, Beeson, Paul B., and Bodley Scott, Ronald (eds.), *The Oxford Companion to Medicine*, 2 vols (Oxford, Oxford University Press, 1986).

Webster, Charles, 'The historiography of medicine', in P. Corsi and P. Weindling (eds.), *Information Sources in the History of Science and Medicine* (London, Butterworth Scientific, 1983), pp. 29–43.

Contemporary research in the history of medicine is comprehensively listed in two ongoing publications: *Bibliography of the History of Medicine*, no. 1– (Bethesda, National Library of Medicine, 1965–), an annual with quinquennial cumulations; and *Current Work in the History of Medicine. An International Bibliography* (Wellcome Institute for the History of Medicine, London, 1954–). A cumulation of *Current Work*, and most secondary literature of the twentieth century until 1977, is listed in the Wellcome Institute for the History of Medicine's, *Subject Catalogue of the History of Medicine*, 18 vols (subject section, 9 vols; biographical section, 5 vols; topographical section, 4 vols) (Munich, Krays International, 1980). Material since 1977 is listed on card files and on computer in the Wellcome Library.

The History of Disease (Chapter 1)

Ackerknecht, Erwin H., *History and Geography of the Most Important Diseases* (New York, Hafner, 1965).

Akroyd, W. R., *Conquest of Deficiency Diseases* (Geneva, World Health Organization, 1970).

Anderson, Roy M., and May, Robert M., *Infectious Diseases of Humans: Dynamics and Control* (Oxford, Oxford University Press, 1991).

Ashburn, P. M., *The Ranks of Death: A Medical History of Conquest of America* (New York, Coward-McCann, 1947).

Burnet, Sir Macfarlane, *Natural History of Infectious Disease*, 3rd edn (Cambridge, Cambridge University Press, 1962).

Cartwright, Frederick F., *Disease and History* (New York, Thomas Y. Crowell, 1972).

Cohen, Mark Nathan, *The Food Crisis in Prehistory: Overpopulation and the Origins of Agriculture* (New Haven and London, Yale University Press, 1977).

Crosby, Alfred W., *Ecological Imperialism: The Biological Expansion of Europe, 900–1900* (Cambridge and New York, Cambridge University Press, 1986).

Further Reading

Crosby, Alfred W., *The Columbian Exchange: Biological and Cultural Consequences of 1492* (Westport, CT, Greenwood Press, 1972).

Dobyns, Henery F., *Their Numbers Become Thinned* (Knoxville, University of Tennessee Press, 1983).

Dubos, René, and Dubos, Jean, *The White Plague: Tuberculosis, Man, and Society* (Boston, Little Brown, 1952).

Fiennes, Richard, *Zoonoses of Primates: The Epidemiology and Ecology of Simian Diseases in Relation to Man* (Ithaca, Cornell University Press, 1979).

Harrison, Gordon A., *Mosquitoes, Malaria, and Man* (New York, Dutton, 1978).

Henschen, Folke, *The History and Geography of Diseases*, transl. by Joan Tate (New York, Delacorte Press, 1962).

Hoeppli, Reinhard, *Parasitic Diseases in Africa and the Western Hemisphere: Early Documentation and Transmission by the Slave Trade* (Basel, Verlag für Recht und Gesellschaft, 1969).

Hopkins, Donald R., *Princes and Peasants: Smallpox in History* (Chicago, University of Chicago Press, 1983).

Kiple, Kenneth F., *The Caribbean Slave: A Biological History* (Cambridge, Cambridge University Press, 1984).

Kiple, Kenneth F. (ed.), *The Cambridge World History of Human Diseases* (Cambridge, Cambridge University Press, 1993).

Livingstone, Frank B., *Abnormal Hemoglobins in Human Populations* (Chicago, Aldine, 1967).

McGrew, Roderick E., *Encyclopedia of Medical History* (New York, McGraw-Hill, 1985).

McKeown, Thomas, *The Origins of Human Disease* (Oxford and New York, Basil Blackwell, 1988).

McKeown, Thomas, *The Modern Rise of Population* (London, Edward Arnold, 1976).

McNeill, William H., *Plagues and Peoples* (Garden City, NY, Anchor Press/Doubleday, 1976).

Ramenofsky, Ann, *Vectors of Death: The Archaeology of European Contact* (Albuquerque, University of New Mexico Press, 1987).

Roe, Daphne A., *A Plague of Corn: The Social History of Pellagra* (Ithaca, Cornell University Press, 1973).

Scrimshaw, Nevin S., Taylor, Carl E., and Gordon, Jack E., *Interactions of Nutrition and Infection* (Geneva, World Health Organization, 1968).

Stannard, David E., *Before the Horror: The Population of Hawaii on the Eve of Western Contact* (Honolulu, University of Hawaii Press, 1989).

Wrigley, Anthony, and Scofield, Roger S., *The Population History of England, 1541–1871* (Cambridge, MA, Harvard University Press, 1981).

Zinsser, Hans, *Rats, Lice, and History*, 4th edn (London, Routledge, 1942).

The Rise of Medicine (Chapter 2)

Cohn, S. K., *The Black Death Transformed* (London, Arnold, 2002).

Edelstein, L., *Ancient Medicine* (Baltimore, Johns Hopkins University Press, 1987).

Estes, J. Worth, *The Medical Skills of Ancient Egypt* (Canton, MA, Science History Publications, 1989).

Jackson, R., *Doctors and Diseases in the Roman Empire* (London, British Museum Publications, 1988).

Jones, Peter Murray, *Medieval Medical Miniatures* (London, British Library, 1984).

Lloyd, G. E. R., *In the Grip of Disease: Studies in the Greek Imagination* (Oxford, Oxford University Press, 2003).

Lloyd, G. E. R., *The Revolutions of Wisdom* (Berkeley, University of California Press, 1987).

Longrigg, J. N., *Greek Rational Medicine* (London, Routledge, 1993).

Nunn, J. F., *Ancient Egyptian Medicine* (London, British Museum Publication, 1996).

Nutton, V., *Ancient Medicine* (London, Routledge, 2004).

Nutton, V., *From Democedes to Harvey* (London, Variorum, 1988).

Rawcliffe, C., *Medicine and Society in Later Medieval England* (Stroud, Alan Sutton, 1994).

Siraisi, N. G., *Medieval and Early Renaissance Medicine* (Chicago, University of Chicago Press, 1990).

Temkin, O., *Hippocrates in a World of Pagans and Christians* (Baltimore, Johns Hopkins University Press, 1991).

Ullmann, Manfred, *Islamic Medicine* (Edinburgh University Press, 1978).

What Is Disease? (Chapter 3)

Balint, M., *The Doctor, His Patient, and the Illness* (London, Pitman, 1957).

Black, Nick, *et al.* (eds.), *Health and Disease: A Reader* (Milton Keynes, Open University Press, 1984).

Bynum, W. F., and Porter, Roy (eds.), *Companion Encyclopedia of the History of Medicine*, 2 vols (London, Routledge, 1993).

Further Reading

Caplan, A. L., Engelhardt, H. T., and MacCartney, J. J. (eds.), *Concepts of Health and Disease* (Reading, MA, Addison-Wesley, 1981).

Currer, Caroline, and Stacey, Meg, *Concepts of Health, Illness and Disease: A Comparative Perspective* (Leamington Spa, Berg, 1986).

Douglas, Mary, *Purity and Danger: An Analysis of Concepts of Pollution and Taboo* (Harmondsworth, Penguin, 1966).

Dubos, René, *The Mirage of Health* (New York, Harper, 1959).

Engelhardt, H. Tristram Jr, 'The concepts of health and disease', in Tristram Engelhardt and Stuart F. Spicker (eds.), *Evaluation and Explanation in the Biomedical Sciences* (Dordrecht, Reidel, 1975), pp. 125–41.

Fee, Elizabeth, and Fox, Daniel M. (eds.), *AIDS, The Burdens of History* (Berkeley, Los Angeles, and London, University of California Press, 1988).

Fee, Elizabeth, and Fox, Daniel M. (eds.), *AIDS: The Making of a Chronic Disease* (Berkeley, Los Angeles, and London, University of California Press, 1992).

Flew, Anthony, *Crime or Disease?* (London, Macmillan, 1973).

Foucault, M., *Naissance de la Clinique: Une Archéologie du Regard Médical* (Paris, Presses Universitaires de France, 1963); transl. by A. M. Sheridan Smith as *The Birth of the Clinic* (London, Tavistock, 1973).

Gilman, Sander L., *Seeing the Insane* (New York, Brunner, Mazel, 1982).

Gilman, Sander, *Disease and Representation: From Madness to AIDS* (Ithaca, Cornell University Press, 1988).

Gilman, Sander L., *Difference and Pathology* (Ithaca, Cornell University Press, 1985).

Helman, C., *Culture, Health and Illness* (Bristol, Wright, 1984).

Illich, I., *Limits to Medicine: The Expropriation of Health* (London, Marion Boyars, 1976; paperback edition, Harmondsworth, Penguin, 1977).

Keele, K., *Anatomies of Pain* (Oxford, Blackwell Scientific Publications, 1957).

King, Lester S., *The Philosophy of Medicine: The Early Eighteenth Century* (Cambridge, MA, Harvard University Press, 1978).

King, Lester S., *The Growth of Medical Thought* (Chicago, University of Chicago Press, 1963).

Kleinman, A., *Social Origins of Distress and Disease: Depression, Neurasthenia, and Pain in Modern China* (New Haven, Yale University Press, 1986).

Parsons, Talcott, *The Social System* (Glencoe, IL, Free Press, 1951).

Riese, Walther, *The Conception of Disease, Its History, Its Versions and Its Nature* (New York, Philosophical Library, 1953).

Further Reading

Risse, G., 'Health and disease: history of the concepts', in W. T. Reich (ed.), *Encyclopedia of Bioethics*, vol. 2 (New York, Free Press, 1978), pp. 579–85.

Rosenberg, Charles E., and Golden, Janet (eds.), *Framing Disease: Studies in Cultural History* (New Brunswick, Rutgers University Press, 1992).

Sacks, Oliver, *A Leg to Stand On* (London, Duckworth, 1984).

Sontag, S., *AIDS as Metaphor* (Harmondsworth, Allen Lane, 1989).

Taylor, F. Kräupl, *The Concepts of Illness, Disease and Morbus* (Cambridge, Cambridge University Press, 1979).

Turner, Bryan S., *Medical Power and Social Knowledge* (London and Beverly Hills, Sage Publications, 1987).

Watts, Geoff, *Pleasing the Patient* (London, Faber, 1992).

Primary Care (Chapter 4)

Beeson, Paul B., and Maulitz, Russell C., 'The inner history of internal medicine', in C. Maulitz and Diana E. Long (eds.), *Grand Rounds: One Hundred Years of Internal Medicine* (Philadelphia, University of Pennsylvania Press, 1988), pp. 15–54.

Bliss, Michael, *The Discovery of Insulin* (Toronto, McClelland and Stewart, 1982).

Brotherston, John, 'Evolution of Medical Practice', in Gordon McLachlan and Thomas McKeown (eds.), *Medical History and Medical Care* (London, Oxford University Press, 1971), pp. 84–125.

Cartwright, Ann, and Anderson, Robert, *General Practice Revisited: A Second Study of Patients and Their Doctors* (London, Tavistock, 1981).

Foster, W. D., *A Short History of Clinical Pathology* (Edinburgh, Livingstone, 1961).

Hodgkin, Keith, *Towards Earlier Diagnosis in Primary Care*, 4th edn (Edinburgh, Churchill Livingstone, 1978; first published 1963).

Johnston, William Victor, *Before the Age of Miracles: Memoirs of a Country Doctor* (Toronto, Fitzhenry and Whiteside, 1972).

King, Lester S., *The Medical World of the Eighteenth Century* (Chicago, University of Chicago Press, 1958).

Koos, Earl Lomon, *The Health of Regionville: What the People Thought and Did about It* (New York, Columbia University Press, 1954).

London, I. S. L., *Medical Care and the General Practitioner, 1750–1850* (Oxford, Clarendon Press, 1986).

Parssinen, Terry M., *Secret Passions, Secret Remedies: Narcotic Drugs in British Society, 1820–1930* (Philadelphia, Institute for the Study of Human Issues, 1983).

Further Reading

Peterson, M. Jeanne, *The Medical Profession in Mid-Victorian London* (Berkeley, University of California Press, 1978).

Porter, Roy (ed.), *Patients and Practitioners: Lay Perceptions of Medicine in Pre-industrial Society* (Cambridge, Cambridge University Press, 1985).

Reiser, Stanley Joel, *Medicine and the Reign of Technology* (Cambridge, Cambridge University Press, 1978).

Rosenberg, Charles, 'The practice of medicine in New York a century ago', *Bulletin of the History of Medicine*, vol. 41 (1967), pp. 223–53.

Rothstein, William G., *American Physicians in the Nineteenth Century: From Sects to Science* (Baltimore, Johns Hopkins University Press, 1972).

Shorter, Edward, *Bedside Manners: The Troubled History of Doctors and Patients* (New York, Simon and Schuster, 1985); republished with a new preface as *Doctors and Their Patients: A Social History* (New Brunswick, NJ, Transaction Publishers, 1991).

Shorter, Edward, *From Paralysis to Fatigue: A History of Psychosomatic Illness in the Modern Era* (New York, Free Press, 1992).

Sneader, Walter, *Drug Discovery: The Evolution of Modern Medicines* (Chichester, Wiley, 1985).

Starr, Paul, *The Social Transformation of American Medicine* (New York, Basic Books, 1982).

Stevens, Rosemary, *Medical Practice in Modern England: The Impact of Specialization and State Medicine* (New Haven, Yale University Press, 1966).

Stevens, Rosemary, *American Medicine and the Public Interest* (New Haven, Yale University Press, 1971).

Taylor, Stephen, *Good General Practice* (London, Oxford University Press, 1954).

Warner, John Harley, *The Therapeutic Perspective: Medical Practice, Knowledge, and Identity in America, 1820–1885* (Cambridge, MA, Harvard University Press, 1986).

Medical Science (Chapter 5)

Booth, Christopher, *Doctors in Science and Society: Essays of a Clinical Scientist* (London, British Medical Journal, 1987).

Brock, Thomas D., *Robert Koch: A Life in Medicine and Bacteriology* (Madison, WI, Science Tech Publishers, 1988).

Bulloch, William, *The History of Bacteriology: University of London. Heath Clark Lectures, 1936* (London, Oxford University Press, 1938); reprinted in 1960 (New York, Dover, 1979).

Further Reading

Bynum, W. F., *Science and the Practice of Medicine in the Nineteenth Century* (Cambridge, Cambridge University Press, 1994).

Bynum, W. F., and Porter, Roy (eds.), *Companion Encyclopedia of the History of Medicine* (London, Routledge, 1993). Various chapters offer the best up-to-date short summaries of particular dimensions of medical science.

Coleman, William, and Holmes, Frederic L. (eds.), *The Investigative Enterprise: Experimental Physiology in Nineteenth-Century Medicine* (Berkeley, Los Angeles, and London, University of California Press, 1988).

Cunningham, George J., *The History of British Pathology* (Bristol, White Tree Books, 1992).

Foster, W. D., *A Short History of Clinical Pathology* (Edinburgh, Livingstone, 1961).

Foster, W. D., *A History of Medical Bacteriology and Immunology* (London, Heinemann, 1970).

Frank, Robert G., *Harvey and the Oxford Physiologists: Scientific Ideas and Social Interaction* (Berkeley, University of California Press, 1980).

Fye, W. Bruce, *The Development of American Physiology: Scientific Medicine in the Nineteenth Century* (Baltimore, Johns Hopkins University Press, 1987).

Goodfield, June G., *The Growth of Scientific Physiology* (London, Hutchinson, 1960).

Hall, Thomas S., *Ideas of Life and Matter: Studies in the History of General Physiology 600 B.C. to 1900 A.D.*, 2 vols (Chicago, University of Chicago Press, 1969).

Harvey, William, *An Anatomical Disputation Concerning the Movement of the Heart and Blood in Living Creatures*, transl. by G. Whitteridge (Oxford, Blackwell Scientific, 1976).

Long, E. R., *A History of Pathology* (New York, Dover Publications, 1965).

Maulitz, Russell C., *Morbid Appearances: The Anatomy of Pathology in the Early Nineteenth Century* (Cambridge and New York, Cambridge University Press, 1987).

Roberts, K. B., *The Fabric of the Body: European Traditions of Anatomical Illustration* (Oxford and New York, Clarendon Press, 1992).

Rothschuh, Karl E., *History of Physiology* (original German edn, 1953); edited and transl. by G. B. Risse (Huntington, NY, Robert E. Krieger, 1973).

Singer, C., and Underwood, E. Ashworth, *A Short History of Medicine* (New York and Oxford, Oxford University Press, 1962).

Further Reading

Hospitals and Surgery (Chapter 6)

Abel-Smith, B., *The Hospitals 1500–1848: A Study in Social Administration in England and Wales* (London, Heinemann, 1964).

Ackerknecht, Erwin H., *Medicine at the Paris Hospital, 1794–1848* (Baltimore, Johns Hopkins University Press, 1967).

Cartwright, F. F., *The Development of Modern Surgery* (London, Arthur Barker; New York, Thomas Y. Crowell, 1967).

Dally, Ann, *Women Under the Knife; A History of Surgery* (London, Hutchinson Radius, 1991; New York, Routledge, 1992).

Freidson, Eliot (ed.), *The Hospital in Modern Society* (London, Collier and MacMillan, 1963).

Gelfand, Toby, *Professionalizing Modern Medicine: Paris Surgeons and Medical Science and Institutions in the 18th Century* (Westport, CT, Greenwood Press, 1980).

Granshaw, Lindsay, *St. Mark's Hospital, London: A Social History of a Specialist Hospital* (London, King's Fund, 1985).

Granshaw, Lindsay, and Porter, Roy (eds.), *The Hospital in History* (London, Routledge, 1989; paperback edition, 1990).

Granshaw, Lindsay, 'The hospital', in W. F. Bynum and Roy Porter (eds.), *Companion Encyclopedia of the History of Medicine* (London, Routledge, 1993), pp. 1173–95.

Haeger, Knut, *The Illustrated History of Surgery* (New York, Bell, 1988).

Hunt, Tony, *The Medieval Surgery* (Woodbridge, Sussex, Boydell Press, 1992).

Hurwitz, Alfred, and Degenshein, George A., *Milestones in Modern Surgery* (New York, Hoeber-Harper, 1958).

Jones, Colin, *The Charitable Imperative: Hospitals and Nursing in Ancien Régime and Revolutionary France*, Wellcome Institute Series in the History of Medicine (London and New York, Routledge, 1989).

Lawrence, Christopher (ed.), *Medical Theory, Surgical Practice: Studies in the History of Surgery* (London and New York, Routledge, 1992).

Lawrence, Ghislaine, 'Surgery (traditional)', in W. F. Bynum and Roy Porter (eds.), *Companion Encyclopedia of the History of Medicine* (London, Routledge, 1993), pp. 957–79.

Nightingale, Florence, *Notes on Hospitals* (London, John W. Parker & Son, 1859).

Pickstone, John, *Medicine and Industrial Society: A History of Hospital Development in Manchester and Its Region 1752–1946* (Manchester, Manchester University Press, 1985).

Further Reading

Pouchelle, Marie-Christine, *The Body and Surgery in the Middle Ages*, transl. by Rosemary Morris (New Brunswick, Rutgers University Press, 1990).

Poynter, F. N. L. (ed.), *The Evolution of Hospitals in Britain* (London, Pitman, 1964).

Ravitch, Mark M., *A Century of Surgery: 1880–1980*, 2 vols (Philadelphia, J. B. Lipincott, 1982).

Risse, Guenter, *Hospital Life in Enlightenment Scotland: Care and Teaching at the Royal Infirmary of Edinburgh* (Cambridge, Cambridge University Press, 1986).

Rosenberg, Charles E., *The Care of Strangers: The Rise of America's Hospital System* (New York, Basic Books, 1987).

Stevens, Rosemary, *In Sickness and in Wealth: American Hospitals in the Twentieth Century* (New York, Basic Books, 1989).

Taylor, Jeremy R. B., *Hospital and Asylum Architecture in England 1840–1914: Building for Health Care* (London and New York, Mansell, 1991).

Thompson, J. D., and Goldin, G., *The Hospital: A Social and Architectural History* (New Haven and London, Yale University Press, 1975).

Tröhler, Ulrich, 'Surgery (modern)', in W. F. Bynum and Roy Porter (eds.), *Companion Encyclopedia of the History of Medicine* (London, Routledge, 1993), pp. 980–1023.

Wallace, Anthony F., *The Progress of Plastic Surgery: An Introductory History* (Oxford, William A. Meeuws, 1982).

Wangensteen, Owen H., and Wangensteen, Sarah D., *The Rise of Surgery: From Empiric Craft to Scientific Discipline* (Minneapolis, University of Minnesota Press, 1978; Folkestone, Kent, Dawson, 1978).

Woodward, J., *To Do the Sick No Harm: A Study of the British Voluntary Hospital System to 1875* (London and Boston, Routledge & Kegan Paul, 1974).

Drug Treatment and the Rise of Pharmacology
(Chapter 7)

Binden, J. S., and Ledniger, D. (eds.), *Chronicles of Drug Discovery* (New York, Wiley, 1982).

Bliss, M., *The Discovery of Insulin* (Toronto, McClelland & Stewart, 1982).

Blunt, Wilfrid, and Raphael, Sandra, *The Illustrated Herbal* (London, Francis Lincoln/Weidenfeld & Nicolson, n.d.).

Holmstedt, B., and Liljestrand, G., *Readings in Pharmacology* (Oxford, Pergamon Press, 1963).

Pagel, W., *Paracelsus: An Introduction to Philosophical Medicine in the Era of the Renaissance*, 2nd rev. edn (Basel, Karger, 1982).

Further Reading

Parascandola, J., *The Development of American Pharmacology: John J. Abel and the Shaping of a Discipline* (Baltimore and London, Johns Hopkins University Press, 1992).

Ross, W. S., *The Life/Death Ratio: Benefits and Risks in Modern Medicines* (New York, Reader's Digest Press, 1977).

Sneader, W., *Drug Discovery: The Evaluation of Modern Medicines* (Chichester, Wiley, 1985).

Weatherall, M., *In Search of a Cure: A History of Pharmaceutical Discovery* (Oxford, Oxford University Press, Oxford, 1990).

Mental Illness (Chapter 8)

Alexander, Franz G., and Selesnick, Sheldon T., *The History of Psychiatry: An Evaluation of Psychiatric Thought and Practice from Prehistoric Times to the Present* (London, Allen & Unwin, 1967).

Barham, Peter, *Closing the Asylum: The Mental Patient in Modern Society* (Harmondsworth, Penguin, 1992).

Feder, L., *Madness in Literature* (Princeton, Princeton University Press, 1980).

Foucault, Michel, *La Folie et la Déraison: Histoire de la Folie à l'Age Classique* (Paris, Librairie Plon, 1961); abridged as *Madness and Civilization: A History of Insanity in the Age of Reason*, transl. by Richard Howard (New York, Random House, 1965).

Howells, John (ed.), *World History of Psychiatry* (New York, Bruner/Mazel, 1968).

Howells, John G., and Osborn, M. Livia, *A Reference Companion to the History of Abnormal Psychology* (Westport, CT, Greenwood Press, 1984).

Hunter, Richard, and Macalpine, Ida, *Three Hundred Years of Psychiatry: 1535–1860* (London, Oxford University Press, 1963).

Ingleby, David (ed.), *Critical Psychiatry: The Politics of Mental Health* (Harmondsworth, Penguin, 1981).

Laing, R. D., *The Divided Self* (New York, Random House, 1969).

Peterson, D. (ed.), *A Mad People's History of Madness* (Pittsburgh, University of Pittsburgh Press, 1982).

Porter, Roy, *Mind Forg'd Manacles: Madness and Psychiatry in England from Restoration to Regency* (London, Athlone Press, 1987; paperback edition, Penguin, 1990).

Porter, Roy, *A Social History of Madness* (London, Weidenfeld & Nicolson, 1987; paperback edition, 1989).

Porter, Roy; *The Faber Book of Madness* (London, Faber, 1991).

Further Reading

Scheff, Thomas, *Being Mentally Ill: A Sociological Theory* (Chicago, Aldine Press, 1966).

Scull, Andrew, *The Most Solitary of Afflictions: Madness and Society in Britain, 1700–1900* (New Haven and London, Yale University Press, 1993).

Scull, Andrew, *Decarceration: Community Treatment and the Deviant – A Radical View*, 2nd edn (Oxford, Polity Press; New Brunswick, Rutgers University Press, 1984).

Sedgwick, Peter, *Psychopolitics* (London, Pluto Press; New York, Harper and Row, 1982).

Simon, Bennett, *Mind and Madness in Ancient Greece* (Ithaca, Cornell University Press, 1978).

Skultans, V., *Madness and Morals: Ideas on Insanity in the Nineteenth Century* (London and Boston, Routledge and Kegan Paul, 1975).

Szasz, Thomas S., *The Manufacture of Madness* (New York, Dell, 1970; London, Paladin, 1972).

Szasz, Thomas S., *The Myth of Mental Illness: Foundations of a Theory of Personal Conduct* (London, Granada, 1972; rev. edn, New York, Harper and Row, 1974).

Szasz, Thomas S., *The Age of Madness: The History of Involuntary Mental Hospitalization Presented in Selected Texts* (London, Routledge and Kegan Paul, 1975).

Medicine, Society, and the State (Chapter 9)

Fox, Daniel, *Health Policies, Health Economics: The British and American Experiences, 1911–1965* (Princeton, Princeton University Press, 1986).

Hollingsworth, J. Rogers, *A Political Economy of Medicine: Great Britain and the United States* (Baltimore, Johns Hopkins University Press, 1986).

Hollingsworth, J. Rogers, Haget, Jerald, and Hanneman, Robert A., *State Intervention in Medical Care: Consequences for Britain, France, Sweden and the United States, 1890–1970* (Ithaca, Cornell University Press, 1986).

Klein, Rudolf, *The Politics of the NHS* (London, Longman, 1983).

Rosen, George, *A History of Public Health* (New York, MD Publications, 1986).

Rosenberg, Charles E., *The Care of Strangers: The Rise of America's Hospital System* (New York, Basic Books, 1987).

Starr, Paul, *The Social Transformation of American Medicine: The Rise of a Sovereign Profession and the Making of a Vast Industry* (New York, Basic Books, 1982).

Further Reading

Stevens, Rosemary, *Medical Practice in Modern England: The Impact of Specialization and State Medicine* (New Haven, Yale University Press, 1966).

Stevens, Rosemary, *In Sickness and in Wealth: American Hospitals in the Twentieth Century* (New York, Basic Books, 1989).

Looking to the Future (Chapter 10)

Austyn, J. M. (ed.), *New Prospects for Medicine* (Oxford, Oxford University Press, 1988).

Helman, C., *Culture, Health and Illness* (Bristol, Wright, 1984).

Illich, I., *Limits to Medicine: The Exploration of Health* (London, Marion Boyars, 1976; paperback edn, Penguin, 1977).

Kennedy, I., *The Unmasking of Medicine* (London, Allen & Unwin, 1981).

McKeown, T., *The Role of Medicine* (Oxford, Blackwell, 1979).

Pietroni, P., *The Greening of Medicine* (London, Gollancz, 1990).

Wilkie, T., *Perilous Knowledge* (London, Faber, 1993).

Index of Medical Personalities

Abel, John Jacob, 1857–1938, American biochemist and pharmacologist, 354

Addison, Thomas, 1793–1860, English physician and medical teacher, 109, 156, 351

Aikin, John, 1747–1822, English physician and writer, 187

Albertus Magnus, St (Count of Bollstädt), c. 1200–1280, German philosopher, theologian, and scientist, 344

Albucasis *see* al-Zahrawi

Alderotti, Taddeo, d. 1295, Italian physician and teacher, 66

Allbutt, (Sir) Thomas Clifford, 1836–1925, English physician, 352

Amyand, Claudius, 1681/6–1740, French surgeon, 347

Aristotle, 384–322 BC, Greek philosopher and naturalist, 52, 53, 55, 57, 63, 80, 90, 239, 244, 343

Arnald of Villanova, 1240?–1311, French physician and teacher, 66

Aselli, Gasparo, 1581–1625, Italian physician and anatomist, 138

Attlee, John, 19th century, English surgeon, 197

Auenbrugger, Leopold, 1722–1809, Austrian physician, 148, 348

Averroës *see* Ibn Rushd

Avicenna *see* Ibn Sina

Baillie, Matthew, 1761–1823, Scottish physician and anatomist, 152, 349

Banting, (Sir) Frederick Grant, 1891–1941, Canadian physiologist, 225, 354

Barker, Lewellys F., 1867–1943, American physician, 125

Barnard, Christiaan Neethling, 1922–, South African surgeon, 2, 356

Battey, Robert, 1828–95, English surgeon, 197

Battie, William, 1704–76, English physician, 185

Bayle, Gaspard-Laurent, 1774–1816, French physician, 154, 155

Bayliss, (Sir) William Maddock, 1860–1924, English physiologist, 168, 353

Beaulieu, Jacques de (Frère Jacques), 1651–1714, French 'stone-cutter', 191

Becquerel, Antoine Henri, 1852–1908, French physicist, 207, 353

Beddoes, Thomas, 1760–1808, English physician and chemist, 92, 150, 188, 198, 349

Behring, Emil Adolf von, 1854–1917, German bacteriologist, 119, 166, 167, 223, 352

Bernard, Claude, 1813–78, French physiologist, 160, 161, 168, 219, 220, 223, 277

Best, Charles Herbert, 1899–1978, Canadian physiologist, 225, 354

Bevis, Douglas Charles Aitchison, 20th century, English physician, 355

Bichat, Marie-François-Xavier, 1771–1802, French pathologist, 152, 153, 160, 192, 349

Bigelow, Jacob, 1786–1879, American physician and botanist, 122

Billroth, Theodor, 1829–94, Austrian surgeon, 200

Black, Joseph, 1728–99, Scottish chemist and physicist, 147, 148

Blackwell, Elizabeth, 1821–1910, English-born American physician, 351

Blalock, Alfred, 1899–1964, American cardiac surgeon, 204, 355

Blane, (Sir) Gilbert, 1749–1834, Scottish physician, 349

Bleuler, Eugen, 1857–1939, Swiss psychiatrist, 256

Boerhaave, Herman, 1668–1738, Dutch physician, 103, 107, 108, 143, 144, 145, 146, 156, 347

Bois-Reymond, Emil Heinrich du, 1818–96, German physiologist, 158, 159, 226

Bonet, Théophile, 1620–89, French anatomist, 151

Bordeu, Théophile de, 1722–76, French physician, 147

Borelli, Giovanni Alfonso, 1608–79, Italian physicist and physiologist, 141

Bostok, Bridget, 18th century, English healer, 76

Bovet, Daniel, 1907–92, Swiss-born Italian pharmacologist, 355

Boyle, Robert, 1627–91, Irish-born British physicist and chemist, 81, 141, 149, 346

Bretonneau, Pierre, 1778–1862, French physician, 350

Bright, Richard, 1789–1858, English physician, 156, 350

Brock, Russell Claude (1st Baron Brock), 1903–80, English surgeon, 204

Broun, Gustav, b. 1829, German physician, 90

Brown, John, c. 1735–88, Scottish physician, 86, 146

Brücke, Ernst Wilhelm von, 1819–92, German physician and physiologist, 158, 159

Brunton, (Sir) Thomas Lauder, 1844–1916, Scottish physician, 119

Buchan, William, 1729–1805, Scottish physician, 104

Buchheim, Rudolph, 1828–79, German physician and pharmacologist, 220

Burnet, (Sir) Frank Macfarlane, 1899–1985, Australian physician and virologist, 301

Burns, John, 1774–1850, Scottish surgeon

Calmette, Albert, 1863–1933, French bacteriologist, 354

Cammann, George P., 1804–63, American physician, 153

Cannon, Walter Bradford, 1871–1945, American physiologist, 161, 170, 227

Carrel, Alexis, 1873–1944, French-born American surgeon and botanist, 201, 202, 354

Cathell, Daniel, 1839–1925, American physician, 109, 110, 115, 125, 128

Caventou, Joseph-Bienaimé, 1795–1877, French pharmacist, 218, 220

Celsus, Aulus Cornelius, 25 BC–AD 50, Roman philosopher and writer, 54, 178, 213, 343

Cerletti, Ugo, 1877–1963, Italian psychiatrist, 355

Chadwick, (Sir) Edwin, 1800–90, English social reformer, 351

Chain, (Sir) Ernst Boris, 1906–79, German-born British biochemist, 355

Index of Medical Personalities

Chamberlen, Peter, 1560–1631, English midwife, 346

Charcot, Jean-Martin, 1825–93, French pathologist and neurologist, 352

Charnley, (Sir) John, 1911–82, English orthopaedic surgeon, 206

Cheselden, William, 1688–1752, English surgeon, 143, 187, 191, 347

Cheyne, (Sir) William Watson, 1852–1932, English surgeon, 200

Chiarugi, Vincenzio, 1759–1820, Italian psychiatrist, 251

Christison, (Sir) Robert, 1797–1882, Scottish pharmacologist, 220

Clarke, William E., 19th century, American dentist, 198

Clay, Charles, 1801–93, English surgeon, 197

Clift, William, 1775–1849, English osteologist and medical draughtsman, 152

Collings, Joseph S., 1866–1950, English physician, 126

Collip, James Bertram, 1892–1965, Canadian biochemist, 225

Colombo, Realdo, c. 1516–c. 1559, Italian anatomist, 140, 346

Comroe, Julius Hiram, 1911–, American physiologist, 323, 324

Constantine the African, c. 1020–87, Latin scholar and translator, 63

Cooper, (Sir) Astley Paston, 1768–1841, English surgeon, 196, 197

Cormack, Allan Macleod, 1924–, South African–born American physicist, 208

Crick, Francis Harry Compton, 1916–, English molecular biologist, 2, 171, 355

Crile, George Washington, 1864–1943, American surgeon and physiologist, 353

Crookes, (Sir) William, 1832–1919, English chemist and physicist, 207

Crowther, Bryan, 19th century, English prison surgeon, 253

Cullen, William, 1710–90, Scottish physician, 146

Curie, Marie (was Marya Sklodowska), 1867–1934, Polish-born French physicist, 207, 208, 353

Curie, Pierre, 1859–1906, French physical chemist, 207, 353

Cushing, Harvey Williams, 1869–1939, American neurosurgeon and physiologist, 169, 202, 354

Dale, (Sir) Henry Hallett, 1875–1968, English physiologist and pharmacologist, 170, 227, 354

Daviel, Jacques, 1696–1762, French oculist, 192

Davy, (Sir) Humphry, 1778–1829, English chemist and science popularizer, 198, 222, 349

Desault, Pierre-Joseph, 1738–95, French surgeon and anatomist, 192, 193

Descartes, René, 1596–1650, French philospher and mathematician, 80, 81, 141, 143, 147, 169, 244, 250, 346

Dietl, Joseph, 1804–78, Austrian physician, 121

Diocles, 4th century BC, Greek physician and anatomist, 52

Dionis, Pierre, 1643–1718, French surgeon, 193

Dioscorides, Pedanius, c. 40–c. 90, Greek physician, 54, 198, 212, 343, 344

Djerassi, Carl, 1923–, Austrian-born American organic chemist, 226

Dobson, Matthew, d. 1784, English physician and anatomist, 150, 349

Dodds, (Sir) Edward Charles, 1899–1973, English physician and biochemist, 355

Doll, (Sir) William Richard Shaboe, 1912–, English cancer researcher and epidemiologist, 175

Domagk, Gerhard, 1895–1964, German bacteriologist and pathologist, 133, 229, 354

Donald, Ian, 1910–87, Scottish obstetrician, 356

Douglass, William, c. 1691–1752, American physician, 109, 347

Dover, Thomas, 1660–1742, English physician, 120, 217

Drinker, Philip, active 20th century, American bioengineer, 354

Dripps, Robert, 1911–73, American medical scientist, 323, 324

Dudley, Harold W., 1887–1935, English pharmacologist, 354

Dupuytren, Guillaume (Baron), 1777–1835, French surgeon and anatomist, 196

Edwards, Robert Geoffrey, 1925–, English reproductive biologist, 206, 356

Ehrlich, Paul, 1854–1915, German medical scientist, 166, 167, 223, 224, 229, 353

Eijkman, Christiaan, 1858–1930, Dutch physician and pathologist, 168

Einthoven, Willem, 1860–1927, Dutch physiologist, 208, 324, 353

Elion, Gertrude Belle, 1919–, American pharmacologist, 232

Ellis, Henry Havelock, 1859–1939, English physician and writer on sex, 353

Elmqvist, Dan Rune, 1935–, Swedish medical engineer, 203

Epicurus, 341–271 BC, Greek philosopher, 74

Erasistratus (of Ceos), active c. 280 BC, Greek physician and anatomist, 52

Erichsen, (Sir) John Eric, 1818–96, English surgeon, 200

Euler, Ulf Svante von, 1905–83, Swedish neurophysiologist, 227

Eustachio, Bartolommeo, 1520–74, Italian anatomist, 138

Fabrizio (or Fabrici), Girolamo (Hieronymus Fabricius ab Acquapendente), 1537–1619, Italian anatomist, 138, 140, 346

Fahrenheit, Gabriel David, 1686–1736, German physicist, 347

Falloppio, Gabriele (Fallopius), 1523–62, Italian anatomist, 138

Farrar, Clarence B., 1874–1970, American psychiatrist, 124

Fauchard, Pierre, 1678–1761, French dentist, 347

Favaloro, Rene, 20th century, American cardiovascular surgeon, 356

Félix, Charles-François, 1635–1703, French surgeon, 193

Ferrier, (Sir) David, 1843–1928, Scottish neurologist, 170

Finlay, Carlos Juan, 1833–1915, Cuban physician and epidemiologist, 164, 165

Finsen, Niels Ryberg, 1860–1904, Danish physician and medical scientist, 207

Fleming, (Sir) Alexander, 1881–1955, Scottish bacteriologist, 354

Flexner, Abraham, 1866–1958, American medical educationalist, 172

Flexner, Simon, 1863–1946, American microbiologist, 172

Florey, Howard Walter (1st Baron Florey), 1898–1968, Australian experimental pathologist, 355

Floyer, (Sir) John, 1649–1734, English physician, 347

Fontanon, Denys, 15th/16th century, French physician, 243

Forlanini, Carlo, 1847–1918, Italian medical scientist, 201

Forssmann, Werner Theodor Otto, 1904–79, German physician, 354

Foster, (Sir) Michael, 1836–1907, English physiologist, 163

Fothergill, John, 1712–80, English physician, 150, 348, 349

Fracastoro, Girolamo (Fracastorius), c. 1483–1553, Italian physician, 87, 345

Freud, Sigmund, 1856–1939, Austrian neurologist and psychoanalyst, 146, 159, 239, 250, 257, 353, 354

Funk, Casimir, 1884–1967, Polish-born American biochemist, 227, 228, 354

Galen of Pergamum, 129–216, Greek physician, anatomist, and physiologist, 54, 80, 103, 343

Gallo, Robert C., 1937–, American virologist, 324

Galvani, Luigi, 1737–98, Italian anatomist and electrophysiologist, 226, 323, 349

Garrod, (Sir) Archibald Edward, 1857–1936, English physician, 171, 353

Gaskell, Walter Holbrook, 1847–1914, English physiologist, 163, 354

Gerard of Cremona, c. 1114–87, Italian scholar, 63, 344

Gibbon, John H. Jr, 1903–73, American surgeon, 355

Gillies, (Sir) Harold Delf, 1882–1960, New Zealand plastic surgeon, 205

Gilman, Alfred, 1908–84, American pharmacologist, 232

Glisson, Francis, c. 1597–1677, English physician and anatomist, 145, 346

Goldberger, Joseph, 1874–1929, Hungarian-born American physician and epidemiologist, 168

Goodman, Louis Sanford, 1906–, American pharmacologist, 232

Graaf, Regnier de, 1641–73, Dutch physician and anatomist, 138, 347

Graham, Evarts Ambrose, 1883–1957, American surgeon, 355

Grassi, Giovanni Battista, 1854–1925, Italian parasitologist, 165

Gray, Alfred L., 1873–1932, American radiologist, 204

Greatrakes (or Greatorex), Valentine, 1629–83, Irish healer, 76

Gregg, (Sir) Norman McAlister, 1892–1966, Australian ophthalmologist, 355

Guérin, Camille, 1872–1961, French bacteriologist, 354

Guy de Chauliac, c. 1300–68, French surgeon, 178, 345

Haffkine, Waldemar Mordecai Wolfe, 1860–1930, Russian-born British bacteriologist, 167

Hahnemann, Christian Friedrich Samuel, 1755–1843, German founder of homeopathy, 349

Haldane, John Scott, 1860–1936, Scottish physiologist, 353

Hales, (Revd) Stephen, 1677–1761, English clergyman, physiologist, and inventor, 157, 347

Haller, Albrecht von, 1708–77, Swiss physiologist, anatomist, and botanist, 145, 146, 147, 348

Halsted, William Stewart, 1852–1922, American surgeon, 199, 200, 352

Haly Abbas *see* al-Majusi

Harvey, William, 1578–1657, English physician and anatomist, 81, 139, 140, 141, 142, 145, 214, 346

Haygarth, John, 1740–1827, English physician, 150

Heberden, William, 1710–1801, English physician, 148

Helmholtz, Hermann von, 1821–94, German physiologist and physicist, 158, 351

Helmont, Johannes (Jean or Jan) Baptiste (or Baptista) van, c. 1579–1644, Flemish chemist and physiologist, 142, 144, 346

Hench, Philip Showalter, 1896–1965, American physician, 355

Henle, Fredrich Gustav Jakob, 1809–85, German pathologist and anatomist, 350

Herophilus, fl. 300 BC, Greek anatomist and surgeon, 52

Herrick, James B., 1861–1954, American physician, 107

Herringham, (Sir) Wilmot Parker, 1855–1936, English physician, 127

Hertzler, Arthur E., 1870–1946, American physician, 106, 115, 117, 122

Hill, (Sir) Austin Bradford, 1897–1991, English epidemiologist, 174, 175, 234, 354

Hippocrates (of Cos), b. c. 460 BC, Greek physician, the 'father of medicine', 78, 212, 343

Hitchings, George Herbert, 1905–, American pharmacologist, 202, 232

Hobbes, Thomas, 1588–1679, English philosopher, 80

Hodgkin, George Keith Howard, active 20th century, English physician, 131

Hodgkin, Thomas, 1798–1866, English physician and pathologist, 155

Hoffmann, Friedrich, 1660–1742, German physician, 144

Holmes Sellors, Thomas, 1902–87, English surgeon, 204

Holmes, Oliver Wendell, 1809–94, American physician and writer, 122, 197

Hooke, Robert, 1635–1703, English physicist, 140

Hopkins, (Sir) Frederick Gowland, 1861–1947, English biochemist, 168, 353

Hounsfield, (Sir) Godfrey Newbold, 1919–, British electrical engineer, 208

Houston, William R., b. 1873, American physician, 125

Howard, John, 1726–90, English prison reformer, 189, 265

Hufeland, Christoph Wilhelm, 1762–1836, German physician, 124, 349

Huggins, Charles Brenton, 1901–, Canadian-born American surgeon, 204

Hunain ibn Ishaq (Johannitius), 808–73, Arab physician, 58, 63, 344

Hunter, John, 1728–93, Scottish anatomist and surgeon, 147, 196, 348

Hunter, William, 1718–83, Scottish anatomist and obstetrician, 152, 348

Huntington, George, 1850–1916, American physician, 172

Huxham, John, 1692–1768, English physician, 149

Ibn an-Nafis, d. 1288, Syrian physician, 59, 344

Ibn Hayyan, Jabir see Jabir ibn Hayyan, Abu Musa

Ibn Ishaq, Hunain see Hunain ibn Ishaq (Johannitius)

Ibn Ridwan, Ali, 11th century, Islamic physician, 59

Ibn Rushd (Averroës), 1126–98, Arab physician, philosopher, and astronomer, 59

Ibn Sina (Avicenna), 980–1037, Islamic physician and philosopher, 59, 63, 64, 178, 213, 344

Jabir ibn Hayyan, Abu Musa, c. 721–c. 815, Arab alchemist and physician, 213

Jenner, Edward, 1749–1823, English physician, 33, 231, 271, 349

Jex-Blake, Sophia Louisa, 1840–1912, English physician and pioneer of medical education for women, 352

Johannitius see Hunain ibn Ishaq

Johnston, William Victor, 1897–1976, Canadian physician, 118, 119

Jones, Warren, 1938–, Australian medical geneticist, 306

Jorden, Edward, 1569–1632, English physician and chemist, 77, 78

Jung, Carl Gustav, 1875–1961, Swiss psychiatrist, 354

Kay, Richard, active 1716–51, English physician, 105, 106, 364

al-Kindi, c. 800–c. 870, Arab philosopher, 63

King, Maurice, 1927–, English epidemiologist, 49, 312, 314

Kitasato, Shibasaburo, 1852–1931, Japanese bacteriologist, 119, 167, 352

Koch, Robert, 1843–1910, German physicist and bacteriologist, 82, 86, 119, 165, 166, 199, 222, 223, 263, 280, 352

Kocher, Emil Theodor, 1841–1917, Swiss surgeon, 201

Kraepelin, Emil, 1856–1926, German psychiatrist, 256

Krafft-Ebing, Richard von (Freiherr), 1840–1902, German psychiatrist, 256

Kühne, Wilhelm, 1837–1900, German physiologist, 167

Kussmaul, Adolf, 1822–1902, German physician, 104, 105, 124

Laënnec, René-Théophile-Hyacinthe, 1781–1826, French physician and medical teacher, 93, 153, 154, 155, 161

Laing, Ronald David, 1927–89, Scottish psychiatrist, 238

Lancisi, Giovanni Maria, 1654–1720, Italian physician, 347

Landsteiner, Karl, 1868–1943, Austrian-born American pathologist, 353, 355

Lane, (Sir) William Arbuthnot, 1856–1943, Irish-born English surgeon, 202

Langley, John Newport, 1852–1925, English physiologist, 163

Larrey, Dominique-Jean (Baron), 1766–1842, French military surgeon, 190, 196

Laveran, Charles-Louise-Alphonse, 1845–1922, French physician and microbiologist, 352

Lavoisier, Antoine-Laurent, 1743–94, French chemist and social reformer, 148, 217, 218, 219, 349

Leeuwenhoek, Antoni van, 1632–1723, Dutch microscopist, 140

Lettsom, John Coakley, 1744–1815, English physician, 150

Lewis, (Sir) Thomas, 1881–1945, Welsh cardiologist and clinical scientist, 116, 173, 174

Liebig, Justus von (Freiherr), 1803–73, German organic chemist, 157, 158, 160, 167, 350

Lillehei, Clarence Walton, 1918–, American thoracic and cardiovascular surgeon, 356

Linacre, Thomas, 1460?–1524, English physician and classical scholar, 345

Lind, James, 1716–94, Scottish naval physician, 167, 217, 227, 234, 348

Lister, Joseph (1st Baron Lister), 1827–1912, English surgeon and bacteriologist, 199, 200, 227, 352

Liston, Robert, 1794–1847, Scottish surgeon, 197, 198

Lizars, John, 1787?–1860, Scottish surgeon, 197

Loewi, Otto, 1873–1961, German-born American pharmacologist, 170, 227

Louis, Pierre-Charles-Alexandre, 1787–1872, French physician and pathologist, 2, 154, 155, 161, 195, 217, 350

Lower, Richard, 1631–91, English physician and physiologist, 140

Ludwig, Karl Friedrich Wilhelm, 1816–95, German physiologist, 158, 159, 277, 351

MacEwen, (Sir) William, 1848–1924, Scottish surgeon, 200

Mackenzie, (Sir) James, 1853–1925, Scottish cardiologist, 116, 121, 173

Macleod, John James Rickard, 1876–1935, Scottish-born Canadian physiologist, 225

Magendie, François, 1783–1855, French anatomist and physiologist, 160, 218, 219, 220

Maimonides see Moses ben Maimon al-Majusi (Haly Abbas), d. 994, Islamic physician, 59, 63

Malpighi, Marcello, 1628–94, Italian anatomist, 141, 143, 347

Manson, (Sir) Patrick, 1844–1922, Scottish physician and parasitologist, 164, 352, 353

Marey, Etienne-Jules, 1830–1904, French physiologist, 351

Martine, George, 1700?–41, Scottish surgeon, 347

Mathews, Joseph, 1847–1928, American physician, 120

Matteucci, Carlo, 1811–68, Italian physiologist, 323

McCollum, Elmer Verner, 1879–1967, American physiologist, 168

McDowell, Ephraim, 1771–1830, American surgeon, 197

Mesmer, Franz, 1734–1815, Austrian physician, 348

Metchnikoff, Elie (Ilya Ilich Mechnikov), 1845–1916, Russian zoologist and bacteriologist, 166, 223, 352, 353

Mondeville, Henri de, b. 1260, French surgeon, 178

Mondino dei Liuzzi, c. 1270–c. 1326, Italian anatomist, 344

Monro, Alexander, *primus*, 1697–1767, Scottish anatomist, 146, 194

Montagnier, Luc, 1932–, French virologist, 324

Morgagni, Giovanni Battista, 1682–1771, Italian physician and anatomist, 151, 152

Morgan, John, 1735–89, American physician, 348

Morison, James, 1770–1840, English drug merchant, 99, 100, 364

Morton, William Thomas Green, 1819–68, American dentist, 198, 351

Moses ben Maimon (Maimonides), 1135–1204, Hispano-Jewish physician and philosopher, 59

Müller, Johannes Peter, 1801–58, German physiologist and comparative anatomist, 158, 159, 160

Murphy, John Benjamin, 1857–1916, American surgeon, 353

Murray, George, 1865–1939, English physician, 224

Murrell, William B., active 19th century, English physician, 119

Naunyn, Bernhard, 1839–1925, German physician, 122, 129

Niccolò da Reggio, active 1305–48, Graeco-Italian scholar, 63

Nightingale, Florence, 1820–1910, English nurse and hospital reformer, 276

Nothnagel, Hermann, 1841–1905, Austrian physician, 123, 124, 126

Oribasius, 325–403, Greek physician, 54

Osler, (Sir) William, 1849–1919, Canadian physician, 10, 122, 124, 125, 219, 352

Palfyn, Jean, 1650–1730, Flemish surgeon, 347

Paracelsus (Philippus Aureolus Theophrastus Bombastus von Honenheim), 1493–1541, Swiss alchemist and physician, 142, 213, 345

Paré, Ambroise, c. 1510–90, French surgeon, 138, 179, 180, 192

Parkinson, James, 1755–1824, English physician, 350

Pasteur, Louis, 1822–95, French chemist and microbiologist, 160, 165, 166, 199, 222, 263, 280, 323, 351, 352, 353

Patin, Gui, 1601–72, French physician, 142

Paul of Aegina (Paulus Aegineta), c. 625–c. 690, Greek physician,

Peabody, Francis Weld, 1881–1927, American physician, 125

Pelletier, Pierre-Joseph, 1788–1842, French pharmacist, 218, 220

Pereira, Jonathan, 1804–53, English physician and chemist, 220

Index of Medical Personalities

Perkin, (Sir) William Henry, 1838–1907, English chemist, 221, 351

Petit, Jean-Louis, 1674–1750, French military surgeon, 192

Pfaff, Philipp, active 18th century, German dentist, 348

Pincus, Gregory Goodwin, 1903–67, American experimental biologist, 226

Pinel, Philippe, 1745–1826, French physician and psychiatrist, 195, 251, 252, 349

Plater, Felix, 1536–1614, Swiss pathologist, 243

Plato, c. 427–347 BC, Greek philosopher, 50

Pott, Percivall, 1714–88, English surgeon, 42, 192, 348

Praxagoras of Cos, active c. 310 BC, Greek physician, 52, 343

Prout, William, 1785–1850, English chemist and physiologist, 350

Pylarini, Giocomo, active early 18th century, Italian physician, 347

Quick, Armand James, 1894–1973, American haematologist, 354

Rau, Johannes, 1668–1719, Dutch surgeon, 191

ar-Razi, Abu Bakr (Rhazes), c. 864–c. 935, Persian physician and alchemist, 59, 344

Réaumur, René-Antoine Ferchault de, 1683–1757, French naturalist and physician, 145, 147, 348

Reid, (Sir) James, 1849–1923, English physician, 84

Reil, Johann Christian, 1759–1813, German physician and psychiatrist, 251

Reverdin, Jacques-L., 1842–1908, French surgeon, 205, 352

Rhazes see ar-Razi

Riva-Rocci, Scipione, 1863–1937, Italian physician, 353

Rivington, Walter, 1835–97, English surgeon, 126, 127

Robinson, George Canby, 1878–1960, American physician, 125

Robiquet, Pierre-Jean, 1780–1840, French chemist, 350

Rokitanski, Carl von (Frieherr), 1804–78, Austrian pathologist, 156

Röntgen, Wilhelm Konrad von, 1845–1923, German physicist, 207, 323, 353

Ross, (Sir) Ronald, 1857–1932, British physician and parasitologist, 165, 173, 281, 353

Roux, Pierre-Paul-Emile, 1853–1933, French physician and parasitologist, 166

Rufus of Ephesus, 1st century BC–1st century AD, Greek anatomist and physician, 54

Ruleau, Jean, active c. 1700, French surgeon, 180

Rumford, Count see Thompson, (Sir) Benjamin

Rush, Benjamin, 1745–1813, American physician and politician, 90, 108, 349

Rutherford, John, 1695–1779, English physician, 187

Sabin, Albert Bruce, 1906–, Polish-born American microbiologist, 43, 356

Sachs, Barney, 1854–1944, American neurologist, 124

Salk, Jonas Edward, 1914–95, American virologist, 43

Sanger, Margaret Louise (née Higgins), 1883–1966, American social reformer and birth-control pioneer, 354

Sargant, William, 1907–88, English psychiatrist, 258

Sauerbruch, Ernst Ferdinand, 1875–1951, German surgeon, 201

Sauvages, François Boissier de, 1706–67, French physician, 146

Scarpa, Antonio, 1752–1832, Italian anatomist, 348

Schafer, (Sir) Edward see Sharpey-Schafer, Edward

Index of Medical Personalities

Schmiedeberg, Oswald, 1838–1921, German pharmacologist, 220

Schönlein, Johannes Lukas, 1793–1864, German physician, 350

Schwann, Theodor Ambroise Hubert, 1810–82, German physiologist, 158, 159, 350

Semmelweis, Ignaz Phillip, 1818–65, Hungarian obstetrician, 199, 351

Senning, Åke, 1915–, Swedish surgeon, 203

Sertürner, Friedrich Wilhelm Adam, 1783–1841, German chemist, 349

Servetus, Michael (Miguel Serveto), 1511–53, Spanish physician and theologian, 139, 345

Sharpey-Schafer, (Sir) Edward Albert, 1850–1935, English physiologist, 163, 169

Sherrington, (Sir) Charles Scott, 1857–1952, English neurophysiologist, 170, 353

Shippen, William, 1736–1808, American physician, 187

Simon, (Sir) John, 1816–1904, English pathologist and public-health reformer, 275

Simpson, (Sir) James Young, 1811–70, Scottish gynaecologist and obstetrician, 198, 351

Sims, James Marion, 1813–83, American surgeon, 197

Škoda, Josef, 1805–81, Austrian physician, 121

Smellie, William, 1697–1763, Scottish obstetrician, 348

Snow, John, 1813–58, English physician, anaesthetist, and epidemiologist, 222, 351

Soranus of Ephesus, fl. AD 110, Greek physician, 54, 178, 343

Souttar, (Sir) Henry Sessions, 1875–1964, English surgeon, 204

Spallanzani, Lazzaro, 1729–99, Italian physiologist, 348

Stahl, Georg Ernst, 1660–1734, German chemist and physician, 144, 146

Starling, Ernest Henry, 1866–1927, English physiologist, 168, 353

Starzl, Thomas E., 1926–, American transplant surgeon, 356

Steptoe, Patrick Christopher, 1913–88, English gynaecologist and obstetrician, 206, 356

Stern, Karl, 1906–75, German physician, 113, 114

Stoerck, Anton, 1731–1803, Austrian physician, 187

Stopes, Marie Charlotte Carmichael, 1880–1958, English birth-control pioneer, 354

Sutleffe, Edward, active early 19th century, English physician, 108

Sydenham, Thomas, 1624–89, English physician and epidemiologist, 148, 149, 150, 347

Sykes, William Stanley, 1894–1960, English physician, 131, 132

Sylvius, Franciscus (Franz de le Boë), 1614–72, German physician, anatomist, and chemist, 138, 142, 147

Szasz, Thomas Stephen, 1920–, Hungarian-born American psychiatrist, 238, 259

Szent-Györgyi, Albert von Nagyrapolt, 1893–1986, Hungarian-born American biochemist, 168, 354

Taussig, Helen Brooke, 1898–1986, American paediatrician, 204

Taylor, ('Chevalier') John, 1703–72, English physician and quack oculist, 192

Tenon, Jacques-René, 1724–1816, French surgeon, 189

Theiler, Max, 1899–1972, South African–born American physician and bacteriologist, 355

Thomas, Edward Donnall, 1920–, American surgeon, 46, 47

Thomas, Lewis, 1913–93, American physician and writer, 8

Index of Medical Personalities

Thompson, (Sir) Benjamin (Count Rumford), 1753–1814, Anglo-American adventurer, social reformer, and physicist, 267

Thomson, Samuel, 1769–1843, American health reformer and herbalist, 98

Trautman, Jeremiah, active early 17th century, German surgeon, 180

Trembley, Abraham, 1700–84, Swiss zoologist, 145

Treviranus, Gottfried Reinhold, 1776–1837, German biologist, 147

Tuttle, Ralph W., active 19th century, American physician, 130

Venel, Jean-André, 1740–91, Swiss orthopaedic surgeon, 193

Vesalius, Andreas, 1514–64, Flemish anatomist, 81, 137, 138, 139, 143, 179, 194, 345

Virchow, Rudolf, 1821–1902, German pathologist, 152, 158, 159, 160, 351

Volhard, Franz, b. 1872, German physician, 113, 114

Waksman, Selman Abraham, 1888–1973, Ukrainian-born American biochemist, 355

Waterhouse, Benjamin, 1754–1846, American physician, 349

Watson, James Dewey, 1928–, American molecular biologist, 2, 171, 355

Welch, William Henry, 1850–1934, American pathologist, 162

Wells, (Sir) Thomas Spencer, 1818–97, English surgeon, 197

Wepfer, Johann Conrad, 1657–1711, German anatomist, 151

Whytt, Robert, 1714–66, Scottish physician, 146, 348

Wiles, John, 20th century, English orthopaedic surgeon, 355

Williams, Daniel Hale, 1858–1931, American surgeon, 352

Willis, Thomas, 1621–75, English anatomist and physician, 140

Wiseman, Richard, 1625–86, English surgeon, 179

Withering, William, 1741–99, English physician, 116, 349

Wöhler, Friedrich, 1800–82, German chemist, 158, 350

Wolff, Caspar Friedrich, 1733–94, German embryologist, 348

Wood, Alexander, 1725–1884, Scottish physician, 117

Woodall, John, 1556?–1643, English surgeon, 179

Wynder, Ernst Ludwig, 1922–, German-born American epidemiologist, 355

Yersin, Alexandre-Emile-John, 1863–1943, Swiss-born French bacteriologist, 166

Young, Thomas, 1773–1829, English physiologist and physicist, 349

al-Zahrawi (Albucasis), c. 976– c. 1013, Spanish Arab surgeon, 60, 178, 344

Zinsser, Hans, 1878–1940, American bacteriologist and immunologist, 355

Zwinger, Theodor, 16th century, Swiss physician, 46, 47

General Index

abortion, 321
abscesses, 177, 200, 229
accoucheurs see mildwives (male)
acetylcholine, 170, 227
acupuncture, 328
acyclovir, 231
addiction, drug, 118
Addison's disease, 156
adrenaline, 171, 227
advertisements for medicines, 264, 281
Africa, 12, 15, 19, 23, 28, 29, 31, 35,
    36, 38, 44, 50, 56, 59, 60, 163, 213,
    220, 260, 284, 296, 312, 314, 340,
    351, 352; slaves, 23
agriculture, 3, 14, 15, 25, 28, 38, 41,
    266
AIDS (acquired immunodeficiency
    syndrome), 5, 43, 44, 87, 88, 89,
    92, 231, 296, 301, 324, 329, 338,
    340, 356, 357; research, 87
alcohol, 99, 116, 162, 198
Alexandria, Egypt, 52, 55, 241
alkaptonuria, 171
allergies, 101
alternative medicine, 98
Alzheimer's disease, 5, 42, 309, 338
ambulances, 196
Americas: indigenous peoples, 28;
    slaves, 28; *see also* United States
amniocentesis, 355
amoebae, 164, 357
amputations, 177, 190, 192

amyl nitrite, 119
anaemias, 38; sickle-cell, 303
anaesthetics, 68, 83, 95, 191,
    196–202, 222
anal fistulae, 66
anatomy, 52, 54, 63, 81, 111, 136,
    137, 138, 139, 140, 142, 143, 144,
    147, 148, 151, 155, 156, 158, 159;
    Enlightenment, 143; Renaissance, 4,
    139; seventeenth century, 142;
    see also dissection
Anderson, Sir Edmund, 77
angina, 119
angioplasty, coronary, 316
animals: 52; dissection, 52, 81;
    domestication, 12; experimentation,
    81; wild, diseases of, 11
anorexia nervosa, 96
anthrax vaccine, 352
antibiotics, 95, 134, 203, 229, 230,
    231, 289, 292, 297, 299, 301, 321;
    resistance to, 231
antibodies, monoclonal, 305–7, 334
anticoagulant drugs, 323
antipsychiatry movement, 238, 258
antipyretics, 117, 221
antisepsis, 4, 196–202
antitoxins, 167, 222
antiviral agents, 231
antivivisection movement, 162
Antonine plague, 20
Apollonia, St, 76

apothecaries, 66, 110, 264, 265, 270, 272; Society of, 110, 272
appendectomy, 202
apprenticeship, 64, 66, 111, 189, 193
Arab medicine, 57–64; 'Medicine of the Prophet', 58, 60
Aristotelianism, 57, 58, 59, 63, 64, 80
armed forces: and disease, 261; health services, 261
arsphenamine (Salvarsan), 224
arthritis, 88, 117, 132, 134, 306, 322, 355
artificial insemination, 320, 321
artists and madness, 246
asbestosis, 41
ascariasis, 357
Asclepius, 46, 50, 51, 55, 181
ascorbic acid (vitamin C) see under vitamins
aspirin family, 117, 118
Assyria, 212
asthma, 117
astrology, medical, 88, 259
asylums, for the insane, 185, 247, 248, 251, 252, 253, 254, 293
Australian Aborigines, 72
Ayurvedic medicine, 9

Babylonia, 47–50, 212
Bach, Johann Sebastian, 347
bacteriology, 4, 88, 95, 160, 164, 279, 323
Baltimore, Maryland: Johns Hopkins University, 219, 279
Banks, Joseph, 203
barber-surgeons, 66, 178, 179, 193; Company of, 193, 194
barbiturates, 118
Bayer Company, 118, 229
'Bedlam' (hospital) see London (hospitals (Bethlem))
bejel (non-venereal syphilis), 25
Belcher, William, 254
beriberi, 39
Bethlem Hospital. see under London
bevacizumab, 334
Bevan, Aneurin, 289
bilharziasis (schistosomiasis), 11, 15

bimaristans, 182
bioethics, 260, 322
biopsy, 85
birth abnormalities, 306, 307
birth control, 310, 312, 314
Black Death, 1, 67, 68, 76, 87, 137, 345
bladder stones, 66, 68, 178, 190, 191
Blake, William, 89, 352
blood, 17, 24; circulation, 59, 81, 157; pressure, 85; transfusions, 75, 89, 140
blood groups, 353
bloodletting, 108; and humoral theory, 108; popular demand for, 109, 113
blue-baby syndrome, 204
Bologna, Italy, 64, 66, 183, 344
bonesetting, 177
Boston, Mass., 35, 186, 196, 198, 298, 299
botanists, medical, 98, 272
botulism, 171
brain, 3, 43, 53, 59, 100, 140, 141, 146, 151, 170, 171, 179, 191, 200, 201, 204, 205, 211, 224, 241, 242, 243, 246, 255, 307, 308, 318, 321, 335, 336
Bright's disease, 156
Britain: friendly societies, 278, 283, 287; market arrangement, 287; National Health Insurance, 283, 284; National Health Service, 5, 126; see also under public health
British Medical Association, 162, 271
British Pharmacopoeia, 215
bronchitis, 47, 131, 153
Brontë, Charlotte, 247
Brown, Charles-Edouard, 201
Brown, Louise, 5, 206
brucellosis, 27, 358
Bruges, Belgium, 67
Brunonians, 86, 146
BSE, 337
buchu, 120
Burke, William, 136, 350
Burney, Fanny, 190
Burton, Robert, 243, 346

bypass surgery, 301, 316, 317
byssinosis, 41
Byzantine Empire, 58

caesarian section, 48, 68, 176, 180, 206
calomel, 108, 120
Cambridge University, 196, 206, 265, 271, 277, 306, 331
Canada, 25, 304, 352
Canary Islands, 23
cancer: breast, 190, 192, 200; chemotherapy, 232, 233; hormone treatment, 204; lung, 112, 131, 175; prostate, 204; radiotherapy, 207; research, 285, 324; scrotal, 42; skin, 42; stomach, 42; surgery, 200, 202
Caribbean, 27, 28, 29, 35, 36
Carrión's disease, 25, 358
CAT (computerized axial tomography), 208, 209, 356
cataract, 60, 178, 192, 355
cautery, 177, 178, 179
cell biology, 4, 82, 324
Chaderton, Laurence, 77
Chagas' disease, 25, 358
charities, medical, 174, 273, 286
chemical industry see dyestuffs; pharmaceutical industry
chemical warfare, 232
chemist and druggist, 265
chemotherapy, 4, 167, 223, 224, 232, 233, 353
Chester Roman hospital, 54
chickenpox, 18, 27, 358
childbirth, 12; anaesthetics, 68, 83; forceps, 68; Greek medicine, 50; medicalization, 95, 96; mortality, 12; puerperal fever, 229; see also birth abnormalities; caesarian section; midwives
childhood diseases, 20, 24
China, 33, 35, 47, 163, 212; traditional medicine, 72, 84, 109, 329
Chiron (centaur), 46
chiropractic, 328
chloral hydrate, 118
chloroform, 198, 222, 350, 351
chlorpromazine (Largactil), 258

cholera, 27, 33, 35–6, 167, 358; bacillus, 82
cholinesterase, 170
Christian Science, 98, 99
Christianity, 55, 73, 74; attitude to body, 75; hospitals, 56; and mental illness, 68, 69; miracles, 55; nursing orders, 181, 188; pilgrimage, 55; religious healing, 55, 75
cinchona (Peruvian bark), 36, 216, 347
cities, 3, 17, 19, 23, 25, 29, 33, 34, 35, 36, 51, 88, 128, 130, 182, 183, 185, 247, 262, 266, 279, 282, 284, 296, 340
Clement VII, Pope, 137
clinical science, 3, 148–9, 172–5
clinics, 118, 128, 286, 295
clots, dissolution of, 134, 301
Clough, Arthur Hugh, 321
codeine, 236, 350
Coleridge, Samuel Taylor, 85
community care, 61, 259, 293
competitive antagonism, 230
complementary medicine, 319, 325, 327, 328, 338
'complexion', 79
computerized axial tomography (CAT), 2
Conan Doyle, Sir Arthur, 120
concentration camps (Nazi), 288
congresses, international, 163, 352
Constantinople, 55, 56, 57, 61, 63, 182, 343, 344, 345, 347
consultants, 127, 128, 270, 284, 286, 290, 323
consumer groups, 293
contact lenses, 355
contagionism, 87
contraception, 312, 321
Cook, Captain James, 32, 348
Cortés, Hernando, 27
Cos, Greece, 51
costs, health care, 209
cretinism, 169, 201
Crusades, 188, 344
Cuba, 36
curare, 161, 219, 236
cystic fibrosis, 172, 302

General Index

Dark Ages, 61
Darwin, Charles, 32, 171, 350, 351, 352
Darwinism, Social, 256
death, 1, 32, 39, 40, 48, 52, 56, 59, 68, 70, 71, 73, 74, 77, 84, 93, 106, 107, 113, 121, 173, 186, 189, 195, 197, 198, 205, 219, 221, 226, 235, 255, 268, 269, 288, 293, 296, 299, 310, 312, 314, 317, 321, 326, 344, 345, 346; *see also* mortality
deficiency diseases, 1, 39, 40, 227, 228; *see also* scurvy
degenerationist theory, 255
degenerative diseases, 299; *see also individual diseases*
dengue, 27, 358
Denmark: bioethics commission, 322
dentistry, 9
Desert Fathers, 73
developing world, 5, 43, 44, 360
Devil, 69, 78, 177
diabetes, 102, 117, 150, 169, 225, 309, 352
diagnosis, 7, 48, 112, 115, 120, 123, 125, 133, 134, 154, 155, 208, 214, 216, 238, 259, 309, 322, 334, 356
dialysis machine, 355
Dickens, Charles, 252
dietetics, 52, 63
digestion, 138, 142, 147, 167, 348
digitalis, 116, 118, 173, 236, 349
diphtheria, 5, 18, 19, 24, 27, 33, 107, 119, 150, 151, 166, 167, 223, 225, 275, 347, 348, 350, 352, 353, 358; antitoxin, 107; history of, 32
disease: Christian conceptions, 55–7, 74; history of, 10–45; /illness distinction, 71–2; mechanical conception, 80–3; medical view of, 78–80; sick role, 95–8; stories of, 91–5
dispensaries, 186, 196, 266
dissection: animal, 52, 81; Greek, 52; medieval, 137; supply of corpses, 350
dissidence, political, 96
DNA, 2, 171, 302, 303, 304, 355
Dorpat (Tartu), Estonia, 220

dracunculiasis, 29, 358
Drinker respirator, 354
dropsy (oedema), 102, 116
drugs *see* pharmacology
dualism, 82
Dubrovnik (Ragusa), Croatia, 183
dyestuffs, 221, 223, 229
Dymphna, St, 62, 247
dysentery, 14, 20, 27, 164, 216, 357

Ebola virus disease, 356, 358
ECT (electroconvulsive therapy), 355
Eddy, Mary Baker, 99
Edinburgh, 104, 136, 146, 155, 163, 185, 187, 194, 197, 198, 220, 265, 347, 352
Edward VII, King of Great Britain, 200
egg donation, 206
Egypt: ancient, 47–50: Hellenistic, 52
electrocardiograph, 127, 173, 208, 353
electroconvulsive therapy, 355
elephantiasis, 164, 358
Eliot, George, 265, 271, 274
embryonic stem cells, 335, 337
emetics, 104
Empiricists, 53
empyema, 106
encephalitis lethargica, 43, 358
endorphins, 3
Enlightenment, 78, 143–8, 152, 155, 185, 186, 193, 244, 250, 256, 264, 273
enzymes, 116, 168
Epicureanism, 74
Epidaurus, Greece, 51
epidemics, 18, 19, 20, 22, 27, 29, 35, 36, 43, 51, 88, 107, 149, 163, 167, 279, 280, 298, 346, 350, 358; *see also individual diseases*
epidemiology applied to clinical problems, 175
epilepsy, 47, 48
equity of health-care provision, 296
ergotism, 19, 358
erysipelas, 27, 131, 151
ether, 197, 198, 222, 351
ethics, 6, 232, 288
eugenics, 171, 281, 320

General Index

euthanasia, 321, 338
evolutionary theory, 171
examination, physical, 83, 84, 85, 112, 113, 115, 121, 195
expectations, patients', 6, 94, 95, 101, 314
experimentation: animal, 81, 162; human patients, 5, 145, 169, 288; self-, 198
expiation, 75, 76
exploration, age of, 22
eye surgery, 208, 356

Fabiola (Roman Christian), 181, 344
feminism, 277
Fendoch Roman military hospital, 54
fertilization, *in vitro*, 206, 320, 356
fetal abnormalities *see* birth abnormalities
fetal tissue transplants, 308
fever: dengue, 27; haemorrhagic, 44; hospital, 266; puerperal, 151, 199, 229; relapsing, 27; rheumatic, 131; scarlet, 27, 32, 33, 122, 131, 347; *see also* yellow fever
fever therapy, 108
fibres, 81, 108, 143, 145, 146, 170, 173
filariasis, 27, 29, 32, 358
Finchale, Co. Durham, 62
flagellants, 76
fleas, prehistoric, 14
Florence, 67, 81, 183, 276, 344
Florentine Health Board, 77
fluoridation of water, 355
foundlings, 186, 347
foxglove, 116, 349
France: bioethics commission, 322; health services, 262; hospitals, 160, 291; medical science, 193; social welfare, 252
friendly societies, 261, 274, 283
Fry, Elizabeth, 350
functional symptoms, 125

G6PD deficiency, 17, 28
Galenic medicine, 56, 58; anatomy, 136; Arab adaptation, 58; Paracelsus' challenge, 214; pharmacology, 136

gall bladder, tumour of, 200, 352
Gama, Vasco da, 31, 345
gangrene, 149, 151, 189
gastroscope, 354
gene therapy, 302, 303, 320, 335, 338
gene-based therapy, 332; personalised medicine, 333
General Medical Council, UK, 110, 215, 351
general practitioners, 103, 110, 111, 118, 120, 126, 127, 128, 194, 272, 283, 285, 289, 290, 291; *see also* primary care
genetics, 2, 82, 171, 281, 289, 334; inherited conditions, 82; *see also* gene therapy
geriatrics, 290
germ theory of disease, 113, 222, 345
German measles (rubella), 355, 360
Germany: chemical industry, 117, 281; health services, 292; laboratory medicine, 118; medical science, 276, 277; Nazi era, 227
Giessen University, 157, 160
glands, 141; *see also* hormones
global warming, 314, 340
glucose-6-phosphate dehydrogenase deficiency, *see* G6PD deficiency
goitre, 169, 201
gout, 93, 94, 95, 148
Granada, Spain, 31
grave-robbing, 273
Greek medicine, 50, 51, 52, 53, 54, 55; anatomy, 52; *see also* Asclepius; Galenic medicine; *Hippocratic Corpus*
guilds, 64, 66
Guineaworm *see* dracunculiasis
gynaecology, 54, 127, 128, 318; *see also* childbirth

haemophilia, 350
haemorrhagic fever, 44, 357, 358
Halle, Germany, 144
Hamburg, Germany, 280
Hammurabi, law code of, 48
Handel, George Frederick, 192
Hare, William, 136, 350
Hartford, Conn., 129

General Index

Harvard University, Mass., 125, 170, 202
Harvey, William, 138
Hawaiian Islands, 32
healing, 2, 4, 9, 46, 47, 48, 51, 55, 60, 62, 66, 67, 70, 72, 75, 76, 78, 98, 99, 100, 122, 123, 155, 177, 181, 184, 186, 189, 194, 209, 247, 260, 325, 327, 329, 338
Health Boards, medieval, 67, 70
health services, 261
health visitors, 280
heart: pacemakers, 2, 203, 205, 356; surgery, 2, 204, 205, 352, 354, 355
heart–lung machine, 355
Hellenistic era, 52
helminthic infestations, 27
Henry VIII, King of England, 183, 184, 345
hepatitis, 25, 356, 359
herbalism, 236, 237
herbals, 212
hereditary disease, 255
hernias, 202, 308
heroic medicine, 109
herpes infections, 231
hip replacement, 355
Hippocratic Corpus, 50, 78, 178, 345
Hippocratic Oath, 50, 79, 177
history-taking, 111, 124, 134
HIV (human immunodeficiency virus), 44, 87, 89, 231, 301, 316, 324
holism, 100
homeopathy, 99, 100, 236, 261, 349
homeostasis, 161
Homo erectus, 12
homosexuality, 257
hookworm, 16, 27, 29, 359
hormones, 4, 201, 204, 225, 226, 305
hospitals: charity, 268; Christian, 56, 57; cost, 209; isolation, 67, 279; medieval, 182, 183; out-patient departments, 126, 128, 130; private patients, 288, 291; specialist, 196, 286; surgery in, 83, 176–210; teaching, 196, 269, 290, 295; traditional, 180–6; women's, 196; *see also* surgery
houseflies, 14, 33

human embryos, 335
Human Genetics Commission (HGC), 334
Human Genome Project, 171, 303, 304, 356
human immunodeficiency virus, *see* HIV
humoral theory, 103, 108; of illness, 85; Renaissance challenge to, 139; and traditional cures, 108
hunter-gatherers, 10, 11, 12, 24, 25, 41
Huntington's chorea, 82, 172, 333
hygiene, 73, 77, 95, 150, 265, 268, 275, 276, 280; *see also* antisepsis; public health
hypertension, 42
hypnosis, 348
hypochondria, 71
hysterectomy, 308
hysteria, 71, 78, 245

iatrochemistry, 141
iatrogenic complaints, 299
iatrophysicists, 141
Illich, Ivan, 8, 94, 95, 298
illness/disease distinction, 71–2
imaging, 2, 134, 307, 336, 356; diagnostic, 134; magnetic resonance imagery (MRI), 336; serial, 336
immunity and immunology, 17, 18, 165, 166, 167, 222; monoclonal antibodies, 305–7
immunization *see* inoculation; vaccination
imperialism, 36, 163–5, 278
impetigo, 131
implantation, surgical, 203
Inchtuthil Roman hospital, 54
incubation (religious healing), 51
India, 9, 10, 18, 33, 36, 39, 47, 59, 163, 329, 345, 346, 347; ancient, 18
Indus Valley culture, 17
Industrial Revolution, 41
infanticide, 12
infectious diseases, 119, 132, 182, 231, 296; *see also individual diseases*
infertility services, 316
inflammation, 43, 84, 115, 117, 139, 160, 268, 306

General Index

influenza, 18, 19, 20, 27, 32, 43, 44, 131, 231, 340, 354, 358, 359; epidemic, 358
inherited conditions, 82
injection of drugs, 225
inoculation, smallpox, 18
inquests, 70
insects, disease-bearing, 11, 14; *see also* houseflies; mosquito; tsetse fly
insemination, artificial, 320, 321
insulin, 225, 257, 354
insurance schemes, 209, 260, 261, 283, 287, 295; private, 287; state, 287
intelligent toilet, 335
intensity of treatment, 133
interferon, 303, 305
interleukin, 303, 305
iodine, 199
ipecacuanha, 216, 218, 236, 252
iron lung, 354
iron medicines, 116
irritability and sensibility, 145
issues, 63, 86, 102, 205, 206, 286, 296, 320, 322
Italy, 28, 53, 56, 61, 62, 63, 64, 66, 67, 68, 76, 87, 137, 141, 178, 184, 213, 251, 254; Health Boards, 67
itinerant practitioners, 191
IVF *see* fertilization, *in vitro*

Jackson, Elizabeth, 77
Japan, 20, 31, 33, 304, 335, 344
Jehovah's Witnesses, 75
Jerusalem, 56, 69, 188
jesters, court, 247
Jews, 23, 56, 60, 64, 66, 70, 73, 345
Job (Biblical figure), 75
Johnson, Samuel, 93, 152, 250
journalism, medical, 150
Judaism, 55, 56, 73
Justinian, 64, 344

Kempe, Margery, 69, 70
Kennedy, Ian, 291, 318
kidneys, 2, 15, 116, 120, 127, 138, 159, 203, 205, 208, 224, 308; artificial, 205
kwashiorkor, 41
kymograph, 159, 351

laboratory medicine, 95
Laing, Jimmie, 258
Lancet, The, 119, 222, 272, 350
Largactil (chlorpromazine), 258
laser technology, 208
lassa fever, 359
Lateran Council, Fourth (1215), 76
laudanum, 213
laxatives, 100, 108, 112, 119, 121
lazarettos, 183
L-dopa, 3, 171, 308
lead poisoning, 41
Lebena, Crete, 51
leeches, 180
Leipzig, Germany, 220
leishmaniasis, 25, 359
Leonardo da Vinci, 137, 345
leprosy, 27, 29, 76, 90, 182, 359; leper houses, 68
leptospirosis (Weil's disease), 11, 359
Lesch-Nyan disease, 303
leukaemia, 160, 232
liberalism, nineteenth-century, 294
lice, 11, 14, 15, 23, 360, 361
licensing: doctors, 111; drugs, 279; midwives, 268
life expectancy, 332
life, prolonging of, 182
life-support systems, 319, 321
limbs, artificial, 66
Lisbon, Portugal, 35, 36
litigation, 5
liver: cirrhosis, 152; transplants, 356
lobotomy, 355
Locke, John, 149, 245, 250, 251, 347
London: Bethlem, 184, 185, 247, 253; Great Plague, 22; Guy's College, 196; Harley Street, 127; King's College Hospital, 196; Medical Society of, 150; Royal Free Hospital, 352; School of Tropical Medicine and Hygiene, 174; St Bartholomew's Hospital, 119, 171, 192; St Giles in the Fields, 183; St Thomas's Hospital, 184, 187, 351; Tavistock Clinic, 354; University College Hospital, 168, 173, 196, 277
London School of Hygiene and Tropical Medicine, 174, 234, 353

General Index

London School of Tropical Medicine, 164

Louis XIV, King of France, 193, 248

Lourdes, 76

Luminal (phenobarbital), 118

lungs, 2, 106, 114, 115, 127, 139, 140, 141, 148, 152, 203, 204, 208, 302

machine, body as, 82, 244

Magellan, Ferdinand, 31, 345

magic, 1, 49, 72, 87, 88, 167, 179, 224, 236

magnetic resonance imagery (MRI), 2, 336

malaria: falciparum, 15, 17, 28, 29; history of, 28, 29, 32; immunity to, 167; quinine, 216; transmission of, 173; vaccine, 339; vivax, 29

malnutrition, 360; *see also* deficiency diseases

mammography, 356

Manchester, 106, 185, 197, 266, 285

mania, 241, 242, 243

manic-depressive conditions, 258

Manichaeanism, 58

marasmus, 41

Marburg virus disease, 356, 359

market competition, 260

Marseilles, France, 183

mastectomy, 200

masturbation, 90

Maya civilization, 25

ME (myalgic encephalomyelitis), 97, 101

measles: history, 15, 16; vaccine, 356

mechanism, 112

Medicaid, 315

medical botanists, 98, 272

Medical Officers of Health, UK, 275, 286

Medical Research Council, 174, 234, 280, 285

medical services, politics of, 263

'medicalization of life', 8, 95

Medizinpolizei, 266

melancholy, 71, 97, 241, 242

meningitis, 1, 68, 107, 131, 348

menopause, 7, 96

menstruation, 96

mental illness, 238, 239, 240, 241, 242, 243, 244, 245, 246; community care, 259; confinement, 246, 247, 248, 249; degenerationist theory, 255–7; delineation and classification of, 257; Devil as cause, 245; improper confinement, 253; medieval, 243–4; modern treatments, 257–8; 'moral treatments', 250; psychoanalysis, 249; psychological and somatic theories, 243; religious madness, 243; in Renaissance, 243–4; schizophrenia, 255–7

mercury, 108, 109, 213, 347

mesmerism, 99, 100

Mesopotamia, 10, 17, 47, 211, 343

metabolism, 17, 158, 231

Methodist Church, 53, 246

Mexico, 27, 29, 35

miasmatism, 88

mice, 14

'Mickey Finn' (chloral hydrate), 118

microscope, 4, 82, 112, 113, 115, 140, 159, 223; electron, 2, 208

Middle Ages, 51, 67, 72, 73, 80, 136, 176, 181, 243; religion and medicine, 72

midwives, 66, 67, 199, 268, 280, 283, 345; licensing of, 67, 268, 280; male, 188, 265

migrations, population, 13, 19, 160

Milan, Italy, 183, 345

minerals, 34, 211, 213

miracles, 55, 75, 181

molecular medicine, 304

monoclonal antibodies, 334

Montpellier, France, 64, 66, 146, 147, 213, 243

morbidity, 339

morphine, 117, 118, 218, 349

mortality, 14, 31, 35, 38, 44, 68, 164, 175, 189, 199, 210, 310, 339

mosquito, 14

MRI (magnetic resonance imagery), 336

mummies, Egyptian, 15

General Index

mumps, 18, 20, 27, 337, 359
Munich, Germany, 157, 267
muscles, 81, 138, 140, 141, 143, 147, 159, 161, 170, 198, 200, 219, 227, 303, 349
muscular dystrophy, Duchenne, 303, 356
mustard plaster,
myalgic encephalomyelitis (ME), 97, 101

Naples, Italy, 183, 345
National Health Service, UK, 3, 96, 103, 210, 261, 263
National Institute for Clinical Excellence (NICE), 337
National Institutes of Health, US, 173, 304, 317, 355
naturopathy, 100
naval medicine, 217, 234
Naturphilosophie, 158
Nazism, 288
negritude, 90
nervous system, neurology, 40, 82, 138, 146, 161, 169, 170, 171, 177, 202, 226, 244, 335; and mental illness, 140, 244
Netherlands, 140
neurasthenia, 97
neuroleptic drugs, 258
neurophysiology, 169
neurosis, 146, 244, 256
neurosurgery, 202
neurotransmitters, 3
New York, 35, 43, 124, 127, 172, 186, 195, 196, 198, 203, 232; Rockefeller Institute for Medical Research, 172, 280
New Zealand, state medical service, 355
niacin, 39, 168, 359
nicotine, 216, 236
nitroglycerine, 119
nitrous oxide, 198, 222, 349, 351
Nobel Prizes, 173, 353
nosology, 86
Nuremberg, Germany, 69, 183
nursing profession, 196, 268, 276, 284

nutrition, 34–5, 38, 40, 41, 167, 168, 280, 285, 296, 360;
hunter-gatherers, 12, 13, 24, 25, 38, 41; *see also* deficiency disease; malnutrition
nymphomania, 90

obstetrics *see* childbirth
occupational diseases, 41
oedema *see* dropsy
Oedipus Complex, 239
older people, 332; morbidity, 332
onchocerciasis, 27, 29, 359
operating theatres, 209
ophthalmoscope, 159, 351
opium, 68, 116, 117, 120, 121, 122, 161, 198, 212, 216, 218; laudanum, 213
Oregon, USA, 315, 316, 337
Oroyo fever *see* Carrión's disease
orthopaedics, 193
osteopathy, 328
ovaries, 90, 138, 169, 197, 226
Oxford University, 175

pacemakers, 2
Padua, Italy, 64, 137, 138, 151
paediatrics, 2, 204
pain, 3, 8, 68, 72, 74, 75, 95, 97, 99, 109, 116, 117, 119, 173, 180, 190, 191, 198, 217, 221, 222, 308, 326, 351
palpation, 113, 114, 115
Panama Canal, 165, 354
pancreas, 161, 168, 169, 224, 225, 352
papyri, Egyptian medical, 177
paralysis of the insane, general, 224
parasites, 82, 231; in prehistroy, 14, 15, 25
Pargeter, William, 246
Paris, 152; Hôpital des Petits Maisons, 182; Hôpital Necker, 153, 195; Hôtel Dieu, 151, 152, 184, 193, 195, 268; Pasteur Institute, 280, 324, 353; Salpêtrière Hospital, 153; surgical academy, 267
Paris school of medical science, 155, 156

Parkinson's disease, 3, 171, 308
Parliament (British): Anatomy Act of
    1832, 136, 269; Apothecaries Act of,
    110; Cruelty to Animals Act (1876),
    162; Madhouses Act of (1774), 253;
    Medical Reform Act of (1858), 215,
    272, 275; National Health Insurance
    Act of (1911), 128; Poor Law
    (1834), 350; Public Health Act of
    (1848), 351; Registration of
    Midwives Act (1902), 353
Parsons, Talcott, 96, 97
pathology, 112, 114, 152, 157, 161,
    195, 214, 279; anatomy, 123
patient, doctor's relationship with, 62,
    71, 84, 97, 103, 104, 115, 119;
    see also under primary care
patient-as-a-person movement, 121,
    122, 123, 124, 125, 126
pellagra, 39, 168, 359
PEM (protein energy malnutrition),
    40, 41
penicillin, 1, 5, 133, 224, 231, 289,
    354, 355
Pepys, Samuel, 85
percussion of chest, 148, 348
Pergamum, Asia Minor, 212
pertussis (whooping cough), 361
Peru, 27, 35, 216
Peruvian bark (cinchona), 216, 218
PET (positron emission tomography),
    85, 209
phagocytosis, 166, 352
pharmaceutical industry, 233
pharmacologists, Arab, 59
pharmacology, 46, 63, 161, 206, 207,
    211–37, 305; alternative treatments,
    222; American drugs, 216; in
    ancient world, 211; Arab, 63;
    drug-resistance, 301, 339; dyestuffs,
    221, 223, 229; epilepsy, 241, 245;
    future drug design, 210, 301, 302,
    305, 318; nineteenth century, 36,
    40, 82; post-war, 174, 289; primary
    care, 9, 103–35; trials, 8, 229, 230,
    234, 235, 237, 282, 301, 355;
    unwanted effects, 235; see also
    Germany (chemical industry)
pharmacopoeias, 70, 215, 216

phenacetin, 118
phenobarbital (Luminal), 118
philosophy, 2, 55, 58, 59, 63, 94,
    98, 101, 123, 140, 141, 144, 155,
    158, 214, 239, 240, 242, 249, 264,
    343
phlebotomy, 85, 180
'phossy jaw', 41
phrenology, 100
phthisis, 153, 154
Physicians, Royal College of (London),
    110, 116, 215, 253, 266, 272
physicians and surgeons, 267
physics, 4, 85, 87, 91, 122, 136, 141,
    158, 236, 265, 304, 323
physiological conception of disease, 83,
    150
physiology, 81, 82, 111, 138, 142,
    146, 148, 156, 158, 159, 160, 161,
    162, 165, 173, 193, 204, 206, 207,
    214, 218, 219, 220, 224, 262, 275,
    305, 348
pilgrimage, 56, 69
pinta, 25
pituitary gland, 169
placebo effect, 83
placenta, 17, 307
plague, 1, 19, 20, 22, 23, 32, 33, 43,
    62, 67, 68, 70, 76, 77, 89, 99, 101,
    107, 150, 167, 183, 359; Black
    Death, 67, 76; bubonic, 22, 27, 67,
    76, 183
Plasmodium, 29, 164, 359
Plymouth, 149; Royal Naval Hospital,
    189
pneumoconiosis, coal workers' 41
pneumonia, 1, 44, 112, 126, 131, 153,
    156, 167, 321
poliomyelitis, 43
politics, 100, 262, 263, 272, 274, 286,
    288, 293, 294
pollution, 42, 89, 90, 101, 319; see also
    miasmatism, 16, 42
polygraph, 173
polyps, nasal, 177
poor, medical services for, 263
population: density, 10; growth, 12,
    19, 33
Portugal, 23, 36, 215, 248, 345

positron emission tomography (PET), 2

possession, diabolical, 77, 87, 245

post-mortem examinations, 83; *see also* dissection

Powell, Enoch, 314

poxes, animal, 15; *see also* smallpox

pregnancy, 68, 334, 355; *see also* childbirth; fertilization

prehistory, 221

primary care, 103–35; drug treatment, 133; general practitioner, 289; home visits, 130; origins of general practitioner, 110; patient–doctor relationship, 103, 111; patients' expectations, 103–5; specialism, 126, 127; technology, 120; traditional medicine, 109

prisons, 247, 254, 265

private medicine, 282

professional identity, 78

prognosis, 48, 112, 123, 255

Prontosil, 133, 229, 354

prostate gland, cancer of, 204

prostitutes, 87, 93, 184, 247, 276

protein energy malnutrition (PEM), 40

prothesis, 203

psoriasis, 317

psychiatry, 5, 9, 118, 251, 256, 257, 259, 277, 284; *see also* mental illness

psychoanalysis, 4, 257

psychology, physicalist, 59

psychoses, 257

psychosomatic illness, 97

psychotropic drugs, 257

public health: scientific basis, 95, 131; state intervention, 262; UK, 262, 265; *see also* hygiene; water supply

public health medicine, 332; tobacco consumption, 332

Puccini, Giacomo, *La Bohème*, 92

puerperal fever, 151, 199

pulse-taking, 49, 52, 84, 85, 112, 115, 149, 173

punishment, illness as, 78

purges, 49; ancient Egyptian, 50

Puritans, English, 77, 78

pus, 33, 49, 106, 160, 166, 177, 178, 190, 229

QALY (quality-adjusted life year), 326

quacks, 47, 79, 178, 192

quality of life, 325, 326, 327

quarantine, 33, 67, 76, 87, 88

quinine, 36, 117, 120, 216, 218, 221

rabbit fever (tularemia), 11, 360

rabies, 62, 352

radionics, 319

radiotherapy, 204, 207

rats, 14, 22

receptors, chemical, 219, 223

records, 48, 96, 149, 211, 212, 217, 253, 309, 336

Red Cross, 163, 351

reflex action, 146, 348

regulation *see* licensing

rehydration, oral, 314

relapsing fever, 27, 360

religious healing: in ancient world, 51; Christian, 55

religious madness, 243, 244, 245, 246

Renaissance, 4, 23, 33, 76, 79, 80, 87, 136, 139, 213, 243–4

repetitive strain injury (RSI), 97

reproduction, 19, 281; *see also* fertilization

research, 2, 5, 40, 43, 82, 83, 85, 102, 118, 122, 130, 134, 137, 138, 141, 143, 150, 153, 157, 158, 159, 160, 162, 163, 165, 168, 171, 172, 173, 174, 175, 206, 223, 225, 227, 228, 229, 231, 232, 233, 244, 255, 280, 281, 285, 292, 293, 295, 298, 301, 317, 322, 323, 324, 335, 338; basic/targeted, 5, 147, 153, 168, 169, 322, 323, 324; funding, 102, 118; pharmaceutical, 134

resistance to disease *see* immunity

respiration, 114, 140, 141, 147, 153, 205, 219

'resurrection men', 136

Retrovir (zidovudine), 231

rheumatic fever, 131, 152

rickets, 180

rickettsias, 15

Rift Valley fever, 360

robotic instrumentation, 334

robotics in surgery, 307, 334

Rocky Mountain spotted fever, 25, 360
Roman Empire, 20, 54, 55, 57, 181,
    182, 343; decline and fall, 28;
    hospitals, 344
Romanticism, 246
Rome, 20, 23, 53, 57, 69, 76, 141,
    181, 183, 212, 213, 344, 345, 356
Roquemadour, France, 62
Rousseau, Jean-Jacques, 250
Royal Society of London, 81, 140,
    215, 346
RSI (repetitive strain injury), 97
rubella, 337, 355, 360
Russia and former USSR, 5

Salerno medical school, 64, 178, 213,
    344
Salmonella, 11, 360
Salvarsan, 119, 224, 353
San Francisco, USA, 163
sanatoria, 280
scabies, 117
scanners, body, 317
scapegoating, 238
scarificators, 108
scarlet fever, 27, 32, 33, 122, 131,
    347, 360
schistosomiasis (bilharziasis), 11, 360
schizophrenia, 5, 256, 257, 337
Schumann, Robert, 246
science, medical: clinical science,
    148–9, 172–5; disease theory,
    149–52; eighteenth century, 143;
    Enlightenment, 143–8; nineteenth
    century, 4, 158, 172; patients'
    attitudes to, 123; seventeenth
    century, 152; tropical medicine,
    163–5; twentieth century, 165–75;
    see also anatomy; technology
scientific materialism, 158
scurvy, 11, 39, 40, 47, 167, 217, 228,
    234, 265, 348, 360
sedatives, 118
selection, natural, 42, 171
self-help groups, 325, 329, 338
sensibility and irritability, 145
septicaemia, 151
serial imaging, 336
serum therapy, 167

setons, 108
sex determination, prenatal, 306
Shakespeare, William, 71, 250, 346
shamans, 177
Shaw, George Bernard, 104
Sheldon, Gilbert, 94
shrines, healing, 62, 181
sick role, 95–8
sickle-cell trait, 17, 28
silicosis, 41
Sin, Original, 73, 74 ;
skin grafting, 205
slaves, 23, 36, 39, 53, 181, 197, 345,
    350
sleeping sickness (African
    trypanosomiasis), 360
smallpox: eradication of, 3, 43, 101;
    history of, 18; inoculation, 75, 150;
    origin of, 27; vaccination, 33, 75
smoking, 175, 216, 302
Smollett, Tobias, 192
Social Darwinism, 256
social welfare, 277, 278
societies, medical, 270, 348
society, medicine and, 260–97
sonography, 208
Soubirous, Bernadette, 76
soul, 73, 75, 79, 81, 93, 142, 143,
    144, 145, 146, 147, 177, 240, 241,
    242, 243, 250
spa resorts, 98
Spain, 22, 23, 31, 36, 53, 59, 60, 63,
    69, 137, 184, 213, 247, 344, 345
specialization, 56, 284
sperm donation, 206, 320
sphygmograph, 351
spiritualism, 100
Spurgeon, Charles Haddon, 74
St Anthony's fire, 40, 358; *see also*
    erysipelas
staphylococci, 133
state intervention, 287; *see also* licensing
stem cells, 335
stems cells, embryonic, 337
sterilization, 199
stethoscope, 84, 85, 113, 120, 153,
    154, 268
stigmatization of illness, 96
Stoicism, 74

Stone, Revd Edmund, 215
streptococci, 229
streptomycin, 1, 174, 234, 355
suicide, 74
sulphonal, 118
sulphonamides, 95, 203, 224, 230, 233
support groups, 328
Surgeons, Company of (London), 110, 194, 266, 347
Surgeons, Royal College of (London), 194, 272
surgery, 307; apprenticeship, 193, 194; artificial organs, 206; cosmetic, 94, 206; GPs perform, 128, 291; guilds, 64, 189, 264, 283; implantation, 203; in hospitals, 176–210; instruments, 55, 334, 358; itinerant practitioners, 191; keyhole, 307–8; market effects, 282; medieval, 60; military, 179; plastic and reconstructive, 2, 203, 205; robotic instrumentation, 334; traditional, 176–80; *see also* anaesthetics; antisepsis; operating theatres; transplant surgery; *and under* heart *and individual operations*
susceptibility, 7, 17, 18, 151, 302
sweating cures, 104
Sweden, 141, 203, 208
Swedenborg, Emmanuel, 99
Swift, Jonathan, 94
symptoms and signs, 112
syphilis, 93, 107; history of, 11, 19, 31, 32, 33, 87, 119, 224; non-venereal, 25, 360; tertiary, 255; treatment of, 119, 353
Syriac medical texts, 57
syringe, hypodermic, 117

Tay-Sachs disease, 303
technology, and primary care, 120–1
telephone, 129, 309, 352
temperaments, four, 212
testicular extract, 201
test-tube babies *see* fertilization (*in vitro*)
tetanus, 11, 167, 171, 352, 360
thalassaemia, 17
thalidomide, 5, 235, 293, 319, 356

Thatcher, Margaret, 259
therapeutic nihilism, 121, 122
thermometer, 347, 352
thiamine, 39, 228, 357
Thomsonians, 98
thyroid gland, 169, 201, 225
Ticehurst House, Sussex, 249
tissues, types of, 336
TNF (tumour necrosis factor), 306
tobacco, 42, 99, 216, 302, 355
tobacco consumption, 332
tonsils, 177
torture, 5
tracers, 2
tracheotomy, 202, 347, 350
trachoma, 27, 360
training: in hospitals, 188; in London, 221; scientific, 153; surgical, 193; *see also* apprenticeship; universities
transmitters, neuro-, 3, 170, 354
transplant surgery, 2, 83, 292, 321
transplantation: foetal tissue, 335; stem cells, 335
trepanation, 46
Treponema, 25, 359
trials, clinical, 3, 155, 167, 174, 217, 235
tribal societies, 9, 77
Tricca, Greece, 51
trichinosis, 11, 25, 360
tropical medicine, 9, 163, 280
Trosse, George, 249
trypanosomiasis, African *see* sleeping sickness
trypanosomiasis, American *see* Chagas' disease
tsetse fly, 360
tuberculosis, 1, 25, 44, 68, 83, 86, 93, 107, 131, 280, 286; bacillus, 86, 280, 352, 360; diagnosis of, 112; history of, 92; of kidneys, 151; and meningitis, 131, 348; modern resurgence of, 5, 296; treatment, 131, 234; vaccine, 1
tularaemia (rabbit fever), 11, 25, 360
tumour necrosis factor (TNF), 306
typhoid fever, 27, 131
typhus, 11, 19, 27, 32, 36, 68, 83, 106, 150, 151, 361

General Index

Udjohorresne, 49
ulcers, peptic, 156, 301
ultrasound, 2, 208, 356
urea, synthesis of, 158
urine inspection (uroscopy), 149
urology, 128, 203
USA: health expenditure, 291;
  hospitals, 195, 209, 288; insurance,
  5; litigation, 5; market situation, 7;
  National Institutes of Health, 304;
  primary care, 110; private medicine,
  315; yellow fever, 35; *see also*
  Americas *and individual places*
uta (mucocutaneous leishmaniasis), 25
uterine prolapse, 52

vaccines and vaccination: malaria, 339;
  measles, 356; polio, 2; smallpox, 33,
  231, 351
valetudinaria (Roman hospitals), 97,
  181
variolation, 33
venereal disease, 185, 296; *see also*
  syphilis, 180
venesection, 85, 180
Venice, Italy, 183
Verdi, Guiseppe, 92, *La Traviata*, 92
Vernon, Admiral Edward, 35
Veronal, 118
verruga Peruana, 25
Victoria, Queen of Great Britain, 84,
  198, 222, 353
Vienna, Austria, 123, 124, 148, 155,
  156, 159, 162, 184, 187, 196, 199,
  200, 268, 351; Allgemeines
  Krankenhaus, 184
viral infections. *see also individual*
  diseases, 10
vitality, 80, 145, 146
vitamins, 4, 34, 168, 227, 228, 237,
  353; vitamin A, 168, 228; vitamin B,
  39; vitamin C (ascorbic acid), 11, 39,
  40, 168, 228, 354, 360; vitamin D,
  168, 228

vivisection, 157, 162, 197, 276,
  277
voluntary associations, 262, 266, 268,
  270, 292
vomiting cures, 104
votive offerings, 76

Walpole, Horace, 93
wars: Crimean, 276, 351;
  Franco-Prussian, 278, 284;
  Peloponnesian, 19; World, First, 8,
  36, 115, 116, 162, 173, 174, 201,
  203, 205, 206, 263, 278, 284, 285,
  286, 288, 354; World, Second, 1, 5,
  123, 134, 203, 205, 210, 232, 234,
  235, 288, 289–94, 355
Washington, George, 349, 351, 353
Washkansky, Louis, 2
Weil's disease, 11, 359
whooping cough, 27, 131, 361
willow bark, 215
witchcraft, 77, 87
women, 50; doctors, 64, 66, 90, 111,
  283; hospitals for, 196; hysteria, 71,
  78; nursing, 283, 284;
  'nymphomania', 90; political
  importance between wars, 286;
  see also midwives
World Health Organization, 3, 43,
  312, 355
worms, parasitic, 14, 17, 358
wound management, 178, 203

X-rays, 4, 42, 153, 207, 208, 209, 307,
  309, 323, 336, 353

yaws, 11, 29
yellow fever, 11, 29, 35–6, 164;
  mosquito-borne, 29, 164; spread,
  35, 36; vaccine, 231
York Retreat, 251

zidovudine, 231
Zovirax, 231

Map Acknowledgements

Every effort has been made to obtain permission to use the copyright material listed below; the publishers apologize for any errors or omissions and would welcome these being brought to their attention.

Maps and Diagrams

1, adapted from 'The bubonic plague' by C. McEvedy; Copyright (1988) *Scientific American* Inc., all rights reserved; **2**, from 'North America' by Frank C. Innes, in *The Cambridge World History of Human Disease* (Cambridge University Press, 1993); **3**, from Paul F. Russell, Luther S. West, and Reginald D. Manwell, *Practical Malariology* (W. B. Saunders, 1946), fig. 128; **4**, from George K. Strode (ed.), *Yellow Fever* (McGraw-Hill, 1951), fig. 67; **5**, adapted from Edward P. Cheyney, *The Dawn of a New Era*, 1250–1453 (Harper & Row, 1962); **6**, reproduced, by permission of WHO, from 'The current global situation of the HIV/AIDS pandemic', *Weekly Epidemiological Record* vol. 70 (2), 8 (1995), map 2; **7**, data from Population Reference Bureau, *World Population Data Sheet*, 1995; **8**, reproduced, by permission of WHO, from 'World malaria situation, 1989, Parts I and II', *Weekly Epidemiological Record* vol. 66 (22–23), 157–63, 167–70 (1991), Map 91363.